Frontiers in Drug Design & Discovery

(Volume 10)

Edited by

Atta-ur-Rahman, *FRS*
Kings College,
University of Cambridge,
Cambridge,
UK

&

M. Iqbal Choudhary
H.E.J. Research Institute of Chemistry,
International Center for Chemical and Biological Sciences,
University of Karachi,
Karachi,
Pakistan

Frontiers in Drug Design and Discovery

Volume # 10

Editors: Atta-ur-Rahman & Muhammad Iqbal Choudhary

ISSN (Online): 2212-1064

ISSN (Print): 1574-0889

ISBN (Online): 978-981-14-2156-3

ISBN (Print): 978-981-14-2155-6

BENTHAM SCIENCE PUBLISHERS LTD.

End User License Agreement (for non-institutional, personal use)

This is an agreement between you and Bentham Science Publishers Ltd. Please read this License Agreement carefully before using the ebook/echapter/ejournal (**"Work"**). Your use of the Work constitutes your agreement to the terms and conditions set forth in this License Agreement. If you do not agree to these terms and conditions then you should not use the Work.

Bentham Science Publishers agrees to grant you a non-exclusive, non-transferable limited license to use the Work subject to and in accordance with the following terms and conditions. This License Agreement is for non-library, personal use only. For a library / institutional / multi user license in respect of the Work, please contact: permission@benthamscience.net.

Usage Rules:

1. All rights reserved: The Work is the subject of copyright and Bentham Science Publishers either owns the Work (and the copyright in it) or is licensed to distribute the Work. You shall not copy, reproduce, modify, remove, delete, augment, add to, publish, transmit, sell, resell, create derivative works from, or in any way exploit the Work or make the Work available for others to do any of the same, in any form or by any means, in whole or in part, in each case without the prior written permission of Bentham Science Publishers, unless stated otherwise in this License Agreement.
2. You may download a copy of the Work on one occasion to one personal computer (including tablet, laptop, desktop, or other such devices). You may make one back-up copy of the Work to avoid losing it.
3. The unauthorised use or distribution of copyrighted or other proprietary content is illegal and could subject you to liability for substantial money damages. You will be liable for any damage resulting from your misuse of the Work or any violation of this License Agreement, including any infringement by you of copyrights or proprietary rights.

Disclaimer:

Bentham Science Publishers does not guarantee that the information in the Work is error-free, or warrant that it will meet your requirements or that access to the Work will be uninterrupted or error-free. The Work is provided "as is" without warranty of any kind, either express or implied or statutory, including, without limitation, implied warranties of merchantability and fitness for a particular purpose. The entire risk as to the results and performance of the Work is assumed by you. No responsibility is assumed by Bentham Science Publishers, its staff, editors and/or authors for any injury and/or damage to persons or property as a matter of products liability, negligence or otherwise, or from any use or operation of any methods, products instruction, advertisements or ideas contained in the Work.

Limitation of Liability:

In no event will Bentham Science Publishers, its staff, editors and/or authors, be liable for any damages, including, without limitation, special, incidental and/or consequential damages and/or damages for lost data and/or profits arising out of (whether directly or indirectly) the use or inability to use the Work. The entire liability of Bentham Science Publishers shall be limited to the amount actually paid by you for the Work.

General:

1. Any dispute or claim arising out of or in connection with this License Agreement or the Work (including non-contractual disputes or claims) will be governed by and construed in accordance with the laws of Singapore. Each party agrees that the courts of the state of Singapore shall have exclusive jurisdiction to settle any dispute or claim arising out of or in connection with this License Agreement or the Work (including non-contractual disputes or claims).
2. Your rights under this License Agreement will automatically terminate without notice and without the

Bentham Science Publishers Pte. Ltd.
80 Robinson Road #02-00
Singapore 068898
Singapore
Email: subscriptions@benthamscience.net

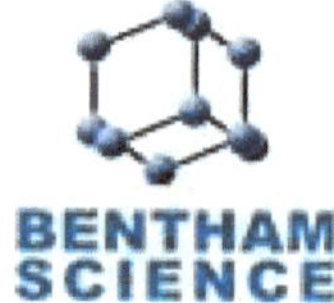

CONTENTS

PREFACE

Development of new therapeutics requires a strong science base in terms of understanding the diseases at the molecular levels, and then identifying new drug leads against novel targets. The world scientific literature is now inundated with a lot of work in this field, and it is often difficult for a researcher to find focused and comprehensive accounts of the topic of his interest. The book series, *"Frontiers in Drug Design and Discovery"* was an attempt to fill this important gap. Volume 10 of the series is a collection of four scholarly written reviews and a research article, contributed by leading experts in the field of drug discovery and development.

Ansari *et al.* have contributed an excellent review on the recent progress made in the research, manufacture, and quality assurance of various classes of industrial, therapeutic and diagnostic proteins. Collectively termed biopharmaceuticals, these proteins are used for the treatment of haemophilia, insulin-dependent diabetes, and various immune and cardiovascular diseases. Recombinant expression systems used in the production of biopharmaceuticals are the focus of this article. Another review by Hefferon *et al.* provides an excellent insight into the emerging field of virus like particles (VLP), various nanoparticles (VNP), and the safe and effective applications in drug delivery and transportation of biomedical agents. Badavath and Jayaparakash have contributed an article on the recent development of monoamine oxidase inhibitors (MOAs) as new and effective antidepressants. Among the MOAs, 4,5-dihydro--H-pyrazole derivatives have special merit due to their interesting molecular architecture, and nanomolar inhibitory potential against MOA enzymes from various sources. Korkotian *et al.* have focused on the problems associated with the treatment of alcohol intoxication. They propose to employ polyphenolic substances of plant origin, collectively called flavonoids, for this purpose. Flavonoids are known to possess a wide range of biological activities. The authors have presented the effects of flavonoids from plants of Scrophulariaceae family on functional properties of rat hippocampal neural cultures in the presence of ethanol. The last review of Barradas *et al.* is an account of the development of novel drug delivery systems, based on smart polymeric scaffolds, for topical applications. Their physicochemical properties, safety, and stimuli-response characteristics as effective drug nanocarriers are presented.

We are extremely grateful to authors for their excellent scholarly contributions, and for the timely submission of their reviews. The 10th volume of the ebook series is the result of the efficient coordination and excellent management Ms. Mariam Mehdi (Assistant Manager Publications), and team leader Mr. Mahmood Alam (Director Publications). We are confident that this volume will receive wide appreciation from students, young researchers, and established scientists.

Atta-ur-Rahman, *FRS*
Kings College
University of Cambridge, Cambridge
UK

&

M. Iqbal Choudhary
H.E.J. Research Institute of Chemistry
International Center for Chemical and Biological Sciences
University of Karachi, Karachi
Pakistan

List of Contributors

Alena Botalova	Department of Immunology, Perm State University, Perm, Russia
Eduard Korkotian	Department of Neurobiology, The Weizmann Institute of Science, Rehovot, Israel Department of Immunology, Perm State University, Perm, Russia
Ghyda Murad Hashim	Department of Cell and Systems Biology, University of Toronto, Toronto, Canada
Henrique de Souza Picciani	Instituto de Macromoléculas Professora Eloisa Mano, Universidade Federal do Rio de Janeiro (IMA/UFRJ), Centro de Tecnologia, Bl. J, Av. Horácio Macedo, 2030, Cidade Universitária, Ilha do Fundão – Rio de Janeiro –, Brazil
Kathleen L. Hefferon	Department of Cell and Systems Biology, University of Toronto, Toronto, Canada
Kazim Husain	Department of Gastrointestinal Oncology, Moffitt Cancer Center and Research Institute, 12902 USF Magnolia Drive, Tampa, FL 33612
Mahbobeh Zamani-Babgohari	Department of Cell and Systems Biology, University of Toronto, Toronto, Canada
Menahem Segal	Department of Neurobiology, The Weizmann Institute of Science, Rehovot, Israel
Mounir G. AbouHaidar	Department of Cell and Systems Biology, University of Toronto, Toronto, Canada
Nasir Mahmood	Department of Cell and Systems Biology, University of Toronto, Toronto, Canada Department of Biochemistry, University of Health Sciences, Lahore, Pakistan
Rais A. Ansari	Department of Pharmaceutical Sciences, College of Pharmacy, Health Professions Division, Nova Southeastern University, 3200 S University Drive, Fort Lauderdale, FL 33328
Sarah Bushra Nasir	Abdus Salam School of Sciences, Nusrat Jahan College, Chenab Nagar, Chiniot, Pakistan
Shakil A. Saghir	Scotts Miracle-Gro, 14111 Scottslawn Road, Marysville, OH 43041 Department of Biological and Biomedical Sciences, Aga Khan University, Karachi, Pakistan
Talita Nascimento	Programa de Pós-graduação em Nanobiossistemas, Universidade Federal do Rio de Janeiro, Av. Carlos Chagas Filho, 373, Cidade Universitária, Ilha do Fundão – Rio de Janeiro, Brazil
Tatyana Bombela	Department of Pharmacognosy, Perm State Pharmaceutical Academy, Perm, Russia

Thaís Nogueira Barradas Instituto de Macromoléculas Professora Eloisa Mano, Universidade Federal do Rio de Janeiro (IMA/UFRJ), Centro de Tecnologia, Bl. J, Av. Horácio Macedo, 2030, Cidade Universitária, Ilha do Fundão – Rio de Janeiro –, Brazil
Universidade Federal de Juiz de Fora. Faculdade de Farmácia Departamento de Ciências Farmacêuticas, Rua José Lourenço Kelmer, s/n. Campus Universitário. São Pedro. Zip Code: 36036-900, Juiz de Fora - MG, Brazil

Venkatesan Jayaprakash Department of Pharmaceutical Sciences and Technology, Birla Institute of Technology-Mesra, Ranchi-835215, Jharkhand, India

Vishnu Nayak Badavath Department of Pharmaceutical Sciences and Technology, Birla Institute of Technology-Mesra, Ranchi-835215, Jharkhand, India

CHAPTER 1

Recombinant Protein Production: from Bench to Biopharming

Rais A. Ansari[1,*], **Shakil A. Saghir**[2,3], **Rebecca Torisky**[2] and **Kazim Husain**[4]

[1] *Department of Pharmaceutical Sciences, College of Pharmacy, Health Professions Division, Nova Southeastern University, 3200 S University Drive, Fort Lauderdale, FL 33328, USA*

[2] *Scotts Miracle-Gro, 14111 Scottslawn Road, Marysville, OH 43041, USA*

[3] *Department of Biological and Biomedical Sciences, Aga Khan University, Karachi, Pakistan*

[4] *Department of Gastrointestinal Oncology, Moffitt Cancer Center and Research Institute, 12902 USF Magnolia Drive, Tampa, FL 33612, USA*

Abstract: The needs for purified proteins in modern medicine, research and industrial application are immense and production of proteins using recombinant technology offers solutions; proteins are used in simple laboratory experiments like protein-protein and protein-DNA interactions and in diagnostic, therapeutic and industrial applications. Some examples of the application of purified recombinant proteins for the treatment of diseases include clotting factors (Factor VIII and IX) for the treatment of hemophilia, insulin-dependent diabetes, and adenosine deaminase for severely compromised immune disease. Recently, human monoclonal antibodies, like anti-tumor necrosis factor-α (Adalimumab) for the treatment of rheumatoid arthritis and Repatha (proprotein convertase subtilisin kexin type 9 or PCSK9) inhibitor antibody for the treatment of and reduction in the risk of myocardial infarction, stroke and revascularization of coronary artery diseases, are produced using protein overexpression methodology described in this chapter. Use of recombinant protein technologies has enabled industries to produce proteins of human significance at a tremendous pace. Production of therapeutic proteins at large scale for millions of individuals to treat diseases is one of the essential needs of mankind. From simple proteins like albumin, growth factors, cytokines, viral vaccines and human monoclonal antibodies, all are being produced utilizing the recombinant protein expression technology and purification processes, whether in a laboratory or biopharming scale in microorganisms, animals and/or plants. This chapter summarizes various recombinant expression systems and their pharmaceutical applications.

[*] **Corresponding author Rais A Ansari:** Department of Pharmaceutical Sciences, College of Pharmacy, Health Professions Division, Nova Southeastern University, 3200 S University Drive, Fort Lauderdale, FL 33328, USA; Tel/Fax: (954) 262-1344/(954) 262-2278; E-mail: ra557@nova.edu

Atta-ur-Rehman and M. Iqbal Choudhary (Eds.)

Keywords: Adenovirus Expression System, Baculovirus-Mediated Expression System, Biopharming, CHO Expression System, Eukaryotic Expression System, Gene of Interest, History of Biopharming, Mammalian Expression System, Possible Contaminants in Expression Systems, Prokaryotic Expression System, Protein Expression System, Recombinant Proteins, Shuttle Vector, Vaccinia Virus Expression System, Yeast Expression System.

INTRODUCTION

Human beings use proteins or smaller peptides in different ways, which could be enzymes added to soap or use of growth hormone for the treatment of pituitary-driven dwarfism. Such proteins can be obtained from various sources. However, yields were previously low and the cost of purifying them was quite high, limiting their production and use. Advancements in the area of recombinant protein production has changed the trend making the yields much higher and the cost much lower, allowing the production of such proteins on industrial scale, opening the door for the treatment of multiple diseases and disorders discussed in this chapter. For example, bovine and porcine insulins had been used for the treatment of insulin-dependent diabetes, and they have now been replaced by human insulin produced in *Escherichia coli* using the recombinant technology. This technology has also enabled us to avoid potential contaminations from pathogens of animal origin, like viruses. By using recombinant protein technology, we can overexpress desired proteins and biopharm them using microorganisms, animals, and/or plants.

BASIC EXPRESSION CONCEPT

In almost all systems for expression of recombinant proteins, either plasmids carry or are used to create the expression viruses with a gene of interest (GOI) which is driven by a promoter from another gene (a heterologous system) which is active in the organism wherein the protein is being expressed. Isolation of proteins and their purity remains the issue; therefore, an affinity tag is added to either the amino-terminal (*N*-terminal) or carboxyl-terminal (*C*-terminal) of the proteins. The tags serve for isolation and purification of the protein and read in frame of the GOI. In order to add the tag at either *N*- or *C*-terminal, 4-6 uncharged amino acids are used between tag and protein (Fig. **1**). Usually, an endopeptidase site is present between the GOI and the tag so that tag can be removed enzymatically. For a majority of tags (*e.g.,* glutathione-S-transferase [GST], maltose binding protein [MBP], chitin, strep-tag, polyarginine [p-Arg], and 6xhistidines [6xHis]) affinity resins are used, while for other tags (*e.g.,* small ubiquitin-related modifier [SUMO], FLAG-tag, c-myc peptide, and 1D4 epitope) (for the list of affinity tags and acronyms, see (Table **1**) antibody-resin affinity columns are employed for purification [1, 2]. A single tag, either at the *N*- or *C*-terminal, is not efficient for obtaining sufficiently quality proteins, therefore, dual tags (one at the N- and the other at the C-terminal or in tandem) are routinely used to further enhance the purity of the proteins. A single step 6xHis tag GOI purification using nickel-nitrilotriacetic acid (Ni-NTA) or other metal-containing resins does not produce a satisfactory purified protein. With dual fusion, one additional affinity purification, following 6xHis-affinity purification, removes the contaminating proteins. To increase the purification further, the dual affinity purified sample is subjected to high pressure liquid chromatography (HPLC) or specific protocols developed for the purification of that GOI.

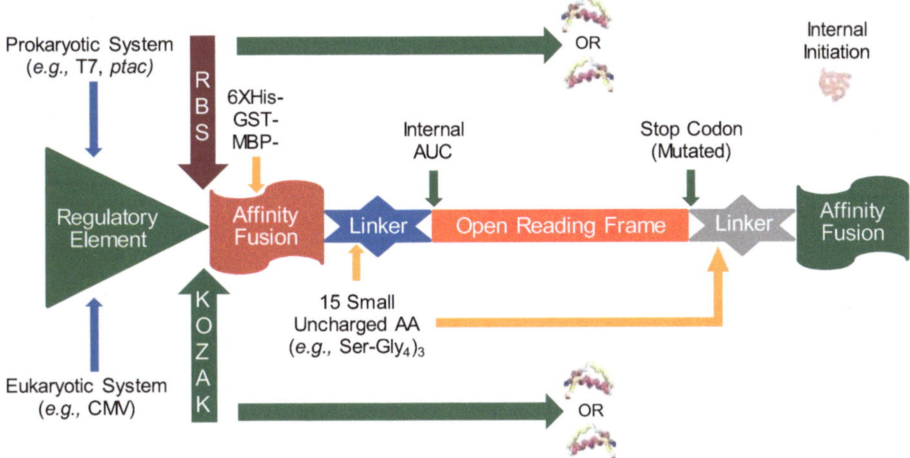

Fig. (1). The basic concept of recombinant proteins and its expression system.

Table 1. List of the affinity/tag.

Polyhistidine (3-10 histidines, usually 6 histines)
Polyarginine (usually 4-5 arginine)
FLAG (N-DYKDDDDK-C)
Metal Affinity Tag (MAT= N-HNHRHKH-C)
Strep-tag (N-WRHPQFGG)
c-MYC peptide (N-EQKLISEEDL-C)
Dual tags with MAT/FLAG and MAT/c-MYC
Hemagglutinin antigen tag (N-YPYDVYA-C)
Calmodulin-binding peptide
Cellolose-binding domain
Acyl carrier protein (8kd)
Small ubiquitin related modifier (SUMO) with 6xHistidines

(Table 1) cont.....

Thioredoxin A (12 kd oxidoreductase)
Ketosteroid isomerase (KSI)
Glutathione-S-transferase (GST)
Maltose binding protein (MBP)

In prokaryotic systems, plasmids directly serve for the expression of GOI in bacteria while viruses (*e.g.,* baculovirus, adenovirus and vaccinia virus) express recombinant proteins by directly infecting the cells. These recombinant viruses when infected to appropriate cells produce the GOI with tag(s). The promoter-derived expression of GOI in a specific cell or organism is either a promiscuous promoter or the promoter of that species-specific gene. Therefore in baculovirus, the polyhedrin gene promoter or the p10 gene promoter which derives expression of the capsid protein is utilized [3, 4]. Similarly, GAL (galactose - inducible gene) promoters which are active in yeast and promoters of other genes like alcohol dehydrogenase (ADH) and glyceraldehyde-3 phosphate dehydrogenase (G3PDH) are used for expression in yeast [5, 6]. Specific viral promoters (T7 and SP6) are also used for driving the gene expression of the GOI [7, 8]. In certain prokaryotic (pET) systems, T7 RNA polymerase remains under the *ptac* promoter and when activated by isopropyl β-D-1-thiogalactopyranoside (IPTG) drives the expression of T7 RNA polymerase, which binds to T7 promoter for driving the expression of the GOI (http://www.emdmillipore.com/US/en/product /pET-Expression-Syst-m-28- Novagen).

The mammalian system includes viruses which infect mammalian cells. The promoters of these viruses utilize the mammalian machinery for replication and production of proteins for viral replication. The two most significant viral expression systems, adenovirus and vaccinia viruses, utilize the cytomegalovirus major immediate early promoter (CMV-MIEP) which is active in most cell types and used for expressing of recombinant proteins [9]. In addition, vaccinia virus utilizes T7 RNA polymerase in trans for the expression of recombinant proteins. For vaccinia virus-based expression, the vaccinia virus T7 RNA polymerase is expressed from vaccinia virus from its promoter (p7.5) which drives the expression of GOI from T7 promoter. The recombinant vaccinia virus with GOI under T7 promoter is produced in thymidine kinase (TK-) cell line and the recombination is achieved at the TK locus which is knocked off in the TK-cells. In order to carry recombination at TK site, the GOI is cloned flanked on both sides with TK gene sequences utilizing the plasmid pGS53. Plasmids are also used for producing a stably transfected cell line deriving GOI expression from CMV-MIEP for the production of recombinant proteins in various mammalian cell lines including Chinese hamster ovary cell line (CHO). In addition to CMV-MIEP, other promoters have also been used [10].

EXPRESSION SYSTEMS

Prokaryotic Expression System

A number of bacterial hosts have been utilized for heterologous protein expression and *E. coli* and *Bacillus subtilis* are the two important and most commonly used prokaryotic expression systems. *E. coli* is the most commonly used prokaryote for the expression and production of recombinant proteins from its gene promoters [11, 12]. Prokaryotes lack post translational modification of proteins. Proteins which lack posttranslational modification, like glycosylation and sumoylation, and are cytosolic in nature, with molecular weight less than 60 kd are easily expressed in a prokaryotic system, especially in *E. coli.* Proteins which are post- translationally modified require expression using eukaryotic and mammalian expression systems. When a prokaryotic system is used for the expression of proteins that require glycosylation, glycosylating enzymes must also be expressed in a prokaryote like *E. coli*. However, when the activity of the protein is linked to glycosylation, inactive proteins may be produced due to differing nature of glycans in prokaryotes. Membrane-bound proteins are not good candidates for expression in prokaryotes due to the association of GOI with lipids, since plasma membranes are absent in *E. coli*. A list of prokaryotic expression systems utilizing various promoters are summarized in Table **2**.

Table 2. List of various promoter systems of prokaryotes and their sources.

Promoter System	**Induction Mechanism**	**System**
lac promoter *tac* promoter *trc* promoter	Isopropyl-β-D-1-thiogalactopyranoside (IPTG)	GE Lifesciences
ara BAD promoter	L-Arabinose	pBAD plasmid, Invitrogen
rha P $_{\mathrm{BAD}}$*tet A* promoter/operator T7 RNA polymerase	L-Rhamnose, Tetracycline, IPTG	pET Plasmid system, Novagen
λPL promoter	Growth at 32°C and induction at 42°C for 1-2 h	SK plasmid system available with NIH repository and Invitrogen

A typical prokaryotic expression system involves a promoter of a prokaryotic gene (*ptac* is a fusion promoter of *ULV5* and *tryp* operon) [13] which is regulated by the addition of a lactose derivative, IPTG. IPTG cannot be metabolized (non-hydrolyzable) by *E. coli* [13] or repressor deactivated by heat when the culturing condition of the heat-inducible promoter is switched from 37°C to 42°C to induce protein expression from lamda phage (λPL) promoter. The λPL promoter utilizes the thermosensitive, λcI repressor protein (cI857) which cannot fold naturally at 42°C and therefore cannot bind to the promoter to repress transcription [14]. Expression from the *ptac* promoter using IPTG results in large amounts of IPTG discharge in the environment; therefore, heat inducible promoters are considered a better choice. In a different set of conditions, when the promoters are from cold shock protein, expression is achieved by reducing temperature. The *ptac* promoter remains under the control of up-mutant (*lacIq*) product which is made operational by adding IPTG. The single gene *lacI* is present in genome and its product cannot efficiently regulate the multi-copy plasmid under the control of *ptac*. Therefore, *lacI* is mutated to produce additional copies of *lacIq* to accommodate the inhibition of multiple copy plasmids deriving the expression from *ptac* promoter. It is evident that in prokaryotes, *lacIq* plays a significant role in the expression of recombinant proteins [15] (Fig. **2**).

The pQE-series of plasmids (Qiagen [16], now Life Sciences) lack the *lac* repressor upmutant (*lacIq)* on the plasmid which is always multiple copy and cannot be completely inhibited from *lacIq* gene product which is present in the *E. coli* genome. The *E. coli* strain DH5α lacks *lacIq* in the genome and when used for cloning GOI in pQE- series plasmids results in clones where the GOI remains constitutively active causing death of positive clones at the expense of excessive expression of GOI (personal observation). Therefore, for GOI to express as 6xHis-fusion using pQE-series plasmids, *E. coli* strain containing *lacIq* in the genome (*Sure* cells) is used for in-frame cloning.

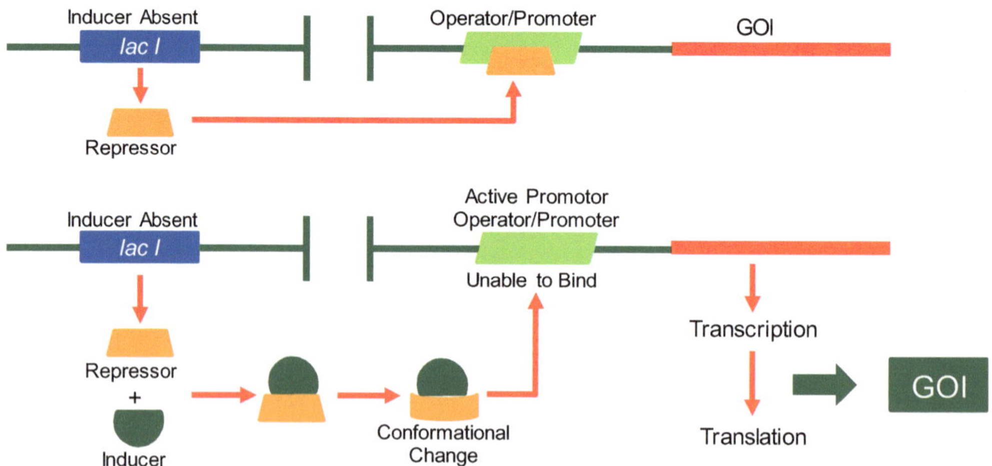

Fig. (2). Mechanism of lac operon based protein expression..

The pET system developed by Novagen is a powerful system that ensures no leaky expression of the recombinant protein. It utilizes a 20-nucleotide long T7 RNA polymerase promoter which cannot be recognized by *E. coli* RNA polymerase. Therefore, in the absence of T7 RNA polymerase, no protein is expressed. A T7 RNA polymerase of DE3 phage is expressed from lacUV5 promoter after induction with IPTG. In the absence of IPTG, T7 RNA polymerase is not expressed due to inhibition by *lacIq*; the promoter upmutant is ten times more effective in carrying out the inhibition. To avoid leaky expression of pET, this system uses T7 lysozyme that inhibits T7 RNA polymerase, which is achieved by introducing another plasmid, pLysS or pLysE. These plasmids carry the T7 lysozyme gene either in silent (pLysS) or expressed (pLysE) orientations in relation to tetracycline responsive promoter (Tc) [17].

The glutathione S-transferase (GST) fusion (pGEX-series) and maltose binding protein fusion (MBP; pMalp2 or pMalc2 series) plasmid (Invitrogen [18], now Thermo Fisher Scientific) carry *lacIq* on the plasmid inhibiting the leaky expression and therefore DH5α is used for cloning the GOI, for both GST and MBP fusions. The MBP fusions are better than GST due to the solubility of MBP [19, 20] than many other fusions proteins (*e.g.*, 6xHis and FLAG-tag fusion proteins). Many other fusion proteins such as metal binding protein, calcium calmodulin binding protein (CaBP), chitin binding protein (CBP) and acyl carrier binding protein (ACP) are also available [21]. Prokaryotic expression systems are easier than other systems as it requires simple culture conditions (*e.g.*, media, additives), low cost, easy scalability, and offers large scale production of recombinant protein in a short period of time (*e.g.*, doubling time of *E. coli* is 20 min). One of the greatest successes of utilizing a prokaryotic system to express proteins is the production of recombinant insulin by Elli Lilly [22].

Eukaryotic Expression System

Shuttle Vectors

A eukaryotic protein expression system involves expression of GOI from a eukaryotic/mammalian promoter. The activity of a promoter is very important as the transcription factors have to find the promoter to drive the expression of GOI. Often the GOI is cloned into a plasmid which is replicated in *E. coli* and later used to stably transfect cells and/or cell lines, like human embryonic kidney-293 (HEK293), human liver (HepG2), Chinese hamster ovary (CHO), HeLa, and baby hamster kidney (BHK) cells. In these situations, a eukaryotic origin of replication which is mostly of viral origin for replication is added to the plasmid. For selecting stably transfected cell lines (*e.g.,* HEK293, HepG2, CHO), a eukaryotic antibiotic resistance gene (*e.g.,* Hygromycin, G418, Puromycin, Zeocin) is also cloned onto the plasmid. Such a plasmid is referred to as "*Shuttle vector*" and is replicated and selected in prokaryotes and eukaryotes. The majority of plasmids used to express the protein in eukaryotic and mammalian cells are shuttle vectors. For lower eukaryotes like yeast, the origin of replication is an autonomously replicating sequence (ARS) derived from the yeast chromosome. The features of shuttle vectors are summarized in the Fig. (**3**). In the proceeding sections, the eukaryotic and mammalian system will be described for the expression of GOI.

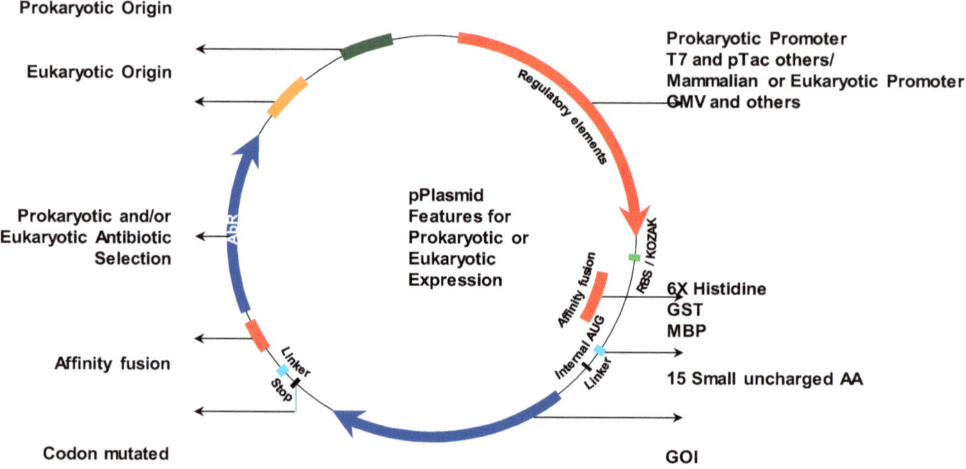

Fig. (3). Features of a shuttle vector.

Yeast Expression System

Primitive eukaryotes which are convenient to grow are utilized for the production of recombinant proteins. Two yeast systems (*Saccharomyces cereviceae* and *Pichia pastoris*) are on the forefront of eukaryotic expression systems. In primitive eukaryotes, proteins can be glycosylated and secreted which is not observed in prokaryotes. The only problem with glycosylation in *S. cereviceae* and *P. pastoris* expression systems is the nature of glycan moiety. For example, in plants and yeasts, glycosylation is of a mannose type whereas animal and human proteins contain glycosylation of galactosamine, sialic acid and glucose. When glycosylation does not affect activity of expressed proteins, lower eukaryotes are used for the expression of human/animal glycosylated proteins. Since the activity of antitrypsin is not affected due to the nature of glycosylation, it is expressed in lower eukaryotes [23]. The cost of expression of proteins in the lower eukaryotes is higher than in the prokaryotes. However, lower eukaryotes can be modified to carry glycosylation-specific genes of mammalian proteins (*i.e.,* humanized proteins) to produce humanized glycoproteins like antibodies [24].

Like prokaryotes, yeast expression systems are also created by cloning GOI into plasmids. Also, as with prokaryotes, yeast-expression plasmids require sequences for maintenance either episomally at the origin of replication or integrated into chromosomes. The plasmids also carry a strong promoter and biomarkers for prokaryotes and eukaryotes for the selection of clones. In yeast expression systems, in addition to integrated plasmids (YIp) and episomal plasmids (YEp), centromeric plasmids (YCp) are also available for expression [25]. The YIp vectors do not replicate autonomously, rather integrate into the chromosome at low frequency providing fewer copies (up to 20) of the GOIs [25]. The YEp vectors carry the natural 2 μm episomal origin of replication providing the ability of plasmids to replicate independently (https://blog.addgene.org). Although YEp plasmids are capable of replicating episomally in the culture, some yeast cells lose the plasmid. Due to loss of YEp plasmid from yeast, large-scale expression of recombinant proteins is not recommended using the YEp plasmid system. Like YEp plasmids, YCp plasmids contain ARS and centromere sequences. YCp-based plasmids tend to be of low copy in yeast cells.

As with prokaryotes, selection of promoters for yeast expression system is achieved by using compatible promoters. In the case of yeast, an inducible promoter such as alcohol dehydrogenase -2 (ADH2), Sucrose -2 (SUC2) and constitutive gene promoter(s) like glyceraldehyde-3-phosphate dehydrogenase (GAPDH) are used. In order to select transformed clones, auxotrophic gene supplementation is used, which is being supplemented when yeast is not transformed and used for selection. The yeast expression systems are shown in Fig. (**4**).

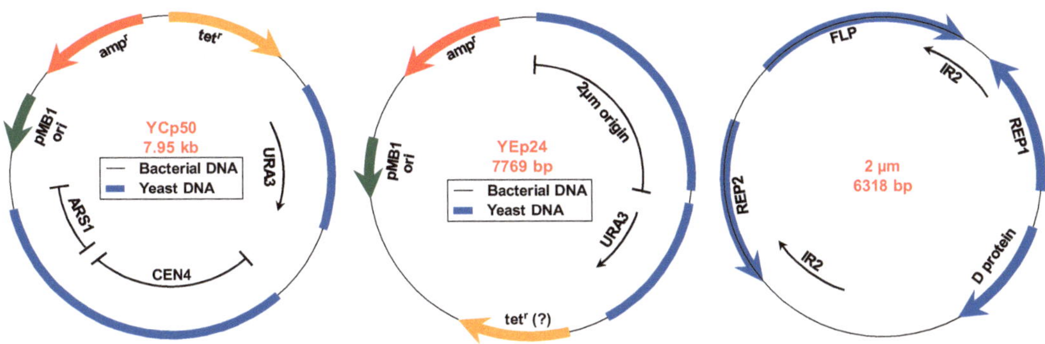

Fig. (4). Expression plasmids for Yeast.

CHO Expression System

For therapeutic proteins to be produced in active form, proper posttranslational modifications and folding are required. Often, it includes posttranslational modification in the form of glycosylation, either *N*-linked to asparagine or *O*-linked to serine/threonine. Glycoproteins are usually produced in mammalian cells, whereas *E. coli* and other prokaryotic systems are deficient in glycosylation. However, attempts to provide specific enzymes for glycosylation into a prokaryotic system to create glycoproteins must take into account their potential adverse biological properties. Therefore, eukaryotic cells derived from rodents and humans (*e.g.,* NIH 3T3, CHO, BHK, HeLa and HepG2) are frequently used for recombinant protein expression from heterologous systems. Despite the availability of many cell lines, the majority of recombinant proteins are produced in CHO cells. The recombinant proteins obtained from CHO cells are biologically active for therapeutic purposes. Additionally, deadly viruses like HIV, influenza, polio, herpes and measles do not replicated in CHO cells, eliminating the possibility of recombinant protein contamination with aforementioned viruses and possible human exposure. A large number of biomoleucles, such as hormones, enzymes and antibodies are produced in CHO cells and cleared for use by US Food and Drug Administration (FDA) [26, 27]. The current global annual sales of biologics produced using CHO cells alone exceed US$30 billion [26].

Although CHO cells are adherent cells, they have been adopted for suspension and thus are scaled up to 10,000 liter capacity for industrial-scale recombinant protein production. The GOI is carried by a shuttle vector which provides both prokaryotic and eukaryotic origins of replication and selection biomarkers for the selection in prokaryotic and eukaryotic (*i.e.,* CHO cells) systems. For a simple GOI expression, CMV-MIEP is used, but a CHO mutant requires dihydrofolate for its growth utilizing expression of GOI from the promoter of dihydrofolate reductase (DHFR) gene [28]. Two DHFR-deficient mutants (DXB11 and DG44) were created from proline auxotroph by Chasin and co-workers and are commonly used today [29 - 31]. The DHFR mutant is transfected with plasmid carrying DHFR gene and GOI under DHFR promoter and grown under the inhibitor, methotrexate (MTX). Inhibition of DHFR metabolism to tetrahydrofolate by methotrexate puts pressure on cell survival inducing the multiplication of DHFR gene which in turns increases the copy number of GOI. This allows increase in copy number of GOI and thus increased expression of recombinant protein as shown in Fig. (**5**).

Baculovirus-Mediated Expression

Baculoviruses are important for the expression of recombinant proteins especially of eukaryotic origin needing posttranslational modification [32]. The proteins are secreted and glycosylated; however, since the proteins are expressed in insect cells, the nature of glycosylation is different than mammalian glycosylation. The baculoviruses are of two types; *Autographa california* (alfalfa looper) nuclear polyhedrosis virus (AcNPV) and *Bombyx mori* (silkworm) nuclear polyhedrosis virus (BmNPV) which have a ~130 kb genome size. Large sections of DNA (up to 30 kb) are inserted into baculovirus expressing genes from late promoters (p10 or polyhedrin gene) which encode architectural proteins. Multiple genes can be expressed in insect cells by infecting them with multiple baculovirus and determining each viral titer in the system.

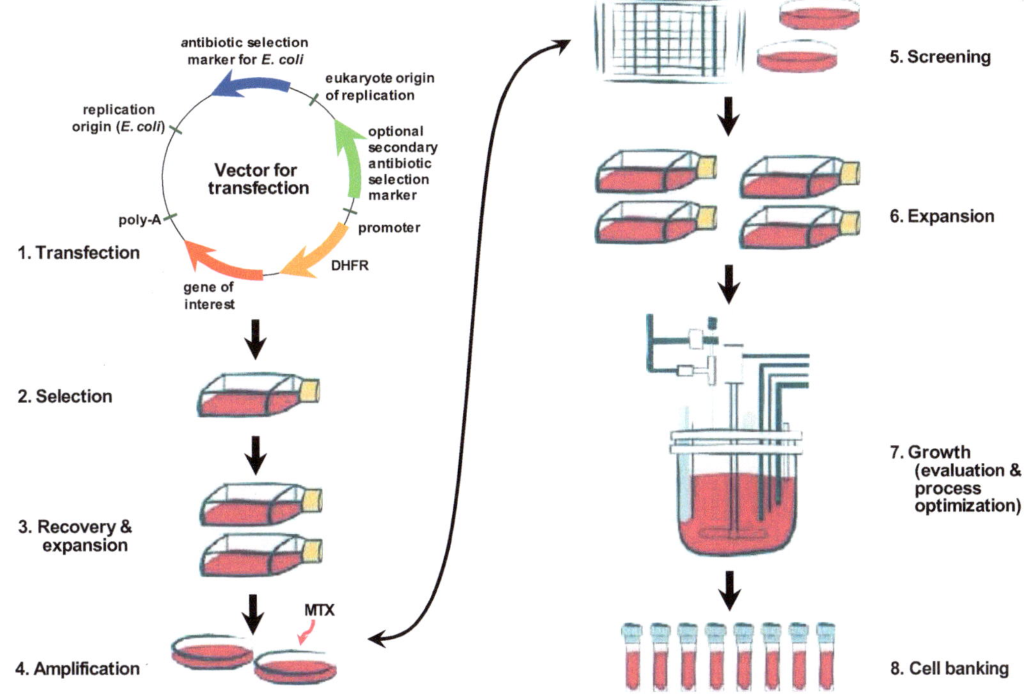

Fig. (5). A schematic presentation of the expression of recombinant protein in CHO cells.

Baculoviruses are produced using a recombination process. Traditionally, the GOI is cloned into a transfer vector which is propagated in *E. coli*. The transfer vector with GOI is transfected into competent DH10BAC *E. coli* cells that contains a *bacmid* and *helper* plasmid. The helper plasmid provides the necessary enzymes for recombination of donor plasmid carrying GOI under the p10 or polyhedrin promoter flanked with recombination sequences to recombine with bacmid. The bacmid is purified and transfected to insect cells. The baculovirus bud out within 3-5 days. These viruses are again used to infect insect cells for further propagation and growth of viruses (Fig. **6**). The plaque forming unit (pfu) activity of viruses are determined for infection of insect cells. A pfu of 3-5/cell is used for expression of recombinant proteins.

The most common cell line used for baculovirus expression system, SF9 cells, is a clonal isolate of the cell line IPLB-SF21-AE *of Spodoptera frugiperda* (fall armyworm). SF9 was originally established from ovarian tissue [13]. In addition to SF9 cells, SF21, Tn-368 and High-Five™ BTI-TN-5B1-4 are also used for the expression of recombinant proteins [33]. There are various claims of better expression of recombinant protein by one or the other cell lines and individual investigators are required to determine the best cell line for the expression of the protein of interest.

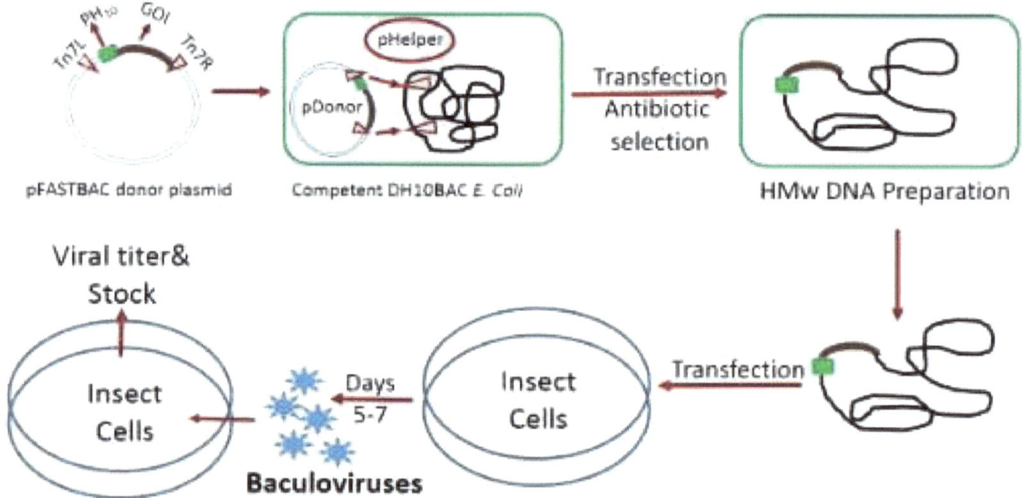

Fig. (6). Baculovirus based expression of GOI.

Because of the nature of infection caused by baculoviruses, there is no possibility of disease(s) from baculovirus infection to humans. Baculovirus-produced recombinant proteins contain high mannose content and therefore the mammalian glycoproteins when expressed in baculovirus may differ in activity. Besides differing in nature of glycosylation, severe acute respiratory syndrome (SARS) virus glycoprotein is produced by the baculovirus expression system [34]. In addition, baculovirus possesses limited capacity to process pro-proteins into active protein as they lack pro-convertase, therefore preprocessing of proteins may be challenging.

Mammalian Expression

Adenovirus Expression System

Several adenoviral expression systems are available which are generated either by cloning or using a process of recombination. The GOI is cloned into a shuttle vector. This shuttle vector carries the GOI to an adenoviral backbone by the process of subcloning or by recombination. The pAdenoX vector is used for the replication of incompetent adenovirus containing and expressing the GOIs. The GOI expression is driven by human CMV immediate-early enhancer/promoter or a promoter of choice (pAd/PL-DEST). Unique enzyme sites are available for excising the GOI and linearizing the plasmid. The GOI of 6.0-7.5 kb size can be carried by adenoviruses. Early passaged HEK293A cells are used for packaging of adenoviruses. The HEK293A cell line contains the E1 gene from adenovirus 5 that is required for the replication of adenoviruses. The adenovirus carrying the GOI is devoid of E1 or E3 gene and therefore, cannot replicate in other cells and is non-oncogenic. The E3 region encodes for proteins involved in evading host immunity and is dispensable. However, the risk of adenoviruses carrying oncogenic genes exists since they are produced in the cell line which carries the gene. The various available adenovirus systems are summarized in Table **3**.

Table 3. Adenovirus virus expression system.

	AdEasy	RAPAd-CMV	Virapower (pAD/CMV/DEST	Adeno-X
Source	Stratagene/Agilent/Qbiogen	Cell Biolab Inc.	Invitrogen	Clonetech
Principle	Homologous recombination in bacteria with AdV backbone	Homologous recombination in HEK-293 cells with AdV backbone	Direct cloning of GOI into AdV backbone plasmid	In vitro direct ligation with AdV backbone
Vector-Shuttle	pShuttle-CMV and various shuttle vectors carrying IRES to express tow genes	pacAd-Ad5-shuttle	No shuttle vector- requires direct ligation into backbone	pCMV-Shuttle2
Vector Backbone	E1 and E3 gene deleted to eliminate recombination competent adenovirus generation	pacAd5 Devoid of left ITR, E1 gene and packaging signal	pAD/DEST, pAD/CMV/V5-DEST, pAD/CMV/V5-GW/LacZ	E1 and E3 gene deleted to eliminate recombination competent adenovirus generation
Process	GOI cloned in pShuttle Homologous recombination in BJ5183 Adenovirus produced in HEK-293	Subcloning in pShuttle vector Homologous recombination in HEK-293 cells Recombinant adenoviruses produced	Subcloning of GOI directly into pAd backbone Bacterail transformation and DNA purification Adenovirus packaged in HEK-293 cells	GOI subcloned into pShuttle Invitro ligation, propagation in bacteria, purify DNA Adenovirus packaged in HEK-293

(Table 3) cont.....

References	(Chabot *et al.*, 2009; Zhang *et al.*, 2008)	(Sutter *et al.*, 2009)	(Li *et al.*, 2008; Lorts *et al.*, 2009)	(Ai et al., 2009; Hirata *et al.*, 2009; Kawanami *et al.*, 2009)

Vaccinia Virus Expression System

Two recombinant vaccinia viruses, one expressing T7 RNA polymerase from p7.5 vaccinia virus promoter and GOI under T7 promoter driven by T7 RNA polymerase are utilized. Usually, both viruses are infected to almost confluent cell lines like HeLa cells at a multiplicity of infection (MOI) of 3-5 viruses/cell. The infection of virus to cells is followed up to 48 h, by which time the majority of the cells are dead but have already expressed proteins of interest. The HIV-gp120 protein has been produced using the vaccinia virus expression system [2, 35]. The overall process of the expression of proteins in vaccinia virus is shown in Fig. (**7**) and the list of proteins expressed in vaccinia virus systems are summarized in Table **4**.

The overall process of the expression of proteins is that the T7 RNA polymerase derives the expression of GOI which is cloned downstream of T7 promoter [36, 37]. Therefore, the vaccinia expression system utilizes two recombinant viruses in which T7 RNA polymerase is first expressed which later derives the expression of GOI [38]. For procedural purposes, the T7 RNA polymerase gene is cloned into pGS53 plasmid which contains P7.5 gene promoter of the vaccinia virus. The promoter is flanked by left (L) and right (R) sequences of TK (thymidine kinase) gene. The TK_L and TK_R sequences are used to recombine with TK gene in vaccinia virus [38]. The process of recombination between plasmid and vaccinia virus results in incorporation of T7 RNA polymerase under P7.5 promoter. Similarly, another recombinant vaccinia virus with GOI under T7 promoter control is produced. The recombined vaccinia virus is grown in TK- cells in the presence of 5-bromouracil. Incorporation of 5-bromouracil in non-recombinant virus is fatal while recombinant viruses survive due to the lack of incorporation of 5-bromouracil. The recombinant viruses are grown and their titer is determined after sucrose gradient purification. In order to carry out vaccinia virus-based expression, two recombinant vaccinia viruses are produced. Viral RNA polymerase (T7 RNA polymerase) processivity is almost 5 times faster than other RNA polymerases; therefore, viral promoters find their utility in successful expression of GOI (Fig. **8**).

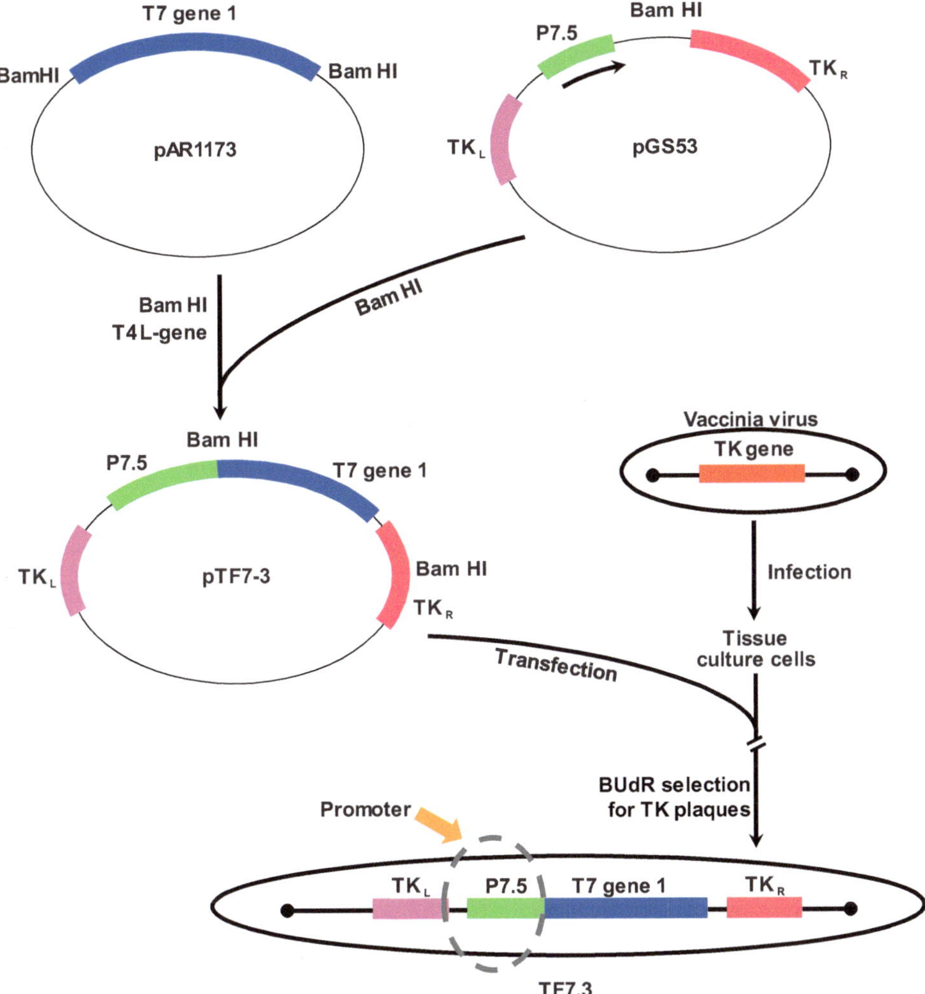

Fig. (7). Vaccinia virus based expression system: Construction of recombinant vaccinia virus.

Table 4. List of protein expressed by Vaccinia virus.

Name of the Protein	Source of Origin	Glycosylation	Cleavage
Factor IX (clotting factor)	Mammalian	Yes	Signal precursor
Preproenkephalin (Interleukin)	Human	Yes	Signal precursor
Hemagglutinin	Influenza	Yes	Signal
Glycoprotein D	Herpes simplex virus I	Yes	Signal
Envelope protein (gp120)	Human immune deficiency virus (HIV)	Yes	Signal
Surface antigens (S, MS, LS)	Hepatitis B	Yes	Secreted

(Table 4) cont.....

Membrane antigen (gp340)	Epstein Barr virus (DNA virus)	Yes	Signal
Glycoprotein	Respiratory syncytial virus	Yes	Signal
Nucleoprotein	Rabies	Yes	Signal

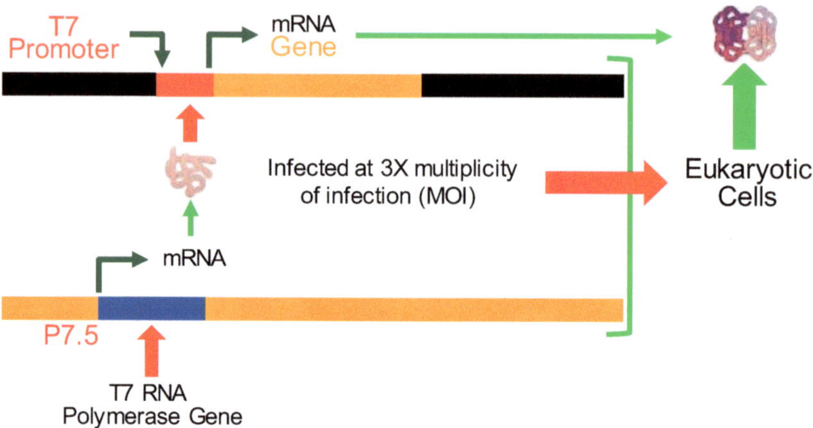

Fig. (8). Vaccinia virus based expression system.

For the expression of proteins, both viruses are infected to almost confluent cell lines like HeLa cells at an MOI of 3-5 viruses/per cell. Vaccinia virus has been used to successfully prepare secreted and glycosylated proteins.

PURIFICATION

Recombinant proteins are purified using affinity tags. A number of affinity tag resins, like Ni-NTA-resin for 6xHis-fusions, reduced glutathione (GSH)-resin for GST-fusion, lentil lectyl-resins for glycosylated proteins are commonly available [2]. Other affinity tags are antibody-resins against various peptides used for purifications. During the purification procedure, the cells expressing the protein are resuspended into phosphate-buffed saline (PBS) in reducing condition (pH 7.4) and broken by sonication and/or two freeze-thaw cycles. Certain proteins, like transcription factors, require salts (*e.g.*, NaCl or KCl) and reducing agents (*e.g.*, dithiothreitol or β-mercaptoethanol) which are added to the buffer. The cells are centrifuged to remove the pellet containing unbroken cells and cell debris while the supernatant containing the expressed protein is further subjected to purification. In the majority of overexpression systems, if the protein is not harmful to the cellular system, it is overexpressed into inclusion bodies which are removed during the first centrifugation step. When inclusion bodies are formed, the pellet is resuspended either in 6M urea or guanidium hydrochloride containing PBS. When expressed protein is dissolved in the aforementioned chaotropic agent, the washing solution used for removing the unwanted bound proteins from affinity resin and elution buffer should also contain chaotropic agents [39]. These chaotropic agents are later removed by dialysis against a buffer. Similarly, Ni-NTA-resin, which binds with 6xHis-fusion proteins, often binds with other proteins as well. In order to avoid the binding of cellular proteins to Ni-NTA resin, the binding of 6xHis-proteins is carried out in a buffer containing 4-6 mM imidazole. Lower level of imidazole is used to avoid binding of histidine-containing proteins of *E. coli* with Ni-NTA resin. However, a higher concentration, *e.g.,* 20 mM, of imidazole is also used for the elution of 6xHis-fusion proteins. In this way, the binding of non-specific cellular proteins is minimized and highly purified 6xHis-fusion protein is prepared; otherwise, a crude mixture with partially purified 6xHis is obtained. In addition to 6xHis affinity, when other affinity proteins like GST or maltose-binding protein (MBP) are used, the Ni-NTA purified proteins are subjected to a second round of affinity binding with GSH or amylose-resins [40]. For the GSH resins, reduced GSH from 10-20 mM is used for elution. Application of higher reduced GSH level in the elution buffer does not give good elution due to the change in the pH of elution buffer resulting in GST-fusion proteins remaining bound with resin. For elution of MBP, maltose is used in elution buffer. For fusions using peptides, there are affinity resins available to bound to antibodies, and a standard protocol is used with a few modifications tailored to the specific proteins. A basic purification protocol is depicted in the Fig. (**9**).

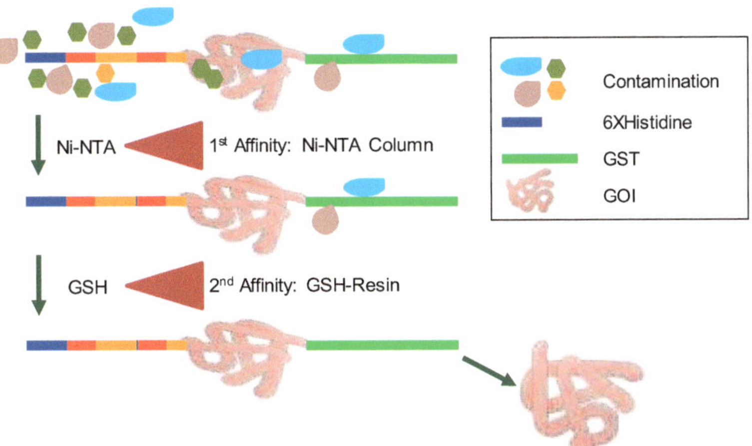

Fig. (9). Typical purification protocol of recombinant proteins.

BIOPROCESS DEVELOPMENT

Industrial scale recombinant protein production requires optimization of protein expression systems in upscaling and downstream processes of purification. High throughput technology (HTP) is used for the manufacturing of proteins. The current HTP requires reducing nutrient volume for maximum protein expression, real time monitoring at micro-scale and providing full automation [41]. The HTP cultivation platforms have been miniaturized where bioreactors utilize from microliter to milliliter volumes. A widely employed platform for microbial screening involves shaken microtiter plates (MTP) which has replaced shaking flasks [42 - 47]. The MTP fails to provide reliable culture performance for upscaling which could be applied for quality control of the processes development. Therefore, bioreactors are used for the optimization of process development where nutrients usage, microbial growth and parameters for efficient sustainable microbial growth are established before the development of large-scale processes. A list of systems for bioreactor application with parameters is provided by Long Q *et al.* [41]. For microbial systems involving *E. coli* or other bacteria, the data generated for nutrient are applied for optimization utilization and accumulation of by-products are applied for optimization of the bioreactor [48]. This optimization is carried out at very small-scale systems using mini-bioreactors available for process optimization. Availability of small-scale bioreactors for microbial growth and recombinant protein production not only solves the problem of process optimization but also offers cost savings [49]. Among various micro-bioreactors, m2p-labs, Inc. Baesweiler, Germany, have introduced BioLector® which contains 48 micro-bioreactors for high-throughput microbial fermentation/screening (https://www.m2p-labs.com). Using BioLector, parameters like biomass, optical density to monitor growth, pH of the nutrient, dissolved oxygen and fluorescence are monitored which makes BioLector easy to use with reproducibile results. It provides computer interface making BioLector a great system for screening bacterial and yeast strains and for the optimization of nutrients and culture conditions. The platform is suitable for aerobic, anaerobic and partial or microaerophilic culture conditions and is used for prokaryotes, eukaryotes, and cells (*e.g.* bacteria [*E. coli*, *B. subtilis*, and *Lactobacillus*], yeasts [*P. pastoris*, *S. cerevisiae*], insects cells [Sf9 and SF 21], and plant cells [*Nicotinum tabacum*]). Other bioreactors, such as advanced micro-bioreactor ambr™ produced by Sartorius (https://www.sartorius.com/us-en), are capable of cell line selection and optimizing nutrient composition and therefore, offer process optimization.

After establishing initial small-scale processes, upscaling is performed for upstream process development where high expression clone(s), nutrient requirements, stable cell line development, through cell line engineering, are critical aspects of upscaling [50 - 54]. Usually, biomanufacturing capacity is increased by using large volume bioreactors, such as 10,000- 25,000 L stainless steel bioreactors. Such a system has been used for producing monoclonal antibodies [55, 56]. In another system, fresh media is continuously perfused to the bioreactor, resulting in significantly higher in cell density when compared with the batch-fed bioreactor [57]. Up to 4-fold higher productivity can be achieved with perfusion at the same bioreactor volume than the batch-fed process [55]. For additional information, readers are advised to check these publications [58 - 61].

BIOPHARMING OF PHARMACEUTICALS

History of Biopharming

Biopharming started in late 1980 (http://www.plantformcorp.com/history-of-bio-pharming.aspx). The concept involves the production of transgenic plants and animals to produce hormones, proteins and antibodies (biologics) by inserting the GOI into a plant or animal species which can be "*farmed*" at large scale to produce biologics given that the laboratory-based production of biologics cannot fulfill all needs, *e.g.,* research and therapy. When scientists reported that antibodies can be produced in tobacco plants, the doors were opened to produce a number of protein- and antibody-based drugs [62, 63]. One example is the replenishment of growth hormones and treatment of immune diseases like rheumatoid arthritis with antibodies [64, 65]. Producing biologics in either plants or transgenic animals are cheaper than producing the products traditionally by chemical or bio-production techniques in laboratories [66]. Fig. (**10**) shows examples of recombinant proteins expressed in various plant and animal systems, along with their advantages and disadvantages.

Biopharming, especially biologics produced in the transgenic plants, require approval from the US Department of Agriculture's Animal and Plant Health Inspection Services (APHIS). The APHIS (https://www.aphis.usda.gov/aphis/ourfocus/biotechnology) is authorized to monitor and provide permission for field trials and development of the biologic pharmaceuticals' production. Farming of transgenic plants for the purpose of biopharming is controversial as well. In 2002, corn plants which were transfected with the gene to make a pig vaccine by ProdiGene, Inc., contaminated adjacent soybean fields in Nebraska [67]. This was due to the lack of specific rules for the containment of transgenic plants, pollen, and seeds. This incident provided fuel to opposition of the GMO (genetically modified organism) industry [68]. With containment strategies in place now to prevent the spread of transgenes to non-targeted plants, biopharming is becoming a reality [69]. Today, transgenic plants are grown in isolated small fields or plant cells are grown in bioreactors to avoid the spreading of transgenes to non-targeted plants and fields.

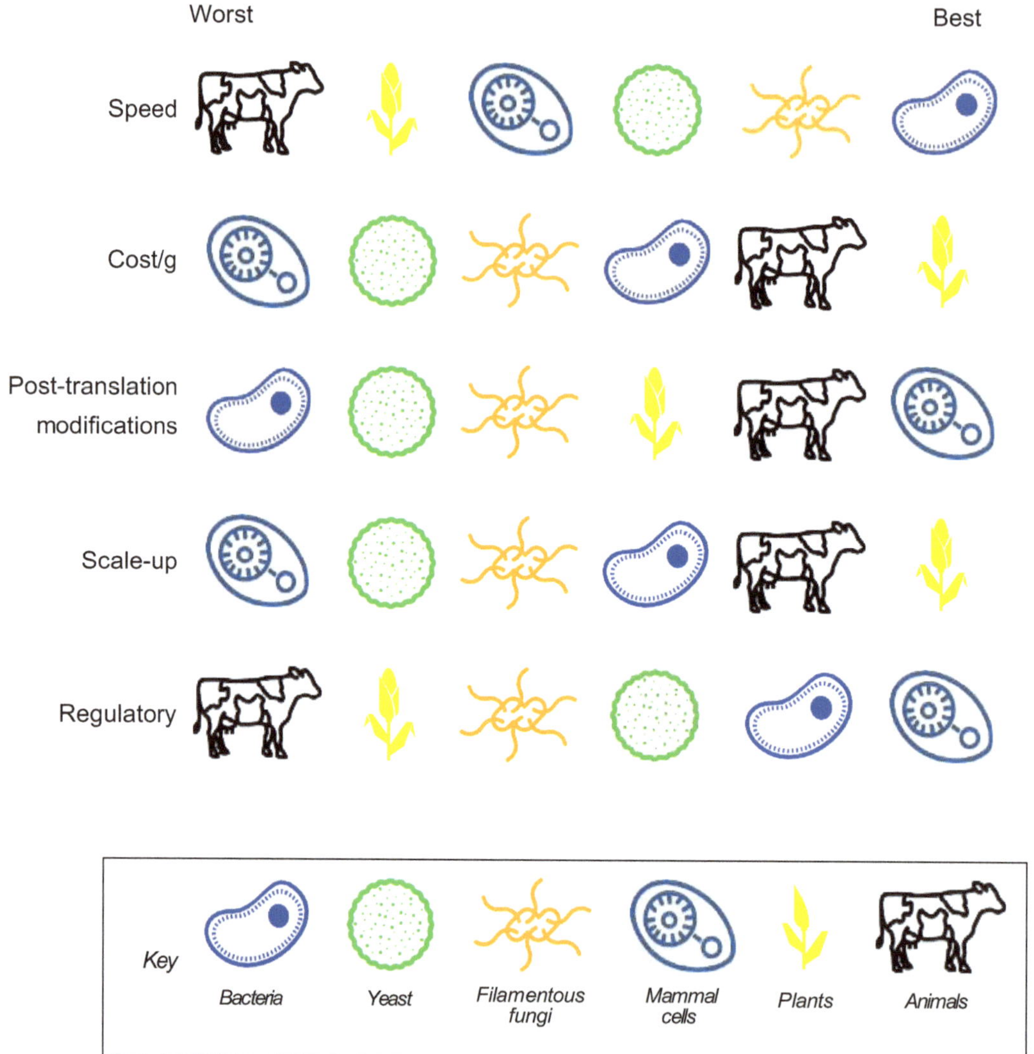

Fig. (10). Relative merits of recombinant protein expressed in various systems.

The first plant-derived product was taliglucerase-alpha which was produced in carrot cells by Protalix Biotherapeutics (Carmiel, Israel) [70]. The FDA approved the drug as "*Elelyso*" for the treatment of Gaucher's disease in 2012. In 2015, the FDA approved *ZMapp*, a plant-produced drug for the treatment of Ebola, a mostly fatal hemorrhagic viral disease. The *ZMapp* was produced by LeafBio Inc. (San Diego, CA, USA) and approved through a fast-track approval process due to the urgency of a treatment for Ebola outbreaks in Africa.

Biologics are beginning to dominate the world pharmaceutical market. The sale of biologics is anticipated to reach US $400 billion by 2020. In 2015, six out of ten drugs marketed globally were biologics. It is anticipated that this trend will continue to rise in the future. The timeline of landmark biopharmaceutical is presented in Table **5**.

Table 5. Time line of pharmaceutical development and biopharming.

Year	Description of Biologics
1982	Using *E. coli* as prokaryotic expression system, human Insulin was produced.
1990	Human serum albumin produced in Tobacco and Potato plants as the 1st plant- derived product.
2006	Tobacco plant made vaccine against Newcastle virus disease produced by Dow Agro Sciences. The vaccine is an injectable and approved in USA.
2012	Elelyso is the enzyme replacement therapy for Gaucher's disease which is being produced in carrot cells by Protalix Pfizer. The Guacher's disease is a rare form of lysosomal storage disease.
2014	Antibodies produced in Tobacco plants by ZMapp for the treatment of human infected with Ebola virus.
2015	US FDA approval of bovine lung Aprotinin production directed by tobacco mosaic virus in tobacco plants. Aprotinin inhibits trypsin and is used to reduce bleeding in surgery.

A CASE OF HUMAN SERUM ALBUMIN AND HUMAN LACTOFERRIN BIOPHARMING

Human serum albumin (HSA) and lactoferrin are important proteins. HSA has many applications and is in short supply. It has been used as a therapeutic since World War II. Its most significant application is for maintaining blood pressure after surgery and in cases of significant blood loss [71]. HSA is also needed in wound healing. In addition, HSA is used as drug and vaccine stabilizer [72] and was the first protein to be used as a blood replacement in the front lines of wars [73].

HSA is not glycosylated and therefore can be expressed in fungi (*e.g., P. pastoris*), plants (*e.g.,* Alfalfa) and animals [73, 74]. Currently, the source of HSA is through ethanol fractionation of human blood. Since HSA is obtained from human plasma, the possibility of contamination with viruses (*e.g.,* HIV, HepC), prion proteins, and other emerging pathogens always exists [73]. One of the major concerns for HSA is that the recombinant HSA (rHSA) has to compete with HSA isolated from human blood or plasma [74]. The rHSA is obtained from bacteria, transgenic plants and animals, and has to be purified to avoid an immune response. A plant-expressed rHSA equivalent to native human serum albumin is available from Akron Biotechnology LLC (Boca Raton, FL, USA), and is devoid of human serum and animal and human viruses. (https://www.akronbiotech.com /product/albumin-recombinant-human/). One attempt to mass produce rHSA was to produce transgenic dairy cattle that could secrete rHSA in milk. The initial attempts were confounded due to contamination with bovine serum albumin (BSA). Tagging HSA coding sequences with affinity proteins will require its removal using proteases which may alter biological activity and immunogenicity - a bottleneck for the development of recombinant proteins at an industrial scale. BSA expression can be deleted during rHSA insertion to produce transgenic cattle for the selective production of human serum albumin using modern transcription activator-like effector nuclease (TALEN) or clustered regularly interspaced short palindromic repeats (CRISPR) technologies [71]. Using somatic cell nuclear transformation (SCNT), transgenic animals, especially cattle, can be produced for the production of recombinant proteins [71].

The initial attempt to produce rHSA in plants was in tobacco leaves and potatoes; however, the yield was less than satisfactory due to proteolytic degradation. An alternative to transgenic whole plants was the utilization of plant cells in culture which can be grown to higher density [74]. A higher yield of rHSA from sugar starvation-induced promoter (alpha Amy3 promoter) was achieved in rice cell cultures [75]. Another approach is the expression of rHSA in the yeast *P. pastoris*. The rHSA expressed in rice or *P. pastoris* exhibits the same amino acid sequence and molecular size (66 kd) as human plasma HSA. The rHSA expressed in these systems shares properties like viscosity, colloidal osmotic pressure and antigenicity with human plasma HSA [76]. The rHSA expressed in Saccharomyces yeast strains is approved by FDA as an excipient in pharmaceutical products like in Recombumin®, which is used in measles, mumps, and rubella vaccines for children (https://albumedix.com/products/recombumin/).

The promising trend to use plants in biotechnology for the expression of recombinant proteins has been demonstrated by obtaining rHSA from fungi. The key advantage with plants is their short life cycle, eukaryotic folding, absence of animal viruses, and low production cost and storage [77].

Lactoferrin (Lf) is an 80 kd globular protein of the transferrin family and is present in secretory fluids such as saliva, tears, milk and colostrum [78]. Its main function is binding and transporting iron for antiviral, antimicrobial, and antiprotozal activities [79]. Expression of Lf has been tried in various species like in *E. coli* [80], *P. pastoris* [81], *S. cerevisae* [82], filamentous fungi [83], and in higher plants like tobacco [84], sweet potato [85] and higher animals like cow [86] and goat [87]. Expression of Lf in cow and goat is fraught with the risk of viral contamination [88], expensive purification and the long life cycle of these animals. The best option for the large-scale Lf protein expression is in higher plants like tobacco [89] utilizing the cauliflower mosaic virus (CaMV35S) promoter. Cultured tobacco cells (Nt-1) are transformed with a plasmid carrying Lf gene controlled by the CaMV35S promoter. One unique property of plant cells is that they can be used to regenerate into whole plants. In this case, transformed cells were used to propagate tobacco plants stably expressing the transgene. Expression of Lf in tobacco plants is between 0.1% and 0.3% of total leaf protein content. Because of the presence of nicotine, nornicotine, and anabasine (nicotine alkaloids), tobacco was not considered a suitable plant for human Lf production.

Therefore, other plant species, like alfalfa was considered; however due to the low expression of Lf, alfalfa was not pursued [90]. Later Lf was expressed in potato by fusing the Lf coding sequences with SEKDEL peptide sequences under control of CaMV35S and auxin-inducible manopine synthase (mas) P2 promoter and achieved an expression level between 0.01 and 0.1% of the total soluble protein [91]. Another species for Lf production is rice. A codon-optimized Lf was expressed between 0.5 and 5.0 g/kg (0.05-0.5%) in the de-husked rice grains [92]. Plant-based glycosylation is different than mammalian glycosylation. The Lf which is expressed in rice is similar in *N*-terminus sequences and activity, like one produced in a mammalian system. Later, Lf was expressed from the glutelin (Gtl) promoter in dehusked rice seeds. Barley and wheat seeds were also used for the expression of Lf as an alternative to rice. The yield of Lf in barley and wheat was lower than in rice. If fast expression is required, *in vitro* cultured plant cells of rice and potatoes can also be used for the production of Lf [93, 94]. A list of human recombinant protein-based drugs is presented in Table **6** along with their manufacturers.

CONTAMINANTS

Residual host-cell proteins (HCPs) are significantly important impurities in recombinant protein biopharmaceuticals and may exhibit immunogenic reactions in humans. The presence of higher levels of HCPs may produce clinically relevant adverse effects. To avoid severe immune reactions, recombinant proteins have to be >99.99% pure. It is recommended that HCPs are reduced to an acceptable level to eliminate an immune response. Removal of HCPs may require salting out, aqueous two-phase extraction, isoelectric focusing and chromatographic purifications. A standard protocol for detection of HCPs is by the ELISA assay, which can detect levels between 1 and 100 ppm, is recommended by the FDA. Another challenge is to identify individual HCPs that can cause allergies at fairly low levels. Similarly, residual DNA presence is another issue with recombinant proteins, especially with rHSA since rHSA is used for the reconstitution of blood. Residual DNA is restricted to 100 pg/dose of purified product [95]. For certain high dose clinical applications, the level of residual DNA was lowerecd to 10 ng/dose in 1997 [96].

Table 6. List of human proteins as recombinant protein available for human use.

Human Proteins as Recombinant	**Source**
Glucocerebrosidase (Ceredase)	Genzyme
Interferon-1βa (Avonex) (Rebif)	Biogenidec Serono
Interferon-1β (Betaseron)	Schering
Erythropoietin	Amgen
Granulocyte colony stimulating factor (GMSF) (Filgrastim) sold as Neupogen	Amgen
α-A galactosidase (Fabrazyme	Genzyme
Tissue plasminogen activator (TPA)	Genentech
Dornase-alpha (DNAse) as Pulmozyme	Genentech
N-acetyl galactosamine-4-sulphatase	BioMarin Pharmaceutical
Nalgazyme ™	
α-L-iduronidase (Aldurazyme)	BioMarin Pharmaceutical and Genzyme

Bacterial derived lipopolysaccharide (LPS), also known as endotoxins, are important contaminants of recombinant protein products when expressed and purified from gram negative bacteria (*e.g., E. coli*). Endotoxins are responsible for the rejection of biopharmaceuticals products when they are present in unacceptable levels. Endotoxins can cause shock, tissue injury and even death. According to the European Pharmacopoeia, endotoxin levels must be lower than 5 endotoxin units/kg body-weight for intravenous injection of rHSA, 10 EU/mg for insulin and 100 EU/mg for interferons [97].

CONCLUSIONS

The demand for high molecular weight recombinant proteins for therapeutic applications in humans is increasing. Significant advances have been made in recent years, in the areas of engineering, microbiology, biochemistry and biotechnology, to produce these proteins, with systems now available using expression systems involving either prokaryotes or eukaryotes. By applying recombinant DNA technology, scientists can manipulate the complementary DNA sequence (cDNA) of human genes to express in prokaryotes and/or eukaryotes. One of the best examples is human insulin produced in *E. coli*. In order to mitigate human needs for the biologically active recombinant proteins, either transgenic animals or plants are produced for biopharming. These genes can be expressed in heterologous systems where promoters are generally species-specific for the production of these recombinant proteins. Animal-based recombinant proteins are costly and may be with possible contaminations for the treatment of human diseases; therefore the FDA has strict guidelines while plant-derived recombinant proteins are cheaper and do not carry animal or human viruses as contaminants.

CONSENT FOR PUBLICATION

Not applicable.

CONFLICT OF INTEREST

The authors declare no conflict of interest, financial or otherwise.

ACKNOWLEDGEMENTS

Declared none.

REFERENCES

[1] Britton ZT, Hanle EI, Robinson AS. An expression and purification system for the biosynthesis of adenosine receptor peptides for biophysical and structural characterization. Protein Expr Purif 2012; 84(2): 224-35.
[http://dx.doi.org/10.1016/j.pep.2012.06.005] [PMID: 22722102]

[2] Young CL, Britton ZT, Robinson AS. Recombinant protein expression and purification: a comprehensive review of affinity tags and microbial applications. Biotechnol J 2012; 7(5): 620-34.
[http://dx.doi.org/10.1002/biot.201100155] [PMID: 22442034]

[3] Knebel D, Lübbert H, Doerfler W. The promoter of the late p10 gene in the insect nuclear polyhedrosis virus Autographa californica: activation by viral gene products and sensitivity to DNA methylation. EMBO J 1985; 4(5): 1301-6.
[http://dx.doi.org/10.1002/j.1460-2075.1985.tb03776.x] [PMID: 3891327]

[4] Possee RD, Howard SC. Analysis of the polyhedrin gene promoter of the Autographa californica nuclear polyhedrosis virus. Nucleic Acids Res 1987; 15(24): 10233-48.
[http://dx.doi.org/10.1093/nar/15.24.10233] [PMID: 3320964]

[5] West RW Jr, Yocum RR, Ptashne M. Saccharomyces cerevisiae GAL1-GAL10 divergent promoter region: location and function of the upstream activating sequence UASG. Mol Cell Biol 1984; 4(11): 2467-78.
[http://dx.doi.org/10.1128/MCB.4.11.2467] [PMID: 6392852]

[6] Mumberg D, Müller R, Funk M. Yeast vectors for the controlled expression of heterologous proteins in different genetic backgrounds. Gene 1995; 156(1): 119-22.
[http://dx.doi.org/10.1016/0378-1119(95)00037-7] [PMID: 7737504]

[7] Högbom E, Magnusson AC, Leanderson T. Functional modularity in the SP6 kappa promoter. Nucleic Acids Res 1991; 19(16): 4347-54.
[http://dx.doi.org/10.1093/nar/19.16.4347] [PMID: 1909431]

[8] Ikeda RA, Lin AC, Clarke J. Initiation of transcription by T7 RNA polymerase as its natural promoters. J Biol Chem 1992; 267(4): 2640-9.
[PMID: 1733960]

[9] Macias MP, Huang L, Lashmit PE, Stinski MF. Cellular or viral protein binding to a cytomegalovirus promoter transcription initiation site: effects on transcription. J Virol 1996; 70(6): 3628-35.
[PMID: 8648697]

[10] Running Deer J, Allison DS. High-level expression of proteins in mammalian cells using transcription regulatory sequences from the Chinese hamster EF-1alpha gene. Biotechnol Prog 2004; 20(3): 880-9.
[http://dx.doi.org/10.1021/bp034383r] [PMID: 15176895]

[11] Hannig G, Makrides SC. Strategies for optimizing heterologous protein expression in *Escherichia coli*. Trends Biotechnol 1998; 16(2): 54-60.
[http://dx.doi.org/10.1016/S0167-7799(97)01155-4] [PMID: 9487731]

[12] Sørensen HP, Mortensen KK. Advanced genetic strategies for recombinant protein expression in *Escherichia coli*. J Biotechnol 2005; 115(2): 113-28.
[http://dx.doi.org/10.1016/j.jbiotec.2004.08.004] [PMID: 15607230]

[13] de Boer HA, Comstock LJ, Vasser M. The tac promoter: a functional hybrid derived from the trp and lac promoters. Proc Natl Acad Sci USA 1983; 80(1): 21-5.
[http://dx.doi.org/10.1073/pnas.80.1.21] [PMID: 6337371]

[14] Valdez-Cruz NA, Caspeta L, Pérez NO, Ramírez OT, Trujillo-Roldán MA. Production of recombinant proteins in *E. coli* by the heat inducible expression system based on the phage lambda pL and/or pR promoters. Microb Cell Fact 2010; 9: 18.
[http://dx.doi.org/10.1186/1475-2859-9-18] [PMID: 20298615]

[15] Calos MP. DNA sequence for a low-level promoter of the lac repressor gene and an 'up' promoter mutation. Nature 1978; 274(5673): 762-5.
[http://dx.doi.org/10.1038/274762a0] [PMID: 355890]

[16] https://www.qiagen.com

[17] Dubendorff JW, Studier FW. Controlling basal expression in an inducible T7 expression system by blocking the target T7 promoter with lac repressor. J Mol Biol 1991; 219(1): 45-59.
[http://dx.doi.org/10.1016/0022-2836(91)90856-2] [PMID: 1902522]

[18] Invitrogen. Available at: https://www.thermofisher.com/us/en/home/brands/invitrogen.html

[19] Fox JD, Waugh DS. Maltose-binding protein as a solubility enhancer. Methods Mol Biol 2003; 205: 99-117.
[PMID: 12491882]

[20] Sun P, Tropea JE, Waugh DS. Enhancing the solubility of recombinant proteins in *Escherichia coli* by using hexahistidine-tagged maltose-binding protein as a fusion partner. Methods Mol Biol 2011; 705: 259-74.
[http://dx.doi.org/10.1007/978-1-61737-967-3_16] [PMID: 21125392]

[21] Terpe K. Overview of tag protein fusions: from molecular and biochemical fundamentals to commercial systems. Appl Microbiol Biotechnol 2003; 60(5): 523-33.
[http://dx.doi.org/10.1007/s00253-002-1158-6] [PMID: 12536251]

[22] Johnson IS. Human insulin from recombinant DNA technology. Science 1983; 219(4585): 632-7.
[http://dx.doi.org/10.1126/science.6337396] [PMID: 6337396]

[23] Arjmand S, Bidram E, Lotfi AS, Shamsara M, Mowla SJ. Expression and purification of functionally active recombinant human alpha 1-antitrypsin in methylotrophic yeast *Pichia pastoris*. Avicenna J Med Biotechnol 2011; 3(3): 127-34.
[PMID: 23408781]

[24] Ward M, Lin C, Victoria DC, *et al.* Characterization of humanized antibodies secreted by *Aspergillus*

niger. Appl Environ Microbiol 2004; 70(5): 2567-76.
[http://dx.doi.org/10.1128/AEM.70.5.2567-2576.2004] [PMID: 15128505]

[25] Gnügge R, Rudolf F. *Saccharomyces cerevisiae* Shuttle vectors. Yeast 2017; 34(5): 205-21.
[http://dx.doi.org/10.1002/yea.3228] [PMID: 28072905]

[26] Zhu MM, Mollet M, Hubert RS, *et al.* Industrial production of therapeutic proteins: cell lines, cell culture, and purification. In: Kent J, Bommaraju T, Barnicki S, Eds. Handbook of Industrial Chemistry and Biotechnology. Springer 2017.
[http://dx.doi.org/10.1007/978-3-319-52287-6_29]

[27] Kim JY, Kim YG, Lee GM. CHO cells in biotechnology for production of recombinant proteins: current state and further potential. Appl Microbiol Biotechnol 2012; 93(3): 917-30.
[http://dx.doi.org/10.1007/s00253-011-3758-5] [PMID: 22159888]

[28] Jayapal KP, Wlaschin KF. Recombinant Protein Therapeutics from CHO Cells-20 Years and Counting, CHO Consortium, SBE Special Section 2007. [https://pdfs.semanticscholar.org/5f96/12ce9170571f296b75246e80cb671bbb886c.pdf]

[29] Graf LH Jr, Chasin LA. Direct demonstration of genetic alterations at the dihydrofolate reductase locus after gamma irradiation. Mol Cell Biol 1982; 2(1): 93-6.
[http://dx.doi.org/10.1128/MCB.2.1.93] [PMID: 6287224]

[30] Urlaub G, Chasin LA. Isolation of Chinese hamster cell mutants deficient in dihydrofolate reductase activity. Proc Natl Acad Sci USA 1980; 77(7): 4216-20.
[http://dx.doi.org/10.1073/pnas.77.7.4216] [PMID: 6933469]

[31] Urlaub G, Käs E, Carothers AM, Chasin LA. Deletion of the diploid dihydrofolate reductase locus from cultured mammalian cells. Cell 1983; 33(2): 405-12.
[http://dx.doi.org/10.1016/0092-8674(83)90422-1] [PMID: 6305508]

[32] van Oers MM, Pijlman GP, Vlak JM. Thirty years of baculovirus-insect cell protein expression: from dark horse to mainstream technology. J Gen Virol 2015; 96(Pt 1): 6-23.
[http://dx.doi.org/10.1099/vir.0.067108-0] [PMID: 25246703]

[33] Wickham TJ, Davis T, Granados RR, Shuler ML, Wood HA. Screening of insect cell lines for the production of recombinant proteins and infectious virus in the baculovirus expression system. Biotechnol Prog 1992; 8(5): 391-6.
[http://dx.doi.org/10.1021/bp00017a003] [PMID: 1369220]

[34] He Y, Li J, Heck S, Lustigman S, Jiang S. Antigenic and immunogenic characterization of recombinant baculovirus-expressed severe acute respiratory syndrome coronavirus spike protein: implication for vaccine design. J Virol 2006; 80(12): 5757-67.
[http://dx.doi.org/10.1128/JVI.00083-06] [PMID: 16731915]

[35] Vasiliver-Shamis G, Tuen M, Wu TW, *et al.* Human immunodeficiency virus type 1 envelope gp120 induces a stop signal and virological synapse formation in noninfected CD4+ T cells. J Virol 2008; 82(19): 9445-57.
[http://dx.doi.org/10.1128/JVI.00835-08] [PMID: 18632854]

[36] Hebben M, Brants J, Birck C, *et al.* High level protein expression in mammalian cells using a safe viral vector: Modified vaccinia virus Ankara Protein Expression Purification 2007; 56(2007): 269-78.
[http://dx.doi.org/10.1016/j.pep.2007.08.003]

[37] Elroy-Stein O, Moss B Gene Expression Using the Vaccinia Virus/T7 RNA Polymerase Hybrid System. Curr Protoc Mol Biol 1998; 16 .19.1-16.19.11.
[http://dx.doi.org/10.1002/0471142727.mb1619s43]

[38] Fuerst TR, Niles EG, Studier FW, Moss B. Eukaryotic transient-expression system based on recombinant vaccinia virus that synthesizes bacteriophage T7 RNA polymerase. Proc Natl Acad Sci USA 1986; 83(21): 8122-6.
[http://dx.doi.org/10.1073/pnas.83.21.8122] [PMID: 3095828]

[39] Penn-Nicholson A, Han DP, Kim SJ, *et al.* Assessment of antibody responses against gp41 in HIV---infected patients using soluble gp41 fusion proteins and peptides derived from M group consensus envelope. Virology 2008; 372(2): 442-56. [http://dx.doi.org/10.1016/j.virol.2007.11.009] [PMID: 18068750]

[40] Chang TL, Kramer MG, Ansari RA, Khan SA. Role of individual monomers of a dimeric initiator protein in the initiation and termination of plasmid rolling circle replication. J Biol Chem 2000; 275(18): 13529-34. [http://dx.doi.org/10.1074/jbc.275.18.13529] [PMID: 10788467]

[41] Long Q, Liu X, Yang Y, Li L, Harvey L, McNeil B, *et al.* The development and application of high throughput cultivation technology in bioprocess development. J Biotech 2014; 192 Pt B: 323-8. [http://dx.doi.org/10.1016/j.jbiotec.2014.03.028]

[42] Duetz W, Chase M, Bill G. Chapter 8 minitiarization of fermentation. AMS Manual of Industrial Microbiology and Biotechnology 3rd ed. 2010; (Electronic)

[43] Duetz WA, Rüedi L, Hermann R, O'Connor K, Büchs J, Witholt B. Methods for intense aeration, growth, storage, and replication of bacterial strains in microtiter plates. Appl Environ Microbiol 2000; 66(6): 2641-6. [http://dx.doi.org/10.1128/AEM.66.6.2641-2646.2000] [PMID: 10831450]

[44] Funke M, Diederichs S, Kensy F, Müller C, Büchs J. The baffled microtiter plate: increased oxygen transfer and improved online monitoring in small scale fermentations. Biotechnol Bioeng 2009; 103(6): 1118-28. [http://dx.doi.org/10.1002/bit.22341] [PMID: 19449392]

[45] Grunzel P, Pilarek M, Steinbrück D, *et al.* Mini-scale cultivation method enables expeditious plasmid production in *Escherichia coli*. Biotechnol J 2014; 9(1): 128-36. [http://dx.doi.org/10.1002/biot.201300177] [PMID: 24130162]

[46] Sohoni SV, Bapat PM, Lantz AE. Robust, small-scale cultivation platform for *Streptomyces coelicolor*. Microb Cell Fact 2012; 11: 9. [http://dx.doi.org/10.1186/1475-2859-11-9] [PMID: 22252012]

[47] Wen Y, Zang R, Zhang X, Yang ST. A 24-microwell plate with improved mixing and scalable performance for high thoughput cell culture. Process Biochem 2012; 47(4): 612-8. [http://dx.doi.org/10.1016/j.procbio.2011.12.023]

[48] Challener C. Fermentation for the future. Biopharm Int 2015; 28: 1. [PMID: 23919241]

[49] Gupta SK, Shukla P. Advanced technologies for improved expression of recombinant proteins in bacteria: perspectives and applications. Crit Rev Biotechnol 2016; 36(6): 1089-98. [http://dx.doi.org/10.3109/07388551.2015.1084264] [PMID: 26384140]

[50] Butler M, Meneses-Acosta A. Recent advances in technology supporting biopharmaceutical production from mammalian cells. Appl Microbiol Biotechnol 2012; 96(4): 885-94. [http://dx.doi.org/10.1007/s00253-012-4451-z] [PMID: 23053101]

[51] Li F, Vijayasankaran N, Shen AY, Kiss R, Amanullah A. Cell culture processes for monoclonal antibody production. MAbs 2010; 2(5): 466-79. [http://dx.doi.org/10.4161/mabs.2.5.12720] [PMID: 20622510]

[52] Rita Costa A, Elisa Rodrigues M, Henriques M, Azeredo J, Oliveira R. Guidelines to cell engineering for monoclonal antibody production. Eur J Pharm Biopharm 2010; 74(2): 127-38. [http://dx.doi.org/10.1016/j.ejpb.2009.10.002] [PMID: 19853660]

[53] Yang. S-T, and Kiu, X. Cell culture processes for biologics manufacturing: recent development and trends. Pharm Bioprocess 2013; 1(2): 133-6. [http://dx.doi.org/10.4155/pbp.13.15]

[54] Zhu J. Mammalian cell protein expression for biopharmaceutical production. Biotechnol Adv 2012; 30(5): 1158-70. [http://dx.doi.org/10.1016/j.biotechadv.2011.08.022] [PMID: 21968146]

[55] Rose S, Black T, Ramakrishnan D. Mammalian cell culture: process development consideration.Handbook of Industrial cell culture. New York, NY: Humana Press 2003.

[56] Yao J, Weng Y, Dickey A, Wang KY. Plants as factories for human pharmaceutical: applications and challenges. Int J Mol Sci 2015; 16(12): 28549-65. [http://dx.doi.org/10.3390/ijms161226122]

[57] Lim J, Sinclair A, Shevitz J, Carter JB. An economic comparison of three cell culture techniques: fed-batch, concentrated fed-batch and concentrated perfusion. Biopharm Int 2011; 24: 54-60.

[58] Gronemeyer P, Ditz R, Strube J. Trends in upstream and downstream process development for antibody manufacturing. Bioengineering (Basel) 2014; 1(4): 188-212. [http://dx.doi.org/10.3390/bioengineering1040188] [PMID: 28955024]

[59] Gupta SK, Shukla P. Sophisticated cloning, fermentation, and purification technologies for an enhanced therapeutic protein production: a review. Front Pharmacol 2017; 8: 419. [http://dx.doi.org/10.3389/fphar.2017.00419] [PMID: 28725194]

[60] Tripathi NK. Production and purification of recombinant proteins from *Escherichia coli.* ChemBioEng Rev 2016; 3(3): 116-33. [http://dx.doi.org/10.1002/cben.201600002]

[61] Tripathi NK, Shrivastava A. Scale up of biopharmaceuticals production.Nanoscale Fabrication, Optimization, Scale-Up and Biological Aspects of Pharmaceutical Nanotechnology. Elsevier Inc. 2018; pp. 133-72. [http://dx.doi.org/10.1016/B978-0-12-813629-4.00004-8]

[62] Düring K, Hippe S, Kreuzaler F, Schell J. Synthesis and self-assembly of a functional monoclonal antibody in transgenic *Nicotiana tabacum*. Plant Mol Biol 1990; 15(2): 281-93. [http://dx.doi.org/10.1007/BF00036914] [PMID: 2129424]

[63] Hiatt A, Cafferkey R, Bowdish K. Production of antibodies in transgenic plants. Nature 1989; 342(6245): 76-8. [http://dx.doi.org/10.1038/342076a0] [PMID: 2509938]

[64] Takeda A, Cooper K, Bird A, *et al.* Recombinant human growth hormone for the treatment of growth disorders in children: a systematic review and economic evaluation. Health Technol Assess 2010; 14(42): 1-209, iii-iv. [iii- iv.]. [http://dx.doi.org/10.3310/hta14420] [PMID: 20849734]

[65] Tanaka T, Hishitani Y, Ogata A. Monoclonal antibodies in rheumatoid arthritis: comparative effectiveness of tocilizumab with tumor necrosis factor inhibitors. Biologics 2014; 8: 141-53. [http://dx.doi.org/10.2147/BTT.S37509] [PMID: 24741293]

[66] Maima AO, Munyendo W. L. L. contemporary advances and precints of biopharming as drugs' production system. J Nat Sci Res 2018; 8(4): 1-9.[ISSN 2225-0921]

[67] Ellstrand NC. Going to "great lengths" to prevent the escape of genes that produce specialty chemicals. Plant Physiol 2003; 132(4): 1770-4. [http://dx.doi.org/10.1104/pp.103.025908] [PMID: 12913134]

[68] Porterfield A. After early struggles, 'biopharming' poised to make big impact on medicine. Genetic Literacy Project 2016. https://geneticliteracyproject.org/2016/01/20/early-struggles-biopharming-poised-make-big-impact-medicine/

[69] Elbehri A. Biopharming and the food system: examining the potential benefits and risks. AgBioForum 2005; 8(1): 18-25. http://www.agbioforum.org

[70] Grabowski GA, Golembo M, Shaaltiel Y. Taliglucerase alfa: an enzyme replacement therapy using

plant cell expression technology. Mol Genet Metab 2014; 112(1): 1-8.
[http://dx.doi.org/10.1016/j.ymgme.2014.02.011] [PMID: 24630271]

[71] Moghaddassi S, Eyestone W, Bishop CE. TALEN-mediated modification of the bovine genome for large-scale production of human serum albumin. PLoS One 2014; 9(2): e89631.
[http://dx.doi.org/10.1371/journal.pone.0089631] [PMID: 24586924]

[72] Alexander MR, Alexander B, Mustion AL, Spector R, Wright CB. Therapeutic use of albumin: 2. JAMA 1982; 247(6): 831-3.
[http://dx.doi.org/10.1001/jama.1982.03320310079043] [PMID: 7057567]

[73] Echelard Y, Williams JL, Destrempes MM, *et al.* Production of recombinant albumin by a herd of cloned transgenic cattle. Transgenic Res 2009; 18(3): 361-76.
[http://dx.doi.org/10.1007/s11248-008-9229-9] [PMID: 19031005]

[74] Chen Z, He Y, Shi B, Yang D. Human serum albumin from recombinant DNA technology: challenges and strategies. Biochim Biophys Acta 2013; 1830(12): 5515-25.
[http://dx.doi.org/10.1016/j.bbagen.2013.04.037] [PMID: 23644036]

[75] Huang LF, Liu YK, Lu CA, Hsieh SL, Yu SM. Production of human serum albumin by sugar starvation induced promoter and rice cell culture. Transgenic Res 2005; 14(5): 569-81.
[http://dx.doi.org/10.1007/s11248-004-6481-5] [PMID: 16245148]

[76] Ohtani W, Nawa Y, Takeshima K, Kamuro H, Kobayashi K, Ohmura T. Physicochemical and immunochemical properties of recombinant human serum albumin from *Pichia pastoris*. Anal Biochem 1998; 256(1): 56-62.
[http://dx.doi.org/10.1006/abio.1997.2480] [PMID: 9466797]

[77] Yao J, Weng Y, Dickey A, Wang KY. Plants as factories for human pharmaceuticals: applications and challenges. Int J Mol Sci 2015; 16(12): 28549-65.
[http://dx.doi.org/10.3390/ijms161226122] [PMID: 26633378]

[78] Gonzalez-Chavez SA, Arevalo-Gallegos S, Rascon-Cruz Q. Lactoferrin research, technology and applications. Int Dairy J 2009; 16(11): 1241-51.
[http://dx.doi.org/10.1016/j.ijantimicag.2008.07.020]

[79] Wakabayashi HYK, Takase M. Lactoferrin research, technology and applications. Int Dairy J 2006; 16(11): 1241-51.
[http://dx.doi.org/10.1016/j.idairyj.2006.06.013]

[80] Tian ZG, Teng D, Yang YL, *et al.* Multimerization and fusion expression of bovine lactoferricin derivative LfcinB15-W4,10 in *Escherichia coli*. Appl Microbiol Biotechnol 2007; 75(1): 117-24.
[http://dx.doi.org/10.1007/s00253-006-0806-7] [PMID: 17225098]

[81] Kruzel ML, Zimecki M. Lactoferrin and immunologic dissonance: clinical implications. Arch Immunol Ther Exp (Warsz) 2002; 50(6): 399-410.
[PMID: 12546066]

[82] Liang Q, Richardson T. Expression and characterization of human lactoferrin in yeast *Saccharomyces cerevisiae*. J Agric Food Chem 1993; 41: 1800-7.
[http://dx.doi.org/10.1021/jf00034a053]

[83] Ward PP, Lo JY, Duke M, May GS, Headon DR, Conneely OM. Production of biologically active recombinant human lactoferrin in *Aspergillus oryzae*. Biotechnology (N Y) 1992; 10(7): 784-9.
[PMID: 1368268]

[84] Salmon V, Legrand D, Slomianny MC, *et al.* Production of human lactoferrin in transgenic tobacco plants. Protein Expr Purif 1998; 13(1): 127-35.
[http://dx.doi.org/10.1006/prep.1998.0886] [PMID: 9631525]

[85] Min WJ Sr, Jeong WJ, Han SK, Lee YB, Liu JR. Production of human lactoferrin in transgenic cell suspension cultures of sweet potato. Biol Plant 2006; 50: 131-4.
[http://dx.doi.org/10.1007/s10535-005-0087-5]

[86] van Berkel PH, Welling MM, Geerts M, *et al.* Large scale production of recombinant human lactoferrin in the milk of transgenic cows. Nat Biotechnol 2002; 20(5): 484-7. [http://dx.doi.org/10.1038/nbt0502-484] [PMID: 11981562]

[87] Han ZS, Li QW, Zhang ZY, *et al.* High-level expression of human lactoferrin in the milk of goats by using replication-defective adenoviral vectors. Protein Expr Purif 2007; 53(1): 225-31. [http://dx.doi.org/10.1016/j.pep.2006.11.019] [PMID: 17208010]

[88] Conesa C, Calvo M, Sánchez L. Recombinant human lactoferrin: a valuable protein for pharmaceutical products and functional foods. Biotechnol Adv 2010; 28(6): 831-8. [http://dx.doi.org/10.1016/j.biotechadv.2010.07.002] [PMID: 20624450]

[89] Mitra A, Zhang Z. Expression of a human lactoferrin cDNA in tobacco cells produces antibacterial protein(s). Plant Physiol 1994; 106(3): 977-81. [http://dx.doi.org/10.1104/pp.106.3.977] [PMID: 7824662]

[90] Stefanova G, Slavov S, Gecheff K, Vlahova M, Atanassov A. Expression of recombinant human lactoferrin in transgenic alfalfa plants. Biol Plant 2013; 57(3): 457-64. [http://dx.doi.org/10.1007/s10535-013-0305-5]

[91] Chong DK, Langridge WH. Expression of full-length bioactive antimicrobial human lactoferrin in potato plants. Transgenic Res 2000; 9(1): 71-8. [http://dx.doi.org/10.1023/A:1008977630179] [PMID: 10853271]

[92] Yemets AI, Tanasienko IV, Krasylenko YA, Blume YB. Plant-based biopharming of recombinant human lactoferrin. Cell Biol Int 2014; 38(9): 989-1002. [PMID: 24803187]

[93] Min SR, Woo JW, Jeong SK, Han YB, Liu JR. Production of human lactoferrin in transgenic cell suspension culture of sweet potato. Biol Plant 2006; 50(1): 131-4. [http://dx.doi.org/10.1007/s10535-005-0087-5]

[94] Suzuki YA, Kelleher SL, Yalda D, *et al.* Expression, characterization, and biologic activity of recombinant human lactoferrin in rice. J Pediatr Gastroenterol Nutr 2003; 36(2): 190-9. [http://dx.doi.org/10.1097/00005176-200302000-00007] [PMID: 12548053]

[95] Acceptability of cell substrates for production of biologicals. Geneva: World Health Organization 1987.https://apps.who.int/iris/handle/10665/38501

[96] Lebron JA, Troilol PJ, Pacchione S, *et al.* Adaptation of the WHO guideline for residual DNA in parenteral vaccines produced on continuous cell lines to a limit for oral vaccines. Dev Biol (Basel) 2006; 123: 35-44. [PMID: 16566435]

[97] Gorbet MB, Sefton MV. Endotoxin: the uninvited guest. Biomaterials 2005; 26(34): 6811-7. [http://dx.doi.org/10.1016/j.biomaterials.2005.04.063] [PMID: 16019062]

CHAPTER 2

Plant Virus Nanoparticles and Virus like Particles (VLPs): Applications in Medicine

Mahbobeh Zamani-Babgohari[1], **Nasir Mahmood**[1,2], **Ghyda Murad Hashim**[1], **Sarah Bushra Nasir**[3], **Mounir G. AbouHaidar**[1] and **Kathleen L. Hefferon**[1,*]

[1] *Department of Cell and Systems Biology, University of Toronto, Canada*

[2] *Department of Biochemistry, University of Health Sciences, Lahore, Pakistan*

[3] *Abdus Salam School of Sciences, Nusrat Jahan College, Chenab Nagar, Chiniot, Pakistan*

Abstract: Both virus like particles (VLPs) and virus nanoparticles (VNPs) are viable platforms for the transportation of drugs, imaging agents, immunogenic ligands and other materials. They can be loaded with genetic material and/or drugs for therapeutic purposes. VLPs possess multivalent molecular settings, which help stimulate various molecular interactions for a potent immune response. VNPs are biodegradable and biocompatible nanoparticles that occur in nature and can be modified with genetic and chemical protocols for therapeutic purposes. There has been considerable research on the use of different VLPs and VNPs as safe and viable platforms for vaccine development, tumor therapy and other medical applications. The following chapter provides insight into applications of plant VLPs and VNPs in medicine.

Keywords: Chimeric VLP, Vaccines, Virus like particles (VLPs), Virus nanoparticles (VNPs), Plant-derived vaccine.

INTRODUCTION

Virus nanoparticles (VNPs) can originate as novel biomaterials from a variety of sources including the structural proteins of viruses infecting plants, animals and bacteria [1]. These biomaterials can self-assemble through noncovalent bonds, resulting in systematic-structured nanoparticles which vary in shape and size [2]. Since the morphology of these complex structures is controlled by genetic variation, it is facile to alter them using synthetic biology [2]. Plant virus nanoparticles ranging from 10-100 nm are a subcategory of these bio-nanoparticles and are expressed in various host systems. The wide variety of plant VNPs provide for a diversity of applications.

[*] **Corresponding author Kathleen L. Hefferon:** Department of Cell and Systems Biology, University of Toronto, Canada; E-mail: kathleen.hefferon@alumni.utoronto.ca

Atta-ur-Rehman and M. Iqbal Choudhary (Eds.)

Virus-like particles (VLPs) are particles that resemble viruses but lack nucleic acid [3]. Changes in ionic strength and pH can be used to disassemble viruses into genetic material and proteins. The resulting coat proteins can self-assemble to form virus-like particles (VLPs) [4] with either single or multiple structural proteins organized in numerous layers [3].

In the following chapter, we describe different types of VLPs, methods for their production and various ranges of VLP applications in medicine. The focus is on VLPs derived from plant viruses; however, to deliver a better overview, non-plant VLPs are also discussed.

VIRUS LIKE PARTICLES (VLPS)

VLPs are complexes of structural proteins that can be expressed in recombinant systems by spontaneous assembly. These structures resemble naturally occurring viruses with respect to conformation and organization but differ as they lack a viral genome [5].

Types of VLPs

VLPs of Structurally Simple Viruses

VLPs of structurally simple viruses consist of non-enveloped viruses that have a nucleocapsid encoded by a single virus encoded protein. Thus, it is easy to generate VLPs of such viruses since the assembly process is dependent on the expression of a single protein. The first single-protein, simple VLPs produced in plants were Norwalk virus (NV) 34 [6]. The Alfalfa mosaic virus (AlMV) coat protein forms VLPs of various shapes and sizes [7]. A modified form of AIMV coat protein bearing HIV-1 and rabies virus epitopes was allowed to express in tobacco plant using a TMV vector. The infected leaf tissue displayed ellipsoid particles of the modified subunits of AlMV [8].

VLPs with Lipid Envelope

Many pathogenic viruses are encapsulated with an envelope derived from the cell membrane of the host. This envelope comprises lipids and proteins of the host cell membrane and viral glycoproteins. The generation of neutralizing antibodies that can target these envelope proteins are essential in vaccine research. Tobacco mosaic virus produces VLPs that are rod-shaped. The first vaccine to have been produced using enveloped VLPs consisted of 17 to 25 nm diameter spherical particles of Hepatitis B surface antigen enveloped with a host cell membrane [9].

VLPs with Multiple-Protein Layers

Numerous non-enveloped viruses consist of several copies of polypeptides within their capsids. These diverse polypeptides are either produced by the processing of polyprotein precursors or by translation from various open reading frames [7]. VLPs of multiple capsid proteins that must interact with one another are more difficult to produce in comparison to those generated by one or two core capsid proteins. One challenge lies in the fact that proteins encoded by numerous discrete mRNAs are liable to be localized differently within the cell, thereby influencing the efficiency of the assembly process [10]. Reoviruses are double-stranded non-enveloped RNA viruses consisting of three spheres bearing four diverse VPs produced by discrete genome segments [7]. VLPs of Cowpea mosaic virus (CPMV) were shown to exhibit antitumor activity against B16F10 lung melanoma [11].

Methods of Production of VLPs

Non-infectious VLPs lacking the viral genome can be produced through the expression of viral proteins in plant hosts. The initial step for VLP production in plants involves the formation of a suitable plasmid for expressing proteins essential for VLP assembly. These proteins include both the capsid/shell and structural proteins of the VLPs [7]. The desired sequence is injected into a suitable vector for steady genetic transformation and utilized for either plasmid or nuclear transformation through standard techniques [12]. The plants at this stage are allowed to regenerate, self-fertilize and generate true-breeds. Plastid transformation is advantageous over nuclear transformation because transgenes encoded by plastids have a low risk of contaminating the environment as they are maternally inherited and not transferred through pollen [7].

The VLPs are expressed transiently through two methods: utilization of replicating plant virus vectors or through a non-replicating binary vector; both can be delivered to the plant by agroinfiltration. A range of plant viruses serve as expression vectors [13] including Potato virus X (PVX) [14], Cowpea mosaic virus (CPMV) [15], and Tobacco mosaic virus (TMV) [16], *etc.*

VLP purification from the plant consists of homogenization of the tissue sample, cell debris removal and plant extract enrichment to obtain the expressed VLPs. The rigid cellulose in the cell wall of the plant cell is removed by either enzymatic degradation or mechanical homogenization. Additional VLP purification is routinely carried out by various methods including tangential flow filtration, ultracentrifugation and chromatography on the basis of affinity, ion exchange and size exclusion [7].

PLANT VIRUS NANOPARTICLES (VNPS)

Classification of Plant Virus Nanoparticles (VNPs)

Depending upon the structure of the original (maternal) viruses, virus nanoparticles are classified into two major groups, enveloped and non-enveloped nanoparticles [17]. (Fig. **1**) depicts the size-structure diagram of icosahedral and helical viruses. There are several characteristics that are common among the plant virus nanoparticles frequently used as nanomaterials. For example, they are non-enveloped, stable at certain conditions, easy to reproduce and purify and possess appropriate structures [18].

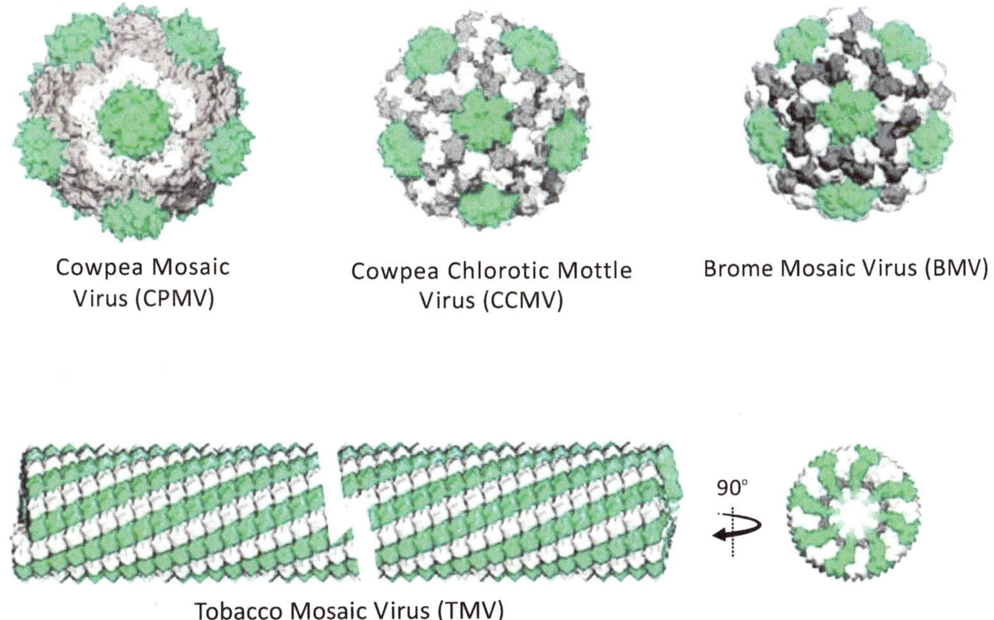

Fig. (1). Schematic pictures of Icosahedral and helical viruses [19].

Filamentous Plant Viruses

The majority of the plant viruses possess filamentous capsids. The genomic material of filamentous viruses are of single-stranded RNA and determines capsid size. The filamentous viruses are categorized into two classes of rigid (rod-shape) and flexible viruses [20].

Potexviruses, Potyviruses and Closteroviruses are categorized as flexible filamentous viruses and are useful for the production of recombinant proteins. It has been reported that flexible viruses can be digested in a human system whereas the rod-shape viruses are not metabolized. Bamboo mosaic virus (BaMV) is one of the flexible filamentous viruses with a diameter of 15 nm× 490 nm and contains a single coat protein species. BaMV VLPs consist of a CP that has been engineered at the N-terminus so that epitopes to Bursal virus and Foot and mouth disease can be inserted for vaccine production [20]. The other group of flexible filamentous viruses are potexviruses (PVX); they also have been useful sources for providing nanoparticle platforms for different applications in medicine. X-ray and EM crystallography have uncovered details of the molecular structure where in contrast to previous opinion, it was recently determined that BaMV possesses a left-handed helical pitch [20].

Rod-like Plant Virus Nanoparticles

Tobacco mosaic virus (TMV) is a rod- shaped virus with dimensions of 18 nm × 300 nm. TMV is the first virus discovered and is often used as a model in virology. The crystallography and study of the atomic structure in rigid viruses is less complex than those of flexible filamentous viruses. For the same reason, TMV has been used as a reference for structural analyses for a number of years [20]. Rod shaped virus nanoparticles are used in metallization and mineralization procedures.TMV nanoparticles are also developed for carrying or decorating metal and other nanomaterials inside or on the surface of the capsid protein [1, 21]. Highly organized nanowires were produced using TMV as the interior surface of the filamentous viruses and are suitable for this purpose. The nanowires are micrometers in length and contain cobalt and nickel. They were produced by filling Pd-activated material into the inner pore of TMV nanoparticles. Manipulation of TMV successfully enabled a lysine residue to be placed at the very end of C-terminus position for biotinylation [3]. There are many examples of chemical use and structural modification of TMV and other filamentous viruses for applications in nano-biotechnology. For instance, TMV has been used for the production of hallow nanotubes by adsorption to AU, silicon and mica [22]. TMV mesostructures were produced using mineralization of silica on the surface of TMV capsid protein [23].

Spherical Plant Viruses

Icosahedral viruses range from 18nm to 500nm in size and are formed from capsomer pentamers and hexamers according to the laws of Caspar and Klug [24]. The symmetric structure of icosahedral viruses favors epitope display. In this way, icosahedral VLPs can load drugs and chemicals that can be carried to specific destinations within the body [25]. Cowpea chlorotic mottle virus (CCMV) is an icosahedral virus from which the derived-VNPs have been used for many applications in medicine [3]. The capsid protein of CCMV has a diameter of 28 nm and is composed of 180 identical coat protein subunits [24]. Different icosahedral virus nanoparticles such as Hibiscus chlorotic ringspot virus (HCRSV), Brome Mosaic virus (BMV), Johnson grass chlorotic ripe mosaic virus (JgCSMV), Cowpea mosaic virus (CPMV), Red clover necrotic mosaic virus (RCMNV) and Physalis Mottle Virus (PhMV) have been manipulated for a variety of applications [23].

Development of Plant Virus Nanoparticles

The fact that virus capsid proteins are actually fundamental subunits of virus nanoparticles, coupled with their ability to self-assemble, is a unique characteristic with tremendous applications. Recent research and development demonstrate the engineering of virus capsid proteins so that the natural process of capsid assembly can be manipulated. Using an *in vitro* self-assembling technique that includes the control of pH and ionic solutions, CCMV nanoparticles can be generated from natural icosahedral structures into tube-shaped, polywalled capsids and hexagonal sheets [26, 27]. The reading frame of Turnip crinkle virus (TCV) coat protein produces VLPs in plant leaves when transiently expressed [28]. Cells of recombinant *Escherichia coli* has been utilized to cultivate VLPs of plant viruses: Rice yellow mottle virus (RYMV) and Cocksfoot mottle virus (CfMV) with ultracentifugation of the bacterial extract to obtain 4–45 mg of VLPs from a 1 litre bacterial culture [29].

Capsid proteins may assemble into common structures along with an external object such as inorganic cargo, or other types of flexible materials. BMV nanoparticles have been reported to self-assemble into structures which contain magnetic cores and quantum dots, so that the resulting nanoparticles displayed properties close to those of the natural form [30, 31]. As another example, RCMNV (Red clover necrotic mosaic virus) was successfully employed to carry quantum dots and nucleic acid functionalized gold nanoparticles, where the presence of oligonucleotides (a genomic sequence) was imperative for proper functionality and assembly of the virus nanoparticles [32, 33].

It is also possible to exploit the diameter of nanoparticles by alternating different degrees of assembly based upon triangulation digits. It has been demonstrated that BMV ligands displayed on the surface of magnetic cargos resulted in the development of virus nanoparticles that are larger than the native virus [30].

Virus capsid proteins can also assemble with flexible substances. Loading virus nanoparticles with negatively charged elements such as electrolytes and anions has been studied in depth. The virus nanoparticles can assemble into functional cargos unless the size of encapsulated materials was the limiting factor. In some cases, it may be possible to achieve different assembled structures besides the native form. For example, encapsulation of polymers for the production of optically active virus CCMV like particles has led to the generation of both spherical (at high ionic solution) and rod-shaped (at low ionic solution) particles [34].

Nanoparticle advancement has led to the successful engineering of fluorescent proteins, mCherry and green fluorescent protein (GFP) into plant virus nanoparticles based on Potato virus X. The resulting cells displayed the fluorescent pigments in optical molecular imaging of human tumor and cancer cells in pre-clinical trials in a mouse model [35].

APPLICATIONS OF VLPS AND PLANT VNPS FOR IMMUNOTHERAPY

VLPs can be used to generate an immune response against epitopes of foreign proteins by fusing portions from different sources to produce a chimeric VLP [24]. An example of a chimeric VLP is the vaccine against HPV in which both major and minor capsid proteins (L1 and L2) are included [36] to provide protection against a larger range of HPV types. VLPs that are used as a vaccine require various modifications in their structure, route of transfer and target host to generate the required immune response [37]. Potato tubers that expressed Norwalk Virus VLPs were given to 20 human volunteers out of which 19 indicated some sort of immune response [38]. Purified particles of AIMV when inserted in mice elicited an immune response resulting in the production of antibodies for virus-neutralization [8]. Similarly, Papaya mosaic virus (PapMV) derived VLPs were seen to possess high immunostimulating potential [39]. Alternanthera mosaic virus (AltMV) derived VLPs were also shown to be highly immunogenic and more stable under a broader range of settings [40].

Alternatively, several capsid proteins that are used to make VLPs such as polyomavirus VP1 and HPV L1 can bind non-specifically to cellular/viral DNA [41] and thus be utilized successfully for gene transfer [42]. Several other studies were also performed to optimize and assess DNA transduction and packaging by

VLPs that were obtained from members of the Polyomaviridae family [43]. SV40-VLPs under 17.7 kb in size and with a highly efficient *in vitro* packaging system [44] have been successfully employed for *in vivo* gene delivery [45].

On the other hand, a number of drugs including small molecules can be conjugated to VLPs, rendering them useful for drug delivery. Another benefit is that the molecule attached to its surface can elicit a stronger immune response due to its presence on the VLP surface. Examples are the development of VLPs which include peptides attached to their surfaces that are derived from the AP205 or Qβ bacteriophage, and which generate an immune response against angiotensin II and nicotine [46].

VLPs can be engineered to present optimized immunogenicity and antigenicity through the presentation of multiple epitopes or peptides [46]. In addition to this, VLPs also offer a number of advantages in the process of vaccine development against some cancers. A number of VLP-based cancer vaccines have the ability to act as self-adjuvants as they contain virus pathogen associated molecular patterns (PAMP) that can improve innate immune response activation through pattern recognition and Toll-like receptor interactions [47, 48]. Several studies have demonstrated that VLPs have the ability to overcome the immunosuppressive microenvironment of the tumor and disrupt self-tolerance to elicit strong cytotoxic activity of lymphocytes. These processes are essential for virus clearance and cancer cell destruction. Together, these unique features of VLPs make them powerful candidates for cancer immunotherapy [46, 49].

The surface of VLPs usually is modified so that they can target specific cell types and reduce immunogenicity [50]. The modification of the outer surface of virus nanoparticle subunits and the resulting desired symmetry controls the multi-valency of ligand display [4]. The interior surface of CCMV has a positive charge useful for the production of structurally distinct nanoparticles by mineralizing nucleation [4]. Using a similar mechanism to CCMV, Red clover necrotic mosaic virus (RCNMV) has also been employed for drug delivery [51]. The multivalency of virus nanoparticles has permitted the combination of multiple therapeutic agents including imaging and ligand/antigen display within a single VNP. In this case, plant VNPs have been employed as a scaffold for MRI and fluorescent techniques [52, 53]. CPMV nanoparticles have been reported to penetrate vascular endothelial cells so that the nanoparticles can be used for imaging. These nanoparticles were used in living mice for imaging blood flow and vasculature [53].

Plant VNPs have also been used for carrying therapeutic agents to target cells. In a study using CCMV nanoparticles, the targeted cells demonstrated an increase in anti-microbial photo-dynamic treatment using a photosensitizer conjugated to a target ligand [4]. Furthermore, the specificity of virus nanoparticles for cell targeting was confirmed using flow cytometry [54]. CCMV nanoparticles exhibited a wide range of distribution in different organs and tissues of mice without any symptoms of toxicity. Plant virus nanoparticles, CCMV specifically, could only survive for about 12 minutes in the blood. It has been suggested that the reticulo-endothelial system in spleen and liver is responsible for this rapid clearance of nanoparticles [4]. On the other hand, PEGylation has enhanced the half-life of nanoparticles over ten times. CCMV has been used as vaccine and pharmaceutical platforms, and no toxicity has been reported [4, 55]. Potato virus X was conjugated to Herceptin, the chemotherapeutic drug for breast cancer. It was shown that conjugation resulted in an enhanced therapeutic capacity of the drug [56].

The shape of virus nanoparticles effects their *in vivo* behaviour especially with respect to its accumulation in tissue and clearance from the system [57]. The filamentous nature of Potato virus X is advantageous as the elongated shape of materials enable them to escape the immune system effectively, thus minimizing the chances of being captured by macrophages [58, 59]. TMV nanoparticles coated with serum albumin (SA) helped to deliver nanoparticle based drugs more effectively *in vivo* by providing a shielding effect against the immune system [60].

Considering the fact that plant virus nanoparticles can trigger an active immune response in animal systems, they can directly be used in medicine as effective adjuvants. However, the route of application (oral or intravenous) may affect the efficacy of the immune response, whereas the intravenous route increases IgG and IgM immune responses [61, 62]. Introducing CPMV into the blood system can increase B-cell proliferation, causing the rapid clearance of nanoparticles. Manipulation of the surface can also affect the immunogenicity of nanoparticles. For example, even minor modifications of the surface of CPMV using PEG and other similar substances resulted in the reduction of an immune response against CPMV [56, 63]. Potato virus X nanoparticles can serve as vaccines since the viral RNA helps to activate Toll-like receptor 7 on the surface of antigen-presenting cells, thereby improving the immune response in a fashion that is similar to adjuvants [64]. Virus like particles produced in different host systems have been used as vaccines for different viral diseases [65]. Gag-VLP produced by a TMV based vector in tobacco plants produced the same immunogenicity profile as Gag-VLP produced in insect cells, suggesting a possible candidate for immunization against HIV [65] Similarly, VLPs containing gp41 protein of HIV and the coat protein of CPMV are known to induce cross-reactive neutralizing antibodies against HIV in a mouse system [65].

TMV rod and spherical nanoparticles have been used to carry doxorubicin to cancer cells, resulting in toxicity that is specific against tumor cells [66]. CMV nanoparticles loaded with doxorubicin could increase the concentration of the drug in ovarian cancer as well as reduce cardio-toxicity in mouse models [67]. The use of PVX nanoparticles resulted in an improvement of drug efficacy in mice suffering from triple negative breast cancer [68]. Plant VLPs are also used for photodynamic therapy (PDT) in cancer and as delivery cargo in infectious disease. PDT creates reactive oxygen species production using different wavelengths, thus delivering PDT by VLP (*i.e.* CCMV) reduces non-target damage [1, 69].

ADVANTAGES OF VLPS AND PLANT VLPS *VS.* SYNTHETIC NANOPARTICLES IN IMMUNOTHERAPY

Plant virus-like particles (VLPs) are powerful tools with multiple functions. Due to their ability to self-assemble, VLPs can be constructed in ample amounts within a short-term period. However, what makes plant virus like particles distinct platforms from other nanoparticles is the fact that they are noninfectious, biodegradable and do not cause toxicity and other adverse reactions. Plant virus nanoparticles behave as nanoscale cargo to deliver medical materials to specific targets. Different shapes and sizes of virus nanoparticles can direct the application for specific cellular uses. For instance, virus nanoparticles with a large mass can be used to target vessel walls while smaller sized rod-shaped nanoparticles are suitable for targeting tumor cells. The atomic structures of many plant virus nanoparticles are known, making it possible to manipulate these platforms for a specific purpose. For some viruses such as TMV, rod shaped viral nanoparticles can be reshaped into the form of spheres [69, 70].

CONCLUSION

Plant virus-like particles have tremendous applications in medicine. Prediction and then production of viable structures of VLPs play a key role in the success and future use of VLPs. The development of customized VNPs suited for defined functions (*i.e.* medical applications) can be made feasible by managing interactions among virus nanoparticles and other substances [3]. Therefore, scientists may need to develop a variety of VLPs derived from the same virus for different applications; which has become quite feasible considering recent developments in imaging and crystallography. In fact, an in depth understanding of the target (*i.e.* a tumor cell or an infectious agent) is essential for the further design of VLPs that will perform the appropriate function. To this end, a multidisciplinary approach will be of significant importance in the years ahead. These are some of the challenges associated with the application of viral nanoparticles with respect to the immune system, which must be addressed in the coming years.

CONSENT FOR PUBLICATION

Not applicable.

CONFLICT OF INTEREST

The authors declare no conflict of interest, financial or otherwise.

ACKNOWLEDGEMENTS

Declared none.

REFERENCES

[1] Steinmetz NF. Viral nanoparticles as platforms for next-generation therapeutics and imaging devices. Nanomedicine 2010; 6(5): 634-41. [http://dx.doi.org/10.1016/j.nano.2010.04.005] [PMID: 20433947]

[2] Lee LA, Wang Q. Adaptations of nanoscale viruses and other protein cages for medical applications. Nanomedicine 2006; 2(3): 137-49. [http://dx.doi.org/10.1016/j.nano.2006.07.009] [PMID: 17292136]

[3] Fuenmayor J, Gòdia F, Cervera L. Production of virus-like particles for vaccines. N Biotechnol 2017; 39(25): 174-80. [http://dx.doi.org/10.1039/c2cs35108k] [PMID: 22880206]

[4] Liu Z, Qiao J, Niu Z, Wang Q. Natural supramolecular building blocks: from virus coat proteins to viral nanoparticles. Chem Soc Rev 2012; 41(18): 6178-94.

[5] Roldao A, Silva A, Mellado M, Alves P, Carrondo M. Viruses and virus-like particles in biotechnology: fundamentals and applications. 2011.

[6] Mason HS, Ball JM, Shi JJ, Jiang X, Estes MK, Arntzen CJ. Expression of Norwalk virus capsid protein in transgenic tobacco and potato and its oral immunogenicity in mice. Proc Natl Acad Sci USA 1996; 93(11): 5335-40. [http://dx.doi.org/10.1073/pnas.93.11.5335] [PMID: 8643575]

[7] Saxena P, Lomonossoff G. Production of virus-like particles in plants. 2015. [http://dx.doi.org/10.1201/b18596-19]

[8] Yusibov V, Modelska A, Steplewski K, *et al.* Antigens produced in plants by infection with chimeric plant viruses immunize against rabies virus and HIV-1. Proc Natl Acad Sci USA 1997; 94(11): 5784-8. [http://dx.doi.org/10.1073/pnas.94.11.5784] [PMID: 9159151]

[9] Gavilanes F, Gonzalez-Ros JM, Peterson DL. Structure of hepatitis B surface antigen. Characterization of the lipid components and their association with the viral proteins. J Biol Chem 1982; 257(13): 7770-. [PMID: 7085648]

[10] Roy P, Noad R. Virus-like particles as a vaccine delivery system: myths and facts. Hum Vaccin 2008; 4(1): 5-12. [http://dx.doi.org/10.4161/hv.4.1.5559] [PMID: 18438104]

[11] Saxena P, Aljabali AA, Saunders K, Evans DJ, Lomonossoff GP. Genetic engineering and

characterization of Cowpea mosaic virus empty virus-like particles. Methods Mol Biol 2014; 1108: 139-53.
[http://dx.doi.org/https://doi.org/10.1371/journal.pone.0183824.]

[12] Scotti N, Rigano MM, Cardi T. Production of foreign proteins using plastid transformation. Biotechnol Adv 2012; 30(2): 387-97.
[http://dx.doi.org/10.1016/j.biotechadv.2011.07.019] [PMID: 21843626]

[13] Gleba YY, Tusé D, Giritch A. Plant viral vectors for delivery by *Agrobacterium*. Curr Top Microbiol Immunol 2014; 375: 155-92.
[http://dx.doi.org/10.1007/82_2013_352] [PMID: 23949286]

[14] Marusic C, Rizza P, Lattanzi L, *et al.* Chimeric plant virus particles as immunogens for inducing murine and human immune responses against human immunodeficiency virus type 1. J Virol 2001; 75(18): 8434-9.
[http://dx.doi.org/10.1128/JVI.75.18.8434-8439.2001] [PMID: 11507188]

[15] Cañizares MC, Liu L, Perrin Y, Tsakiris E, Lomonossoff GP. A bipartite system for the constitutive and inducible expression of high levels of foreign proteins in plants. Plant Biotechnol J 2006; 4(2): 183-93.
[http://dx.doi.org/10.1111/j.1467-7652.2005.00170.x] [PMID: 17177795]

[16] Lindbo JA. TRBO: a high-efficiency tobacco mosaic virus RNA-based overexpression vector. Plant Physiol 2007; 145(4): 1232-40.
[http://dx.doi.org/10.1104/pp.107.106377] [PMID: 17720752]

[17] Kushnir N, Streatfield SJ, Yusibov V. Virus-like particles as a highly efficient vaccine platform: diversity of targets and production systems and advances in clinical development. Vaccine 2012; 31(1): 58-83.
[http://dx.doi.org/10.1016/j.vaccine.2012.10.083] [PMID: 23142589]

[18] Culver JN, Brown AD, Zang F, Gnerlich M, Gerasopoulos K, Ghodssi R. Plant virus directed fabrication of nanoscale materials and devices. Virology 2015; 479: 200-12.

[19] Zhang Y, Dong Y, Zhou J, Li X, Wang F. Application of plant viruses as a biotemplate for nanomaterial fabrication. Molecules 2018; 23(9): 2311.
[http://dx.doi.org/10.3390/molecules23092311] [PMID: 30208562]

[20] DiMaio F, Chen CC, Yu X, *et al.* The molecular basis for flexibility in the flexible filamentous plant viruses. Nat Struct Mol Biol 2015; 22(8): 642-4.
[http://dx.doi.org/10.1038/nsmb.3054] [PMID: 26167882]

[21] Bruckman MA, Niu Z, Li S, *et al.* Development of nanobiocomposite fibers by controlled assembly of rod-like tobacco mosaic virus. NanoBiotechnology 2007; 3: 31-9.
[http://dx.doi.org/10.1007/s12030-007-0004-4]

[22] Fujikawa S, Kunitake T. Surface fabrication of hollow nanoarchitectures of ultrathin titania layers from assembled latex particles and tobacco mosaic viruses as templates. Langmuir 2003; 19: 6545-52.
[http://dx.doi.org/10.1021/la026979e]

[23] Fowler CE, Shenton W, Stubbs G, Mann S. Tobacco mosaic virus liquid crystals as templates for the interior design of silica mesophases and nanoparticles. Adv Mater 2001; 13: 1266-9.
[http://dx.doi.org/10.1002/1521-4095(200108)13:16<1266::AID-ADMA1266>3.0.CO;2-9]

[24] Zandi R, Reguera D, Bruinsma RF, Gelbart WM, Rudnick J. Origin of icosahedral symmetry in viruses. Proc Natl Acad Sci USA 2004; 101(44): 15556-60.
[http://dx.doi.org/10.1073/pnas.0405844101] [PMID: 15486087]

[25] Hefferon KL. Repurposing plant virus nanoparticles. Vaccines (Basel) 2018; 6(1): 11.
[http://dx.doi.org/10.3390/vaccines6010011] [PMID: 29443902]

[26] Tang J, Johnson JM, Dryden KA, Young MJ, Zlotnick A, Johnson JE. The role of subunit hinges and molecular “switches” in the control of viral capsid polymorphism. J Struct Biol 2006; 154(1): 59-67.

[http://dx.doi.org/10.1016/j.jsb.2005.10.013] [PMID: 16495083]

[27] Lavelle L, Gingery M, Phillips M, *et al.* Phase diagram of self-assembled viral capsid protein polymorphs. J Phys Chem B 2009; 113(12): 3813-9.
[http://dx.doi.org/10.1021/jp8079765] [PMID: 19673134]

[28] Castells-Graells R, Lomonossoff GP, Saunders K. Production of mosaic turnip crinkle virus-like particles derived by coinfiltration of wild-type and modified forms of virus coat protein in plants methods in molecular biology. New York, NY: Humana Press 2018; 1776.
[http://dx.doi.org/10.1007/978-1-4939-7808-3_1]

[29] Balke I, Resevič̌a G, Zeltins A. Isolation and characterization of two distinct types of unmodified spherical plant sobemovirus-like particles for diagnostic and technical uses. Methods Mol Biol 2018; 1776: 19-34.
[http://dx.doi.org/10.1007/978-1-4939-7808-3_2] [PMID: 29869232]

[30] Huang X, Bronstein LM, Retrum J, *et al.* Self-assembled virus-like particles with magnetic cores. Nano Lett 2007; 7(8): 2407-16.
[http://dx.doi.org/10.1021/nl071083l] [PMID: 17630812]

[31] Dixit SK, Goicochea NL, Daniel MC. Quantum dot encapsulation in viral capsids. Nano Lett 2006; 6: 1993-9.

[32] Loo L, Guenther RH, Basnayake VR, Lommel SA, Franzen S. Controlled encapsidation of gold nanoparticles by a viral protein shell. J Am Chem Soc 2006; 128(14): 4502-3.
[http://dx.doi.org/10.1021/ja057332u] [PMID: 16594649]

[33] Loo L, Guenther RH, Lommel SA, Franzen S. Encapsidation of nanoparticles by red clover necrotic mosaic virus. J Am Chem Soc 2007; 129(36): 11111-7.
[http://dx.doi.org/10.1021/ja071896b] [PMID: 17705477]

[34] Ng BC, Chan ST, Lin J, Tolbert SH. Using polymer conformation to control architecture in semiconducting polymer/viral capsid assemblies. ACS Nano 2011; 5(10): 7730-8.
[http://dx.doi.org/10.1021/nn202493w] [PMID: 21942298]

[35] Shukla S, Dickmeis C, Fischer R, Commandeur U, Steinmetz NF. In planta production of fluorescent filamentous plant virus-based nanoparticles. Methods Mol Biol 2018; 1776: 61-84.
[http://dx.doi.org/10.1007/978-1-4939-7808-3_5] [PMID: 29869235]

[36] Grgacic EV, Anderson DA. Virus-like particles: passport to immune recognition. Methods 2006; 40(1): 60-5.
[http://dx.doi.org/10.1016/j.ymeth.2006.07.018] [PMID: 16997714]

[37] Wakabayashi MT, Da Silva DM, Potkul RK, Kast WM. Comparison of human papillomavirus type 16 L1 chimeric virus-like particles versus L1/L2 chimeric virus-like particles in tumor prevention. Intervirology 2002; 45(4-6): 300-7.
[http://dx.doi.org/10.1159/000067921] [PMID: 12566713]

[38] Tacket CO, Mason HS, Losonsky G, Estes MK, Levine MM, Arntzen CJ. Human immune responses to a novel norwalk virus vaccine delivered in transgenic potatoes. J Infect Dis 2000; 182(1): 302-5.
[http://dx.doi.org/10.1086/315653] [PMID: 10882612]

[39] Lebel MÈ, Langlois MP, Daudelin JF, *et al.* Complement component 3 regulates IFN-α production by plasmacytoid dendritic cells following TLR7 activation by a plant Virus-like Nanoparticle. J Immunol 2017; 198(1): 292-9.
[http://dx.doi.org/10.4049/jimmunol.1601271] [PMID: 27864474]

[40] Ekaterina K, Pechnikova Evgeniya V , Mishyna Maryia Yu , *et al.* Structure and properties of virions and virus-like particles derived from the coat protein of Alternanthera mosaic virus. PLoS ONE 2017; 12(8): e0183824.
[http://dx.doi.org/https://doi.org/10.1371/journal.pone.0183824]

[41] Forstová J, Krauzewicz N, Sandig V, *et al.* Polyoma virus pseudocapsids as efficient carriers of

heterologous DNA into mammalian cells. Hum Gene Ther 1995; 6(3): 297-306. [http://dx.doi.org/10.1089/hum.1995.6.3-297] [PMID: 7779913]

[42] Tegerstedt K, Franzén AV, Andreasson K, *et al.* Murine polyomavirus virus-like particles (VLPs) as vectors for gene and immune therapy and vaccines against viral infections and cancer. Anticancer Res 2005; 25(4): 2601-8. [PMID: 16080500]

[43] Kimchi-Sarfaty C, Gottesman MM. SV40 pseudovirions as highly efficient vectors for gene transfer and their potential application in cancer therapy. Curr Pharm Biotechnol 2004; 5(5): 451-8. [http://dx.doi.org/10.2174/1389201043376670] [PMID: 15544493]

[44] Arad U, Zeira E, El-Latif MA, *et al.* Liver-targeted gene therapy by SV40-based vectors using the hydrodynamic injection method. Hum Gene Ther 2005; 16(3): 361-71. [http://dx.doi.org/10.1089/hum.2005.16.361] [PMID: 15812231]

[45] Ambühl PM, Tissot AC, Fulurija A, *et al.* A vaccine for hypertension based on virus-like particles: preclinical efficacy and phase I safety and immunogenicity. J Hypertens 2007; 25: 63-72. [http://dx.doi.org/10.1097/HJH.0b013e32800ff5d6]

[46] Ong HK, Tan WS, Ho KL. Virus like particles as a platform for cancer vaccine development. PeerJ 2017; 5e4053 [http://dx.doi.org/10.7717/peerj.4053] [PMID: 29158984]

[47] Crisci E, Bárcena J, Montoya M. Virus-like particles: the new frontier of vaccines for animal viral infections. Vet Immunol Immunopathol 2012; 148(3-4): 211-25. [http://dx.doi.org/10.1016/j.vetimm.2012.04.026] [PMID: 22705417]

[48] Rynda-Apple A, Patterson DP, Douglas T. Virus-like particles as antigenic nanomaterials for inducing protective immune responses in the lung. Nanomedicine (Lond) 2014; 9(12): 1857-68. [http://dx.doi.org/10.2217/nnm.14.107] [PMID: 25325241]

[49] Jennings GT, Bachmann MF. The coming of age of virus-like particle vaccines. Biol Chem 2008; 389(5): 521-36. [http://dx.doi.org/10.1515/BC.2008.064] [PMID: 18953718]

[50] Rohovie MJ, Nagasawa M, Swartz JR. Virus-like particles: Next-generation nanoparticles for targeted therapeutic delivery. Bioeng Transl Med 2017; 2(1): 43-57. [http://dx.doi.org/10.1002/btm2.10049] [PMID: 29313023]

[51] Loo L, Guenther RH, Lommel SA, Franzen S. Infusion of dye molecules into Red clover necrotic mosaic virus. Chem Commun 2008; (): 88-90. [http://dx.doi.org/10.1039/B714748A]

[52] Lewis JD, Destito G, Zijlstra A, *et al.* Viral nanoparticles as tools for intravital vascular imaging. Nat Med 2006; 12: 354. [http://dx.doi.org/10.1038/nm1368]

[53] Allen M, Bulte JW, Liepold L, *et al.* Paramagnetic viral nanoparticles as potential high-relaxivity magnetic resonance contrast agents. Magnetic Resonance in Medicine: An Official J Int Soc Magn Res Med 2005; 54: 807-12. [http://dx.doi.org/10.1002/mrm.20614]

[54] Suci PA, Varpness Z, Gillitzer E, Douglas T, Young M. Targeting and photodynamic killing of a microbial pathogen using protein cage architectures functionalized with a photosensitizer. Langmuir 2007; 23(24): 12280-6. [http://dx.doi.org/10.1021/la7021424] [PMID: 17949022]

[55] Grill LK, Palmer KE, Pogue GP. Use of plant viruses for production of plant-derived vaccines. Crit Rev Plant Sci 2005; 24: 309-23. [http://dx.doi.org/10.1080/07352680500253180]

[56] Esfandiari N, Arzanani MK, Soleimani M, Kohi-Habibi M, Svendsen WE. A new application of plant

virus nanoparticles as drug delivery in breast cancer. Tumour Biol 2016; 37(1): 1229-36. [http://dx.doi.org/10.1007/s13277-015-3867-3] [PMID: 26286831]

[57] Lee KL, Shukla S, Wu M, *et al.* Stealth filaments: Polymer chain length and conformation affect the *in vivo* fate of PEGylated potato virus X. Acta Biomater 2015; 19: 166-79. [http://dx.doi.org/10.1016/j.actbio.2015.03.001] [PMID: 25769228]

[58] Arnida , Janát-Amsbury MM, Ray A, Peterson CM, Ghandehari H. Geometry and surface characteristics of gold nanoparticles influence their biodistribution and uptake by macrophages. Eur J Pharm Biopharm 2011; 77(3): 417-23. [http://dx.doi.org/10.1016/j.ejpb.2010.11.010] [PMID: 21093587]

[59] Vácha R, Martinez-Veracoechea FJ, Frenkel D. Receptor-mediated endocytosis of nanoparticles of various shapes. Nano Lett 2011; 11(12): 5391-5. [http://dx.doi.org/10.1021/nl2030213] [PMID: 22047641]

[60] Hu H, Yang Q, Baroni S, Yang H, Aime S, Steinmetz NF. Polydopamine-decorated tobacco mosaic virus for photoacoustic/magnetic resonance bimodal imaging and photothermal cancer therapy. Nanoscale 2019; 11(19): 9760-8. [http://dx.doi.org/10.1039/C9NR02065A] [PMID: 31066418]

[61] Kaiser CR, Flenniken ML, Gillitzer E, *et al.* Biodistribution studies of protein cage nanoparticles demonstrate broad tissue distribution and rapid clearance *in vivo.* Int J Nanomedicine 2007; 2: 715.

[62] Singh P, Prasuhn D, Yeh RM, *et al.* Bio-distribution, toxicity and pathology of cowpea mosaic virus nanoparticles *in vivo.* J Control Release 2007; 120(1-2): 41-50. [http://dx.doi.org/10.1016/j.jconrel.2007.04.003] [PMID: 17512998]

[63] Raja KS, Wang Q, Gonzalez MJ, Manchester M, Johnson JE, Finn MG. Hybrid virus-polymer materials. 1. Synthesis and properties of PEG-decorated cowpea mosaic virus. Biomacromolecules 2003; 4(3): 472-6. [http://dx.doi.org/10.1021/bm025740+] [PMID: 12741758]

[64] Kong Q, Richter L, Yang YF, Arntzen CJ, Mason HS, Thanavala Y. Oral immunization with hepatitis B surface antigen expressed in transgenic plants. Proc Natl Acad Sci USA 2001; 98(20): 11539-44. [http://dx.doi.org/10.1073/pnas.191617598] [PMID: 11553782]

[65] Kushnir N. Virus-like particles as a highly efficient vaccine platform: Diversity of targets and production systems and advances in clinical development. Vaccine 2012; 17. 31(1): 58-83.

[66] Bruckman MA, Czapar AE, VanMeter A, Randolph LN, Steinmetz NF. Tobacco mosaic virus-based protein nanoparticles and nanorods for chemotherapy delivery targeting breast cancer. J Control Release 2016; 231: 103-13. [http://dx.doi.org/10.1016/j.jconrel.2016.02.045] [PMID: 26941034]

[67] Zeng Q, Wen H, Wen Q, *et al.* Cucumber mosaic virus as drug delivery vehicle for doxorubicin. Biomaterials 2013; 34(19): 4632-42. [http://dx.doi.org/10.1016/j.biomaterials.2013.03.017] [PMID: 23528229]

[68] Le DH, Lee KL, Shukla S, Commandeur U, Steinmetz NF. Potato virus X, a filamentous plant viral nanoparticle for doxorubicin delivery in cancer therapy. Nanoscale 2017; 9(6): 2348-57. [http://dx.doi.org/10.1039/C6NR09099K] [PMID: 28144662]

[69] Plummer EM, Manchester M. Viral nanoparticles and virus-like particles: platforms for contemporary vaccine design. Wiley Interdiscip Rev Nanomed Nanobiotechnol 2011; 3(2): 174-96. [http://dx.doi.org/10.1002/wnan.119] [PMID: 20872839]

[70] Carignan D, Thérien A, Rioux G, *et al.* Engineering of the PapMV vaccine platform with a shortened M2e peptide leads to an effective one dose influenza vaccine. Vaccine 2015; 33(51): 7245-53. [http://dx.doi.org/10.1016/j.vaccine.2015.10.123] [PMID: 26549362]

CHAPTER 3

MAO Inhibitory Activity of 4, 5-Dihydro-1 H-Pyrazole Derivatives: A Platform To Design Novel Antidepressants

Vishnu Nayak Badavath* and **Venkatesan Jayaprakash**

Department of Pharmaceutical Sciences and Technology, Birla Institute of Technology-Mesra, Ranchi-835215, Jharkhand, India

Abstract: Emergence of treatment-resistant depression is the new challenge before us. As antidepressants currently existing in the market are of little or no use, clinicians are looking for newer and effective antidepressants to handle situations. Inhibition of Monoamine oxidase, an effective strategy discontinued a few decades before due to selectivity related issues. Technological advancement in chemistry and biology interface is now availing hopes of achieving the design and synthesis of novel, isoform-selective and tissue-specific inhibitors. This has renewed the interest in re-exploring the MAO inhibitors in the past decade. Under this background, the chapter reviews MAO inhibitory activity and antidepressant activity of 4, 5-dihydro-1*H*-pyrazole derivatives reported to date. Since different sources of enzymes (rat, bovine, human, *etc.*) were used by different groups to evaluate the newly synthesized compounds, any discussion on structure-activity-relationship may not be justified. Hence, the authors made an attempt to summarize the literature based on the chemical architecture of the compounds that may help the medicinal chemists to further explore the unexplored chemical space. Further, efforts by the scientific community to report the effect of chirality of compounds on activity and selectivity, experimentally or through computational simulations are also documented.

Keywords: 4, 5-Dihydro-1*H*-Pyrazole Derivatives, Antidepressant Activity, Chiral Separation and Computational Studies, MAO Inhibitory Activity.

INTRODUCTION

According to the WHO, depression is a common mental disorder, characterized by loss of interest or pleasure, sadness, low self-worth or feelings of guilt, appetite or disturbed sleep, poor concentration and feelings of tiredness.

* **Corresponding author Dr. Vishnu Nayak Badavath:** Department of Pharmaceutical Sciences & Technology, Birla Institute of Technology, Mesra, Ranchi-835215, Jharkhand, India; Tel: +91-9430316423; E-mail: drvishnuchem@gmail.com

Atta-ur-Rehman and M. Iqbal Choudhary (Eds.)

Depression can be long-lasting or recurrent, substantially impairing an individual's ability to function at work or school or cope with daily life. At its most severe , depression can lead to suicide. When mild, people can be treated without medicines but when depression is moderate or severe, they may need medication and professional counseling. Depression can be easily diagnosed and treated by non-specialists as a part of primary health care. Only a small proportion of individuals who do not respond to first-line treatment approaches specialists for treatment of complicated depression.

As per the WHO report, globally there are more than 350 million people of all age groups suffering from depression. It is a leading cause of disability worldwide which affects women more than men. There are nearly one million deaths every year globally due to depression leading to suicides. In India, around 36% of the population is suffering from Depression (Source: WHO factsheet, date of citation 15/04/2019). Geo-political and socio-economic conditions play a major role in the onset and progression of depressive illness. Counseling and appropriate treatment at the right time may effectively prevent the progression of depression. Treatment generally aimed at restoring the level of Noradrenaline and Serotonin in the brain. One of the successful approaches is to inhibit the Monoamine oxidase-A (MAO-A), the enzyme responsible for the degradation of Noradrenaline and Serotonin [1].

Monoamine oxidases (MAO) are responsible for maintaining the level of neurotransmitters (Noradrenaline and Serotonin) in the central nervous system (CNS). Increased activity of MAO-A is responsible for depression, while the increased activity of MAO-B causes neurodegenerative disorders such as Parkinson's and Alzheimer's disease [2]. Therefore, Monoamine oxidases are valid drug targets for designing drugs for the treatment of depression, Parkinson's and Alzheimer's disease. MAO inhibitors, introduced into clinical practice during the 1960s, were abandoned due to adverse effects, such as hepatotoxicity and the so-called "cheese reaction", which was characterized by hypertensive crisis [3]. Further, it was understood that most of the adverse effects were due to non-selective inhibition of MAO-isoforms [4]. This led to an intensive search for novel MAO inhibitors (MAOIs), selective towards isoforms and this effort has increased considerably in recent years. Selective MAO-A inhibitors such as Clorgyline (irreversible) and Moclobemide (reversible, efficacy moderate) are effective in the treatment of depression [5]. Similarly, selective and irreversible MAO-B inhibitors such as Selegiline and Rasagiline are useful in the treatment of Parkinson's and Alzheimer's diseases [6, 7]. Most of the inhibitors in the clinical practice are either selective and irreversible or non-selective reversible. The reported literature stated that, selective and reversible MAOIs can reduce the adverse effects, (such, as hepatotoxicity and the so-called "cheese reactio", which is characterized by hypertensive crisis) caused by non-selective and irreversible MAO inhibitors [4].

Monoamine Oxidases Enzyme and their Mechanism of Action

Monoamine oxidases are FAD containing enzymes bound to the outer mitochondrial membrane and are responsible for the oxidative deamination of neurotransmitters and dietary amines [8] to produce the corresponding aldehyde, ammonia and hydrogen peroxide using oxygen as an electron acceptor [9]. This led to the rapid degradation of these molecules and ensures the proper functioning of synaptic neurotransmission, regulation of emotional behavior and other brain functions.

$$RCH_2NH_2 + FAD + O_2 + H_2O \longrightarrow RCHO + FADH_2 + H_2O_2 + NH_3$$

Increased activity of MAO enzymes due to their over expression may cause low level of neurotransmitter and higher oxygen consumption (local hypoxia). Decreased level of neurotransmitter led to the behavioral disturbances (Depression). On the other hand the byproduct of MAO-mediated reactions encompasses several chemical species (H_2O_2 generated Reactive Oxygen Species (ROS)) with potential neurotoxic property leading to the onset and progression of neurodegenerative disorders (Fig. **1**) [2].

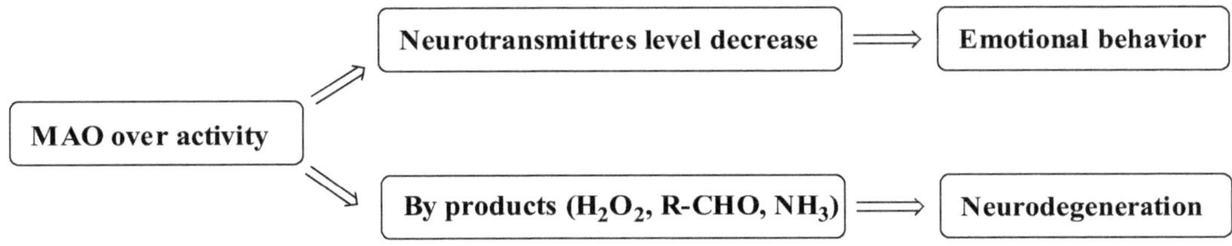

Fig. (1). Schematic diagram on pathological outcome due to overexpression of MAO.

Mary Bernheim discovered MAO enzyme for the first time in the liver [10]. They exist as two different isoforms, hMAO-A and hMAO-B, which differ by their sequence (70% sequence identity as deduced from their cDNA clones) [11], specificity towards their substrate and selective inhibitors [8, 12]. Both hMAO-A and hMAO-B are found in astroglia and neurons, although the brain exhibits high concentration of MAO-A and MAO-B, their regional and cell specific localization are quite different. MAO-A is predominantly found in catecholaminergic neurons, mammilary complex and coerulus hypothalamus, while MAO-B is found serotonergic neurons, astrocytes and histaminergic cells. MAO-A is also found outside the central nervous system (lung, liver, small intestine, and placenta), while lowest levels are found in the spleen and brain micro vessels [13]. Similarly, high level of MAO-B is found in liver, small intestine and platelets, while its presence is poor in spleen, lung, pancreas and skin fibroblast [13, 14].

Monoamine Oxidase Inhibitors (Maois)

The discovery of MAOIs resulted from a search for derivatives of isoniazid (isonicotinc acid hydrazide) with antitubercular activity [15]. During clinical trials with this hyrdrazine derivative, a rather consistent beneficial mood elevation was noted in depressed patients with tuberculosis. Although no longer clinically used, iproniazid, the first derivative to be synthesized was found to be hepatotoxic. However, this lead to the search for other newer MAOIs relatively less toxic than iproniazid [16]. MAOIs cause a rapid and sustained increase in 5-HT (most), norepinephrine and dopamine (least) content in nerve terminals, by inhibiting MAO thereby preventing degradation of these amines. This increase in the cytoplasmic concentration of amines enhances the rate of spontaneous leakage of amines and also their release (indirectly through sympathomimetic amines) [16]. Some early MAOIs were abandoned from clinical practice due to their adverse effects mainly attributed to non-selective inhibition of isoforms. MAO inhibitors currently available in the market for the treatment of depression are presented in Tables **1** and **2**. "Cheese reaction" was mainly due to the non-specific inhibition of MAO-A in the gut (peripheral) that warranted brain-specific MAO inhibitors, while brain specific inhibitor reduces "cheese reaction", isoform selective inhibitors are to be developed for their therapeutic potential in treatment of depression (MAO-A selective) and neurodegenerative disorders (MAO-B selective) [4]. Development of new generation of MAO inhibitors that specifically inhibits brain-MAO in isoform selective and reversible mode has renewed the research interest on MAO-inhibitors [17, 18]. MAO inhibitors are classified as reversible or irreversible, according to their interaction with the isoform. MAO irreversible inhibitors previously have been used as clinical drugs. However, this type of inhibition has been shown to induce significant toxic effects, mainly provoked by the inhibition of the peripheral MAO located in gut, liver and endothelium. On the other hand, competitive reversible inhibitors have less influence in the enzyme recovery after withdrawal since the ingested tyramine is able to displace the inhibitor from the MAO active site and be metabolized in the normal way by peripheral enzyme in gut and liver [19]. Besides, the slow and variable enzyme recovery following the withdrawal of irreversible inhibitors is a disadvantage in clinical use, since the turnover rate for MAO biosynthesis in the human brain seems to require about 40 days. Thus, the reversible MAO inhibitors may have a value in this aspect.

Table 1. Selective MAO-A inhibitors in clinical use.

Moclobemide	Eprobemide	Pirlindole
Tolaxatone	Befloxatone	Metralindole
Bifemelane	Brofaromine	Clorgyline
Esuprone	Curcumin	

Table 2. Selective MAO-B inhibitors in clinical use.

Selegiline	Rasagiline
Ladostigil	Safinamide

In humans, Moclobemide is rapidly and almost completely absorbed and totally metabolized *via* the liver [20], about 44% of the drug is lost due to the first pass metabolism in liver [21]. The elimination half-life is around 2 h [22]. Selegiline, being fat soluble has a low oral bioavailability that may be increased to moderate level by taking the pill with a high-fat meal [23]. Selegiline oral bioavailability is drastically increased in females taking oral contraceptives (10- to 20-fold) [24]. This could lead to loss of MAO-B selectivity in favor of an MAO-A selectivity, which in turn would make patients susceptible to the usual risks of unselective MAOIs such as tyramine-induced hypertensive [24]. Due to this, search for newer inhibitors with favorable pharmacokinetic profile is till on.

Importance of 4, 5-Dihydro-1H-Pyrazoles (Pyrazolines)

4,5-dihydro-1H-pyrazole derivatives have been studied for their anti-inflammatory [25], antimicrobial [26], antitubercular [27], antiviral [28], cerebro protective [29], analgesic [30], anticancer [31] and anticonvulsant activity [32] *etc*. Chalcone derived nitrogen containing heterocyclic compounds were designed and screened for their antidepressant/MAO inhibitory activity. They were designed to mimic iproniazid and pyrazoline were designed as cyclic analogue of Iproniazid Fig. (**2**).

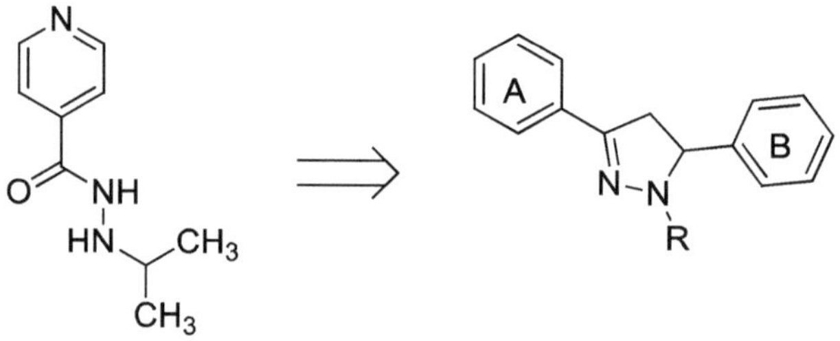

Iproniazid **Pyrazoline**

Fig. (2). Cyclic hydrazides (pyrazolines) as MAO inhibitors.

Pyrazolines are also having the proficiency of binding to MAO enzyme and its subtypes reversibly or irreversibly. Hence, they are now becoming elegant pharmacophore for developing the new drug entities targeting MAO for the treatment of depression and neurodegenerative disorders [33]. Chemical stability, opportunity for carrying out modifications at multiple sites (N1, C3 & C5) and stereoisomerism (C5) on pyrazolines led researchers to enlarge their contribution in developing of new molecules against monoamine oxidase isoforms (MAO-A and MAO-B) [34]. We made an attempt to summarize the modifications at different sites on pyrazolines scaffold. The classification is based on substitution pattern and hence multiple substitution patterns reported by the same group in a manuscript is placed under respective class. This is to quickly identify the number of compounds reported in a particular substitution pattern that will help a medicinal chemist to identify the unexplored chemical space within the substitution pattern. Due to this and other reasons listed below:

(i) Literature covering *in-vitro* enzyme assay and animal studies are covered.

(ii) Literature covering non-specific inhibition to specific inhibition of MAO isoforms.

(iii) Source of enzyme were different (bovine liver, rat liver, rat brain, human *etc.*).

(iv) Assay methodology were different (colorimetry, fluorimetry *etc.*).

we did not attempt to present SAR under each class. Readers are thus advised to refer respective manuscript for getting information on SAR of the compound series reported by the research group.

MAO INHIBITORY ACTIVITY OF PYRAZOLINES

3-Benzyl-5-Aryl-*N*1-Phenyl Pyrazoline Derivatives

Parmar *et al.,* synthesized nine derivatives with 4-chlorobenzyl substitution at the 3rd position of pyrazoline. One of the compound (**1**) having 4-hydroxy-3-methoxy phenyl substitution at the 5th position of pyrazoline was found to inhibit MAO enzyme in rat liver homogenate to the extent of 90.00±1.25% [35].

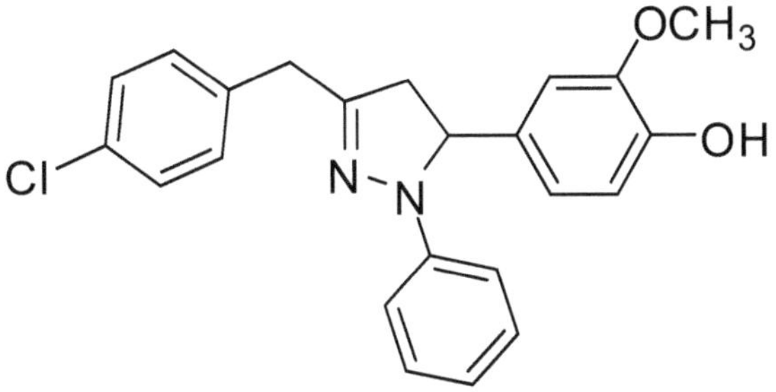

OCH_3

OH

Cl

N

N

1

1, 3, 5-Triaryl Pyrazolines

Parmar *et al.,* synthesized a series of six novel 1*N*-phenyl-3-(2,3,4-trihydroxy phenyl)-5-aryl pyrazoline derivatives and evaluated them for MAO inhibitory activity using rat brain homogenate. Compound (**2**) having 3,4-dimethoxy phenyl substitution at 5th position of pyrazoline was found to have 74.28±0.98% inhibition [35].

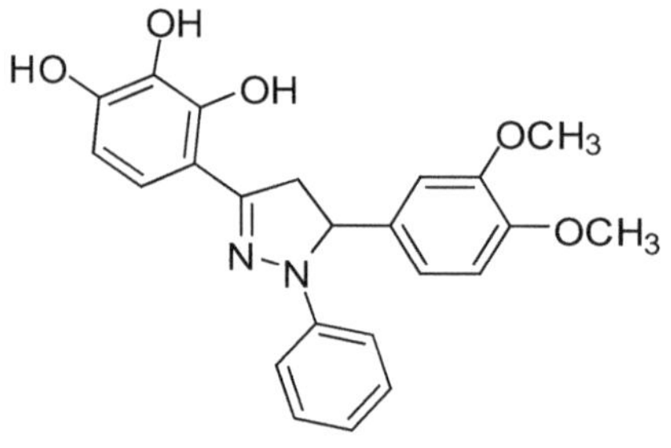

2

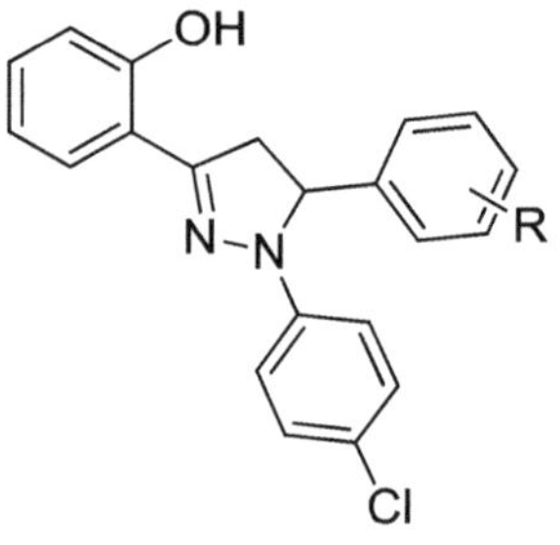

3

Manna *et al.,* found that the selectivity bovine MAO and bovine serum oxidase (BSAO) inhibition is purely dependent on substitution of phenyl ring at 5th position of 4,5-dihydro-(1*H*)-pyrazole. All the compounds, triphenyl pyrazolines (**3**) reported were found to be selective towards BSAO [36].

Chimenti *et al.,* reported the synthesis of a series of twenty-one novel *N1*(4-chloro phenyl)-3-(2-hydroxy phenyl)-5-aryl pyrazolines. The compounds were tested for their inhibitory activity against bovine brain mitochondrial MAO-isoforms. Compound (**4**, bMAO-A:IC_{50} = $9.7x10^{-5}$ ± 0.25 μM; bMAO-B: IC_{50} = 2.5 x 10^{-5} ± 0.10 μM) with 2-nitrophenyl substitution at 5th position was found to be selective towards bMAO-B, while the compound (**5**, bMAO-A: IC_{50} = $1.3x10^{-5}$ ± 0.01 μM; bMAO-B: IC_{50} = 3.8 x 10^{-3} ± 0.02 μM) with 3-nitrophenyl substitution was found to be selective towards bMAO-A [37].

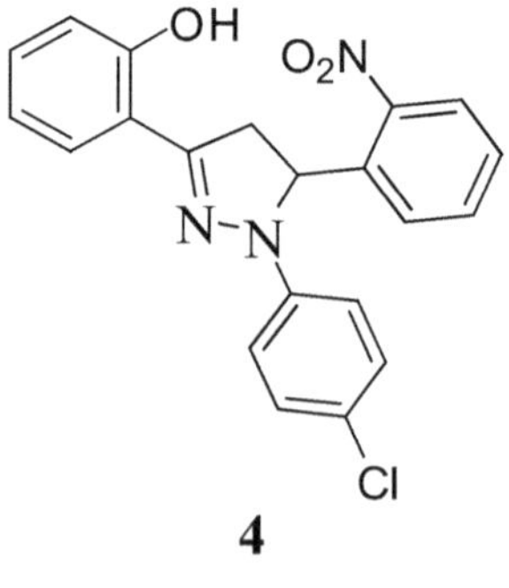

4

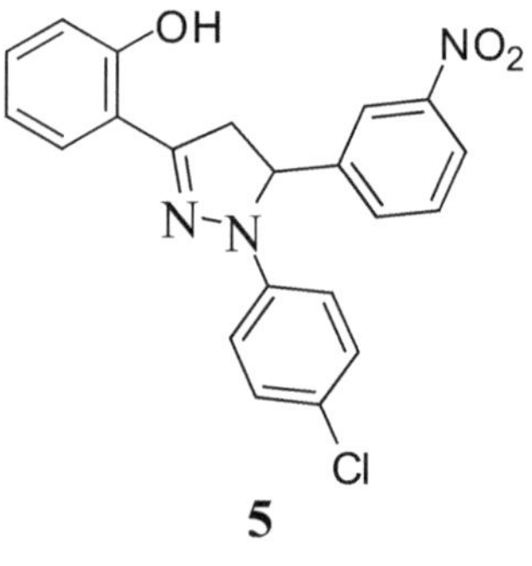

5

N1-Acyl-3, 5-Diaryl-Pyrazolines

Manna *et al.,* synthesized six novel *N*1-acetyl-3,5-diaryl pyrazoline derivatives and they were tested for their selectivity amongst bovine brain mitochondrial MAO, BSAO and porcine kidney amine oxidases (PKDAO). All the compounds were found to be selective towards bMAO. Compound (**6**) with of 2,4-dimethoxyphenyl substitution at 5th position of pyrazoline exhibited Ki value of $8.0x10^{-6}$ M towards MAO and no inhibition at all towards BSAO and PKDAO [38].

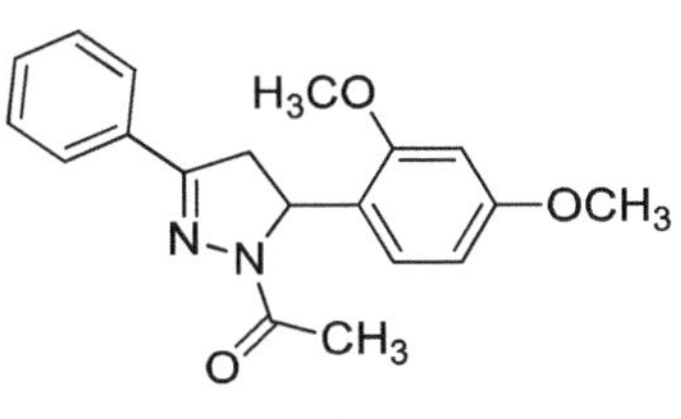

6 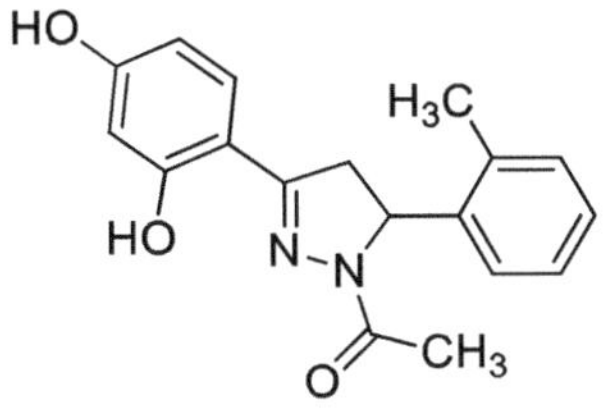 **7** 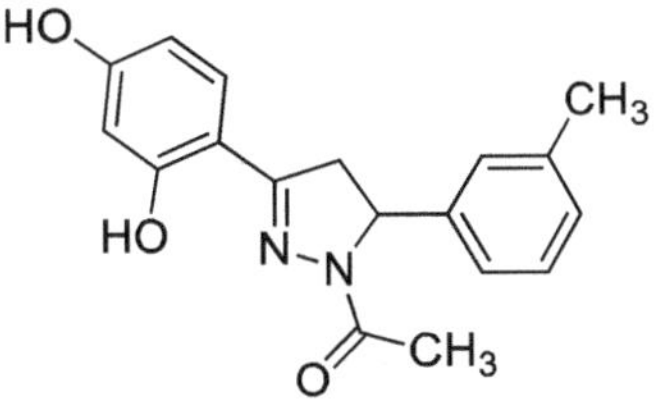 **8**

Manna *et al.,* reported a series of six novel 1*N*-acetyl-3,5-diaryl-pyrazoline derivatives and were tested against bovine brain mitochondrial MAO-isoforms. Two compounds carrying 2,4-dihydroxyphenyl at 3rd position of pyrazolines were found to be potent amongst the six. Within the two, compound (**7**, bMAO-A: K*i* = $5.2x10^{-8}$ ± 1.40 μM; bMAO-B: K*i* = 3.0 x 10^{-8} ± 1.20 μM) carrying 2-methylphenyl at 5th position of pyrazoline inhibited bMAO-B selectively while the compound (**8**, bMAO-A: K*i* = $1.3x10^{-8}$ ± 0.30 μM; bMAO-B: K*i* = 3.8 x 10^{-8} ± 0.35 μM) carrying 3-methylphenyl, bMAO-A [39].

Chimenti *et al.,* synthesized and screened a series of twelve and later thirty-two novel *N*1-acetyl-3,5-diaryl pyrazoline derivatives for their bovine brain mitochondrial MAO-isoform inhibitory activity. All were found to inhibit bMAO-A selectively. Compound (**9**, bMAO-A: IC_{50} = $8.0x10^{-9}$ ± 0.01 μM; bMAO-B: IC_{50} = 1.3 x 10^{-4} ± 0.03 μM) having 2-methoxypheyl substitution at 5th position of pyrazoline was found to be potent amongst the twelve with best selectivity index [37, 40].

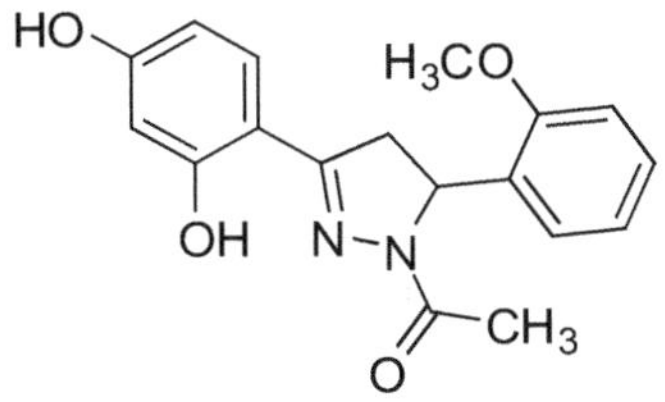

9 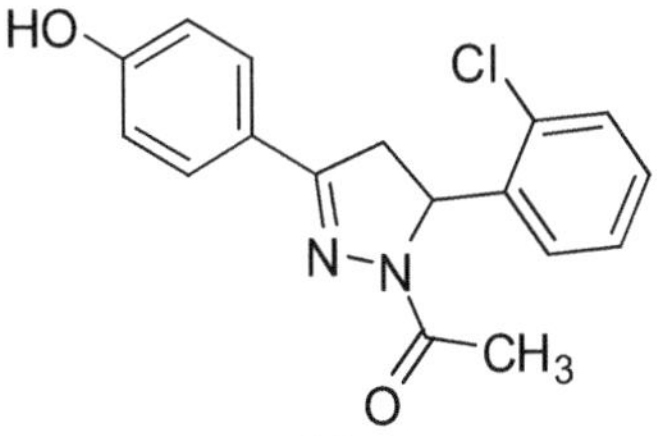 **10** 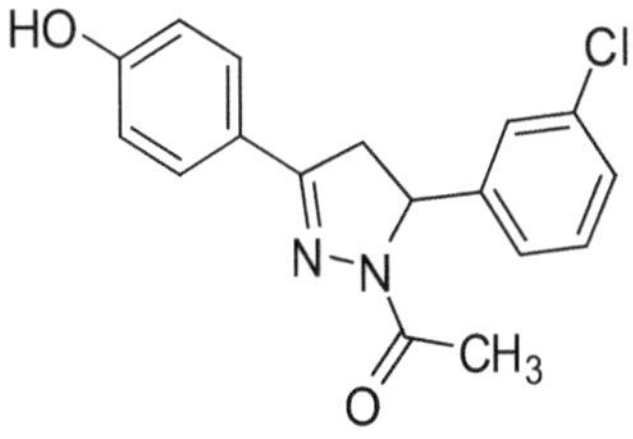 **11**

Cirilli *et al.,* investigated the novel series of 1-acetyl-3-(4-hydroxy- and 2,4-dihydroxyphenyl)-5-phenyl-4,5-dihydro-(1H)-pyrazole derivatives against bovine brain mitochondria MAO-isoforms [41]. Compound (**10**, bMAO-A: IC_{50} =8.6x10^{-9} ± 0.4 M; bMAO-B: IC_{50} =8.7x10^{-5} ± 0.4 M) having 2-chlorophenyl substitution at 5th position of pyrazoline exhibited best selectivity towards bMAO-A. While, compound (11, bMAO-A: IC_{50} =1.0x10^{-8} ± 0.3 M; bMAO-B: IC_{50} =2.3x10^{-5} ± 0.2 M) having 3-chlorophenyl was found to be potent bMAO-A inhibitor.

Chimenti *et al.,* have reported bovine brain mitochondrial MAO-isoform inhibitory activity of fourteen *N*1-acetyl-3,5-diarylpyrazoline derivatives. All the compounds were found to be potent and highly selective towards bMAO-A inhibitors [42]. Compound (**12**) having 2-hydroxyphenyl substitution at 3rd position and 2,3-dimethoxy substitution at 5th position of pyrazoline exhibited best potency and selectivity towards bMAO-A.

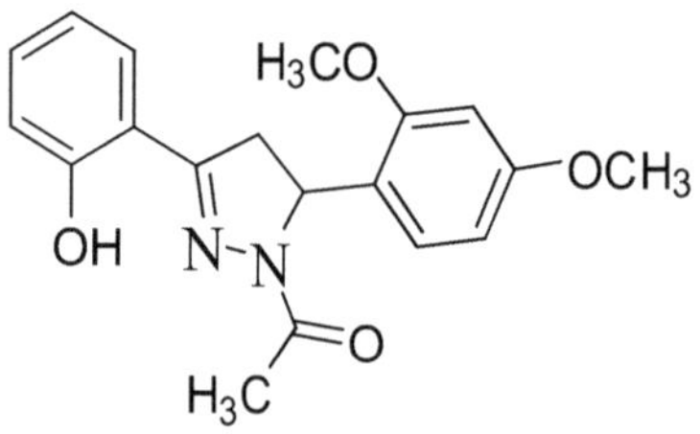

H3CO OCH3 OH N N O H3C

12

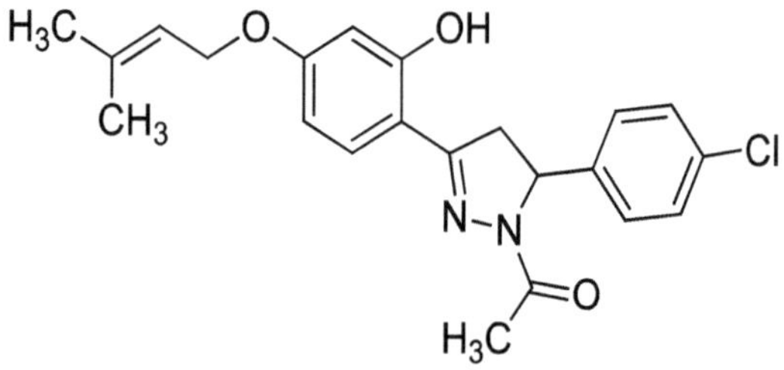

H3C O OH CH3 Cl N N O H3C

13

A series of five *N*-acetyl-3-[(2'-hydroxy-4'-prenyloxy)-phenyl]-5-aryl-pyrazoline derivatives were reported for their hMAO-inhibitory activity by Fioravanti *et al.* Two compounds were found to be inactive against both the isoforms, while one was non-selective and other two were selective towards hMAO-B [43]. Compound (**13**) having 4-chlorophenyl substitution at 5th position of pyrazoline was found to be the best amongst the two [43].

Guglielmi *et al.,* reported the effect of substitution pattern at N1, C3 and C5 on potency and selectivity of MAO isoform for already reported series of 1-acetyl-(**14**)/1-thiocarbamoyl- (**15**) 3,5-diphenyl-4,5-dihydro-(1*H*)-pyrazoles. The study revealed that bulky aromatic groups at C5 were makes compounds potent and selective towards MAO-A. Compounds having *p*-prenyloxyaryl moiety at C3 shifts the selectivity towards MAO-B [44].

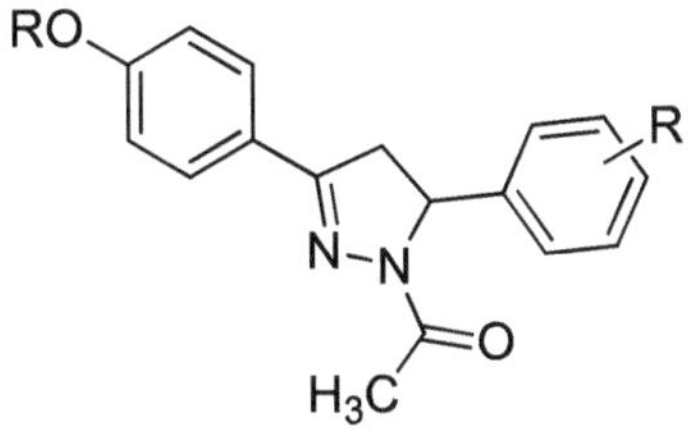

14 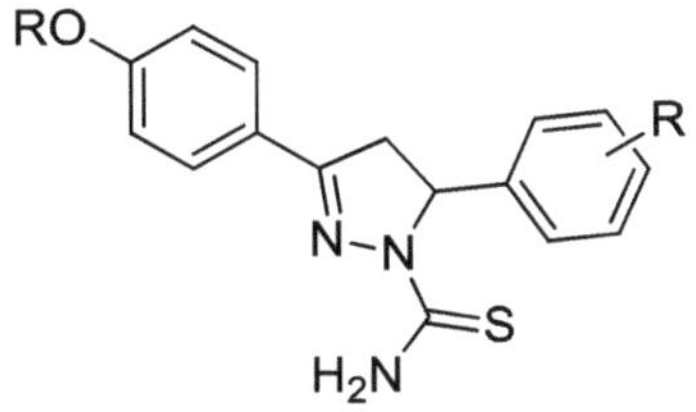 **15**

Chimenti *et al.,* evaluated the bovine brain mitochondrial MAO inhibitory activity of a series of twenty-five 1*N*-propanoyl-3,5-diaryl-pyrazoline derivatives. Twenty compounds were found to be selective towards bMAO-A, while the rest five were selective towards bMAO-B. But, the best selectivity index was found to be 2.7 (**16**) and -1.82 (**17**) for bMAO-A and bMAO-B, respectively [45]. Hence, the compounds in this series may be considered to be non-selective.

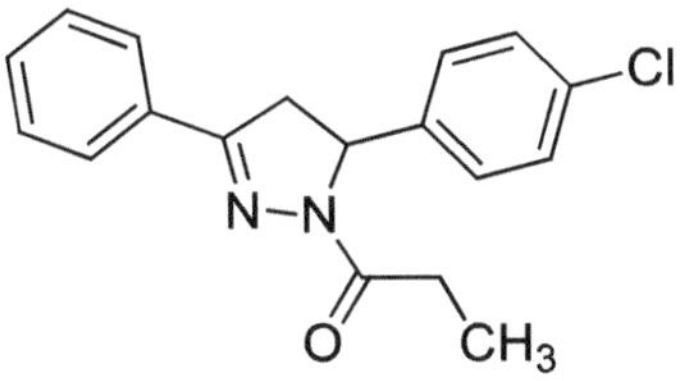

16 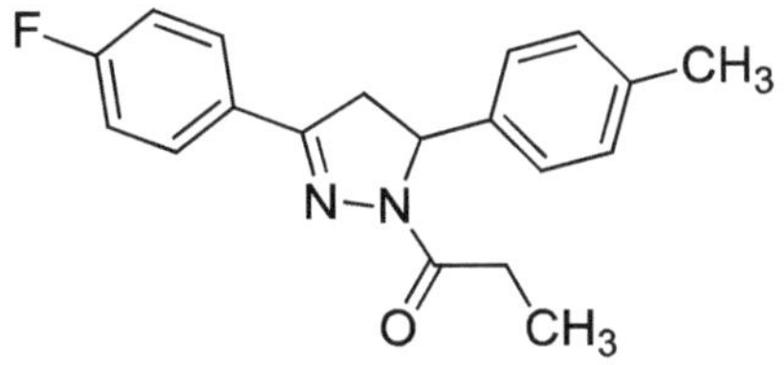 **17**

Goksen *et al.,* reported the hMAO inhibitory activity of series of 1-[2-(-5-methyl/chloro)-2-benzoxazolinone-3-yl) acetyl]-3, 5-diaryl-4, 5-dihydro--H-pyrazole derivatives. They found new selective, competitive and reversible inhibitors of MAO-A isoform, some of them were more selective than the standard drug Moclobemide. Compound (**18**, hMAO-A: IC_{50}=0.003±0.00001µM) having unsubstituted benzoxazolinone was found to be potent within the series reported [46].

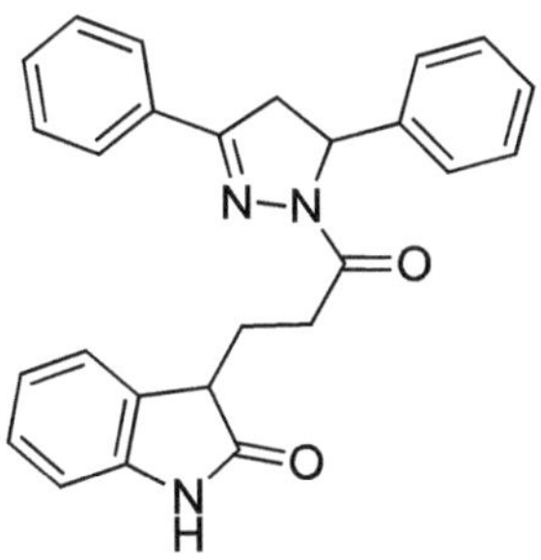

18 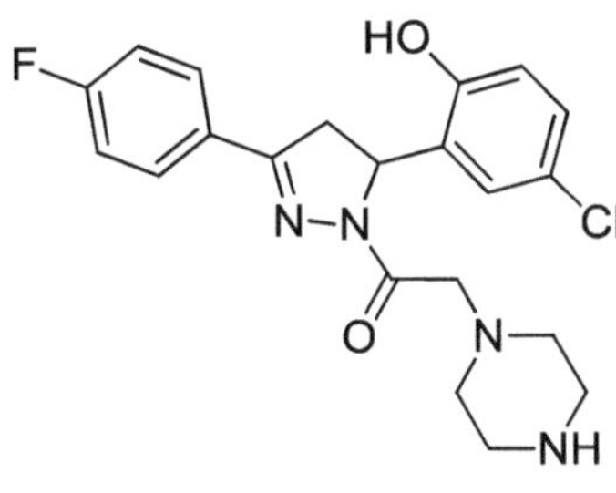 **19**

Tong *et al.,* designed, synthesized and evaluated hMAO inhibitory activity of twenty-six novel 1*N*-acyl-3,5-diaryl pyrazoline derivatives. They introduced piperidine, morpholine, piperazine and imidazoline rings in 1*N*-acetyl group. Three compounds were found to be inactive against both the isoforms, nine against hMAO-B and three against hMAO-A at 60 μM concentration. Except one compound all others were found to be selective against hMAO-A. Compound **19** was found to be potent amongst the series. X-ray crystal structure for one compound was solved, but no information regarding chiral separation and configuration of C5 carbon was discussed [47].

Sahoo *et al.,* reported the synthesis and rat liver MAO-isoform inhibitory activity of two 1*N*-benzoyl-3-(2-hydroxy phenyl)-5-aryl pyrazolines (**20**, **21**). Both are found to be selective towards rat liver MAO-A. The compound (**20**, rMAO-A: K*i*= 0.80 μM; rMAO-B: K*i*= 99230 μM) having 2-hydroxy phenyl substitution at 5th position was found to be 7-fold better than its 4-hydroxy phenyl counterpart (**21**, rMAO-A: K*i*= 5.77 μM; rMAO-B: K*i*= 20330 μM) [48].

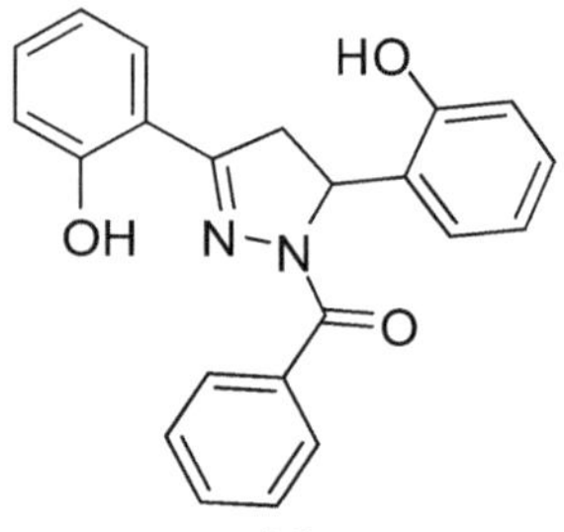

20 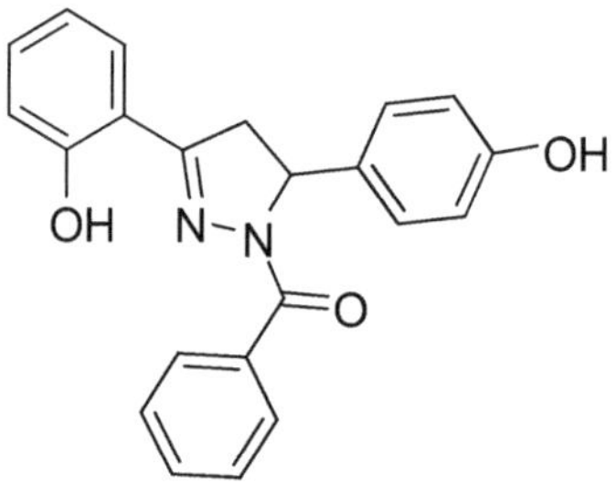 **21** 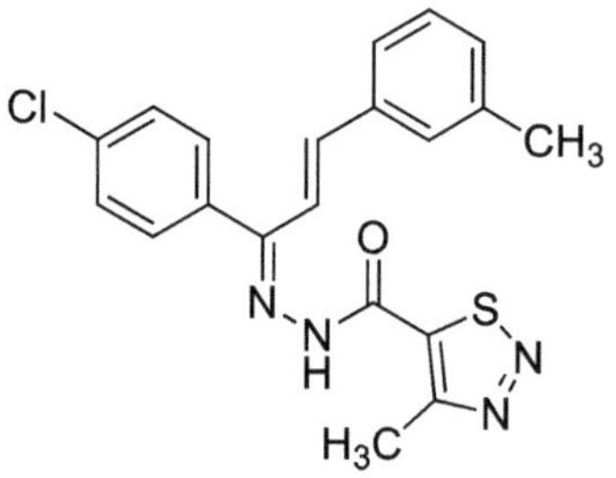 **22**

Evranos-Aksoz *et al.,* synthesized a novel series of 2-pyrazoline and hydrazone derivatives and evaluated for hMAO inhibitory activity. Two hydrazones (**22**, **23**) were found to be potent, competitive and reversible hMAO-A, while one pyrazoline (**24**) having thiophene-2-carbonyl substitution at 1N was reported be selective inhibitor of hMAO-B [49].

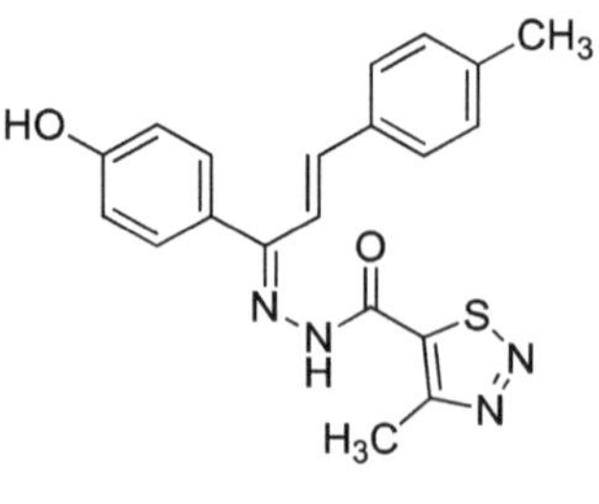

23 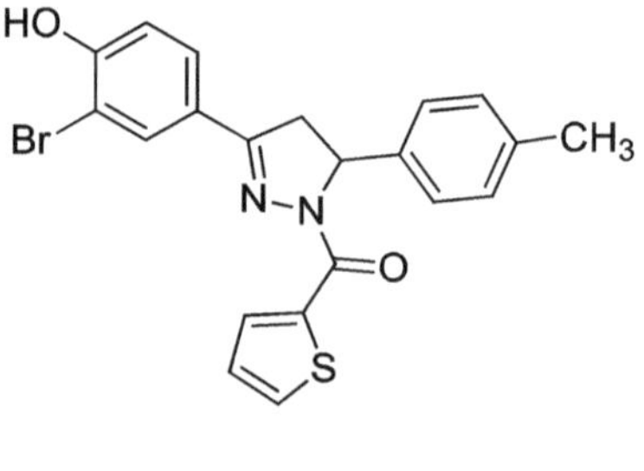 **24** 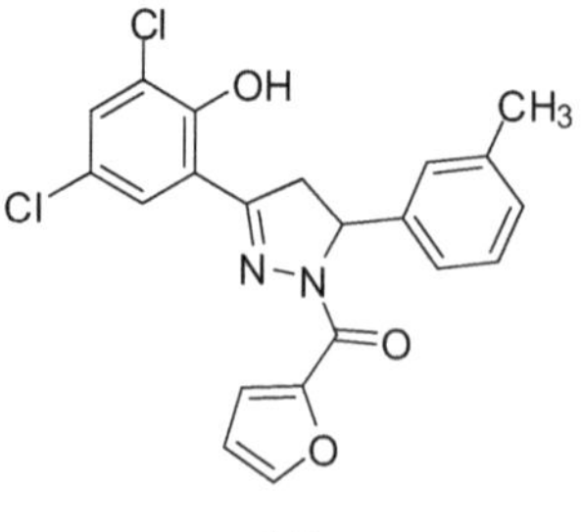 **25**

Evranos-Aksoz*et al.,* reported the synthesis and hMAO inhibitory activity of ten 3,5-diaryl-2-pyrazoline derivatives, among them compound **25** having furan--carbonyl substitution at 1N showed higher selectivity toward hMAO-A than the standard drug Moclobemide [50].

N1-Thiocarbomoyl-3, 5-Diaryl Pyrazolines

Chimenti *et al.,* reported the synthesis and MAO inhibitory activity of *N*1-thiocarbomoyl-3-aryl/heteroaryl, 5-aryl/heteroaryl pyrazoline derivatives using bovine brain mitochondrial MAO-isoform. Amongst four compounds having substituted 3,5-diphenyl substitution, three compounds were found to be selective towards bMAO-A, while the other was found to be bMAO-B selective. The most potent compound **26** [bMAO-A, K*i*= M (±SD) 6.0 x10^{-9} (±0.03), bMAO-B,K*i*= M (±SD) 1.0 x10^{-6} (±0.04)] was having 4-fluro phenyl and 4-chloro phenyl at 3rd and 5th position of the pyrazoline, respectively. They also reported compound with heteroaryl substitution at 3rd or 5th position of pyrazoline. Compound **27** [bMAO-A,K*i* M (±SD) 4.0 x10^{-9} (±0.01), bMAO-B,K*i* M (±SD) 1.7 x10^{-7} (±0.02)] having furan-2-yl substitution at 5th position were found to be selective towards bMAO-A, while compound **28** [bMAO-A,K*i*= M (±SD) 4.1 x10^{-8} (±0.07), bMAO-B,K*i*= M (±SD) 6.0 x10^{-9} (±0.01)] having thiophen-2-yl substitution at 3rd position was found to be selective towards bMAO-B. Substitution of chlorophenyl group at 5th position shifts selectivity towards bMAO-B (not true for compound having flurophenyl substitution at 3rd position (**27**)). Heteroaromatic (furan-2-yl) substitution at 5th position favors selectivity towards bMAO-A and also improves potency in comparison with their phenyl counterparts. Whereas, substitution of heteroaromatics (thiophen-2-yl) at 3rd position shifts selectivity towards bMAO-B [51].

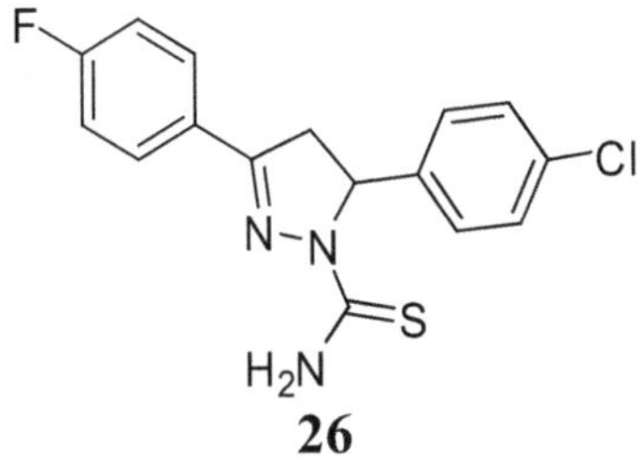

F, N-N, Cl, S, H_2N **26** | H_3C, N-N, O, S, H_2N **27** | S, Cl, N-N, S, H_2N **28**

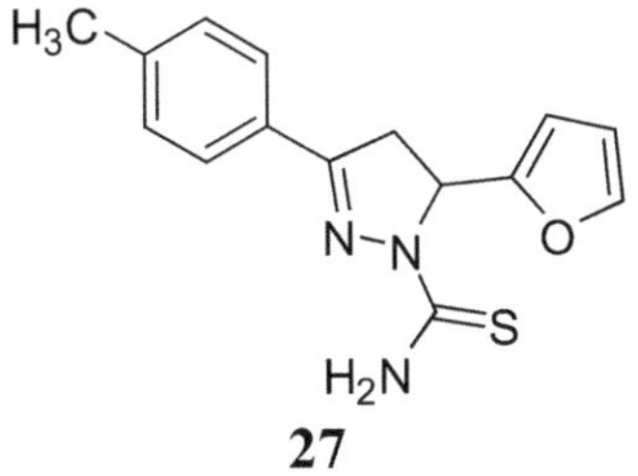

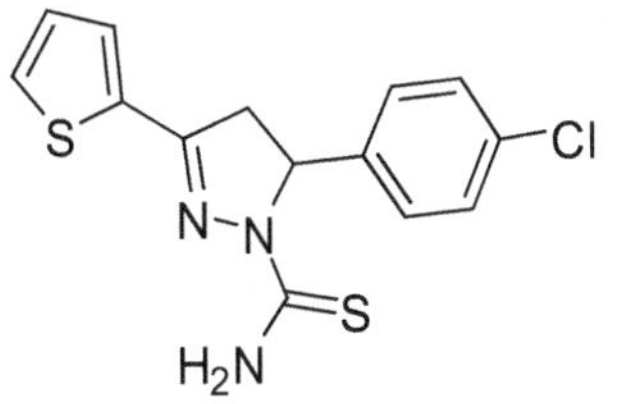

Palaska *et al.,* reported the rat liver MAO inhibitory activity of a series of ten 1*N*-thiocarbamoyl-3,5-diaryl pyrazoline derivatives. Compounds having phenyl substitution at 3rd position were found to be inactive. Compounds having 4-chloro, 4-bromo and 4-methoxy phenyl substitution at 3rd position of pyrazolines were selective towards rMAO-A, amongst them 4-methoxy phenyl derivatives are found to be potent. Compound **29** (rMAO-A, IC_{50} =4.80±l 0.73 μM) and **30** (rMAO-A, IC_{50} =3.14±0.83 μM) were found to be selective towards rMAO-A [52].

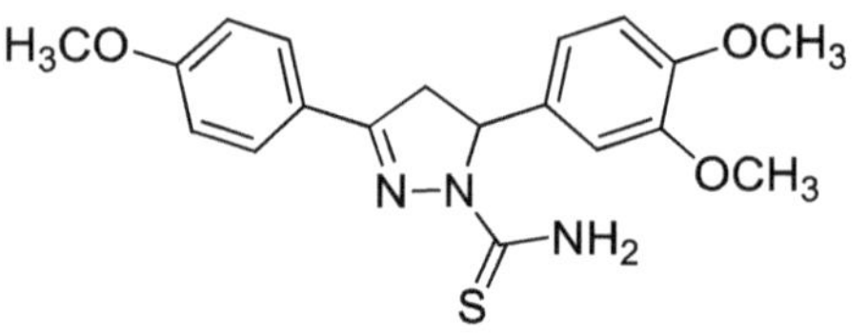

29 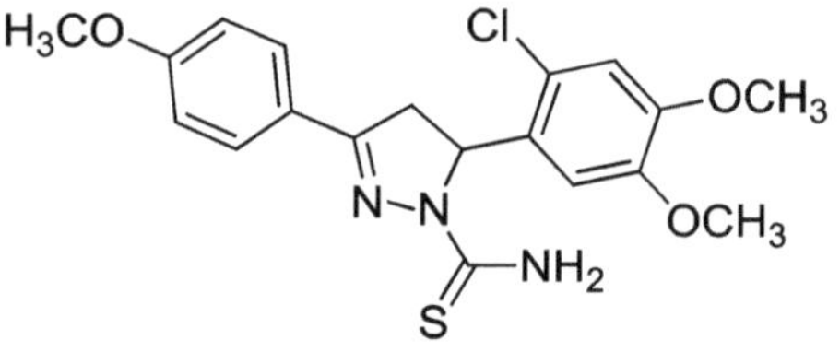 **30**

Chimenti *et al.,* reported the hMAO-isoform inhibitory activity of two *N1*-thiocarbamoyl-3-aryl-5-(thiophen-2-yl)-pyrazolines. Both were found to be inactive against hMAO-A at 100μM concentration, but inhibited hMAO-B at lower μM concentration. One which was having 4-methyl phenyl substitution at 3rd position of pyrazoline **31** (hMAO-B, IC_{50} = 18.26±0.98 μM) was found to be potent than 4-fluoro phenyl substitution **32** (hMAO-B, IC_{50} = 23.21±1.07 μM) [53].

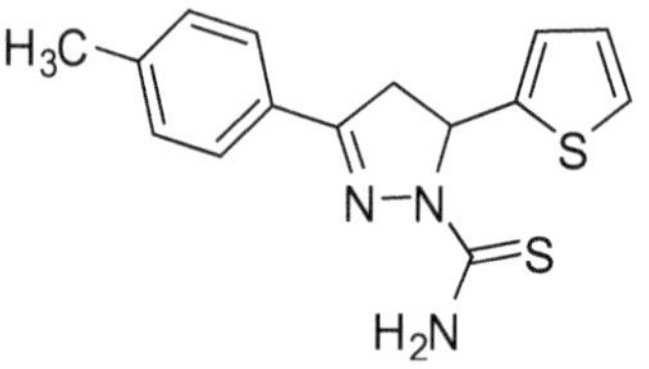

31 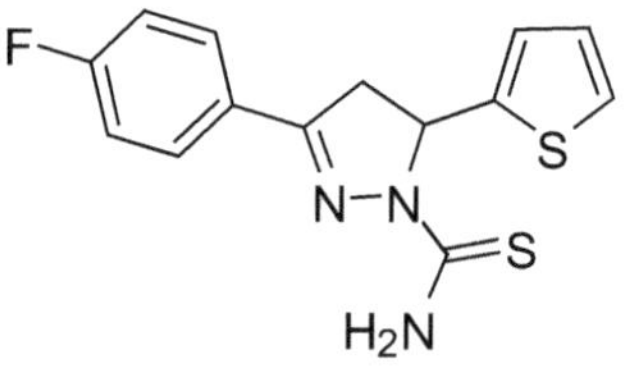 **32**

Chimenti *et al.,* reported bovine brain mitochondrial MAO-isoform inhibitory activity of *N1*-thiocarbamoyl-3,5-heteroaryl-pyrazolines. Two compounds with thiophen-2-yl at 5th position of the pyrazoline were found to be inactive at the maximum concentration studied. The other two with pyrrol-2-yl [(**33**, bMAO-B, IC_{50}=69.38±4.23 μM) and furan-2yl (**34**, bMAO-B, IC_{50}=33.26±1.99 μM)] at 5th position were found to be selective towards bMAO-B with poor selectivity index [53].

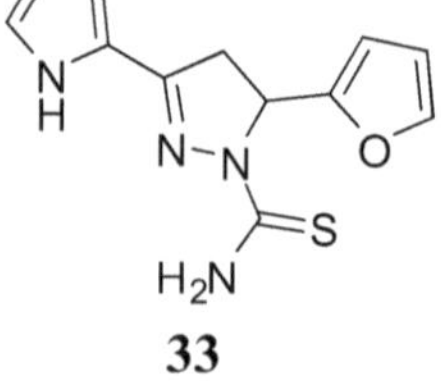

33 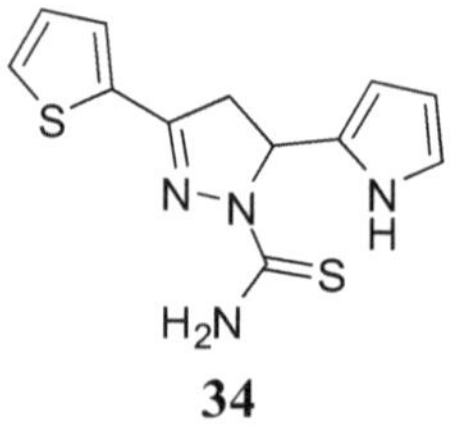 **34**

Chimenti *et al.,* reported the hMAO-isoform inhibitory activity of *N*1-thiocarbamoyl-3-phenyl-5-(furan-2-yl)-pyrazoline **35** (hMAO-A, IC_{50}=54.65±3.12 μM, hMAO-B, IC_{50}=32.48±1.64 μM). It was found to be selective towards hMAO-B with low selectivity index of 1.7 [53].

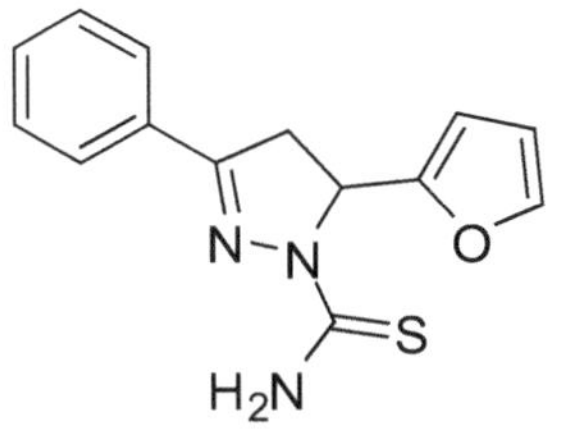

35 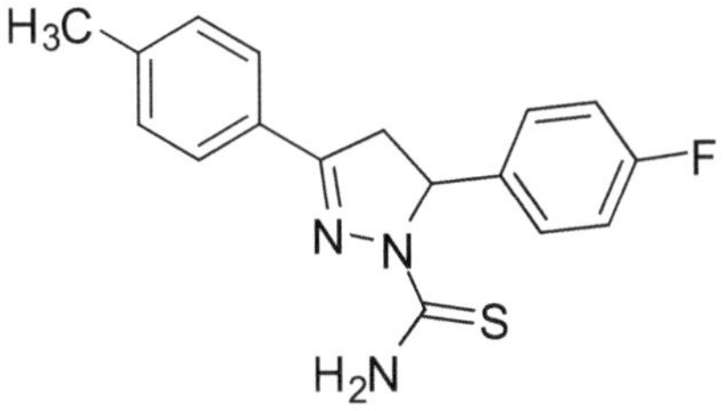 **36**

Chimenti *et al.,* evaluated the hMAO inhibitory activity of a series of seven 1*N*-thiocarbamoyl-3,5-diaryl-pyrazoline derivatives. Six compounds were found to be inactive against hMAO-A up to 100μM concentration, while the rest one was found to be selective towards the hMAO-B in μM range. Compound **36** (hMAO-B, IC_{50} =7.18±0.55 μM) having 4-methyl phenyl and 4-fluro phenyl substitution at 3rd and 5th position of pyrazoline, respectively was found to be potent inhibitor of hMAO-B amongst the seven [53].

Gokhan *et al.,* reported the bovine liver mitochondrial MAO-isoform inhibitory activity for a series of nine *N*1-(alkyl/allyl thiocarbomoyl)-3-aryl-5-(thiophen-2-yl)-pyrazoline derivatives. Six compounds were found to be non-selective while three compounds with 4-methoxy phenyl substitution at 3rd position of the pyrazoline **37** (MAO-B, IC_{50} =43.0 ± 10.0 μM) and **38** (MAO-B, IC_{50} =22.0 ± 0.9 μM), were found to be selective towards bMAO-B [54].

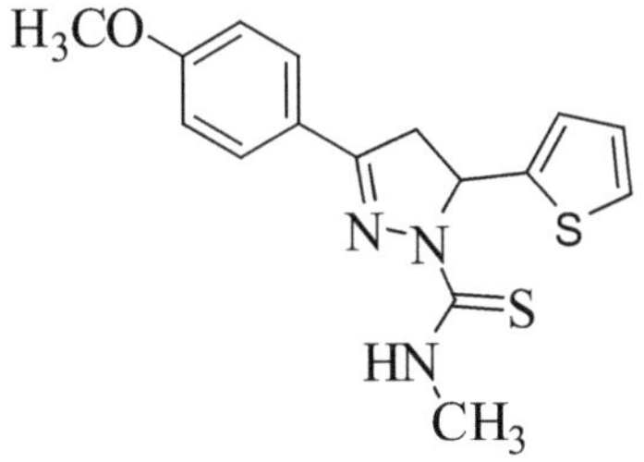

37 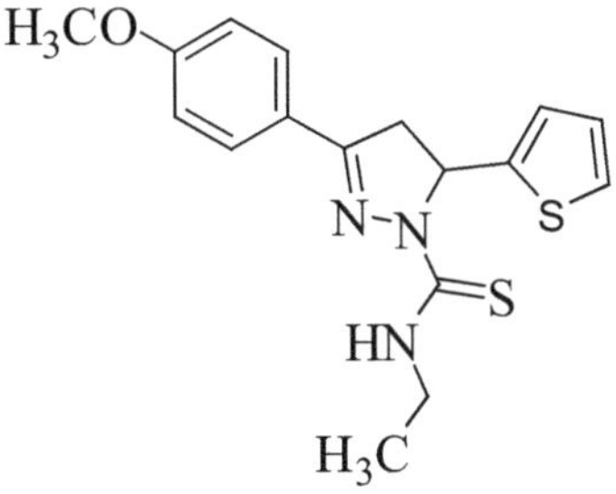 **38**

Gokhan *et al.,* reported the bovine liver mitochondrial MAO-isoform inhibitory activity for a series of three *N*1-(phenyl thiocarbomoyl)-3-aryl-5-(thiophen-

2-yl)-pyrazoline derivatives. Two compounds were found to be non-selective while one compound with 4-methoxy phenyl substitution at 3rd position of the pyrazoline (**39,** MAO-B, IC_{50} =91.5± 1.1 μM) was found to be selective towards bMAO-B [54].

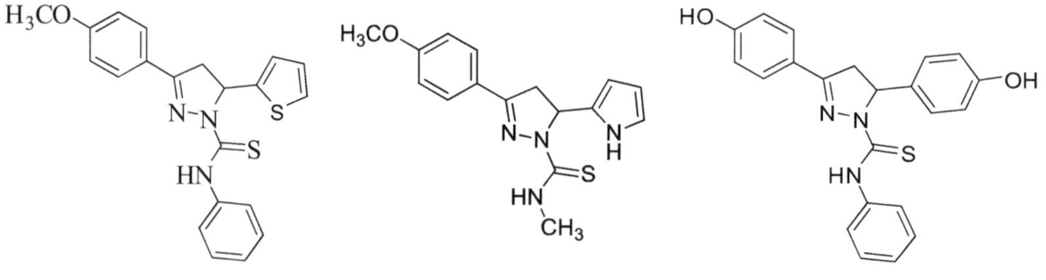

39 **40** **41**

Ucar *et al.,* reported the MAO inhibitory activity associated with rat liver semicarbazide-sensitive amine oxidase (SSAO) activity of some pyrazoline derivatives containing a thienyl ring *i.e.*, 1-*N*-substituted thiocarbamoyl-3-phen-l-5-thienyl-2-pyrazoline (**40**, IC_{50}= 70.11±6.34 μM, 0 min, IC_{50}= 42.10± 4.26 μM, 60min) against SSAO [55].

Jayaprakash *et al.,* reported the rat liver MAO-isoform inhibitory activity of 1*N*-thiocarbomoyl-3-(2-hydroxy phenyl)-5-(4-hydroxy phenyl)-pyrazoline. Compound **41** [rMAO-B, IC_{50}=45.13± 3.20 μM (0 min), rMAO-B, IC_{50} =19.45 ± 1.2 μM (60 min)] was found to be selective towards rMAO-B [56].

Inhibitory activity of *N*1-(phenyl thiocarbomoyl)-3-(2-hydroxy phenyl)---(thiophen-2-yl)-pyrazoline against rat liver MAO-isoform was reported by Jayaprakash *et al.,* (2008). Compound **42** [rMAO-A, IC_{50} =31.20 ± 2.35 μM (0 min), rMAO-A, IC_{50} =5.56 ± 0.45 μM (60 min)] was found to inhibit rMAO-A selectively [56].

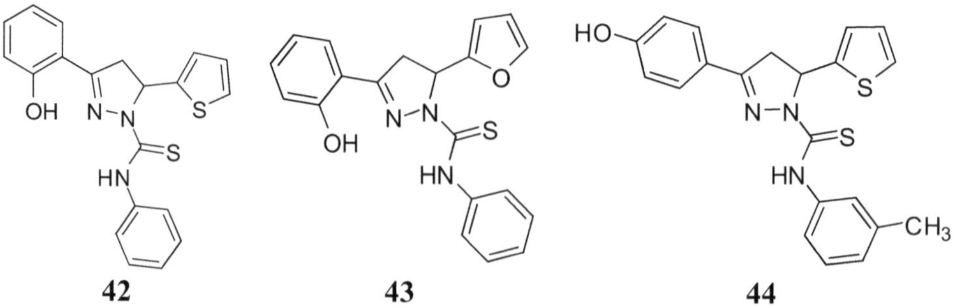

42 **43** **44**

Inhibitory activity of *N*1-(phenyl thiocarbomoyl)-3-(2-hydroxy phenyl)-5-(fur-n-2-yl)-pyrazoline against rat liver MAO-isoform was reported by Jayaprakash *et al.,* (2008). Compound **43** [rMAO-A, IC_{50}=74.12±5.37 μM (0min), rMAO-A, IC_{50}=33.41±2.85 μM (60 min)] was found to inhibit rMAO-A selectively [56].

Karuppasamy *et al.,* evaluated the rat liver MAO-isoform inhibitory activity of a series of seven *N*1-(aryl thiocarbamoyl)-3-aryl-5-(thiophen-2-yl)-pyrazoline derivatives. All were found to be selective towards rMAO-A. Compound having 3-methyl phenyl thiocarbamoyl substitution at *N*1-position of the pyrazoline **44** (rMAO-A, K*i*=150.10±10.05 nM, rMAO-B, K*i*=22,10,000±110.000 nM) was found to be potent amongst the seven [57].

Karuppasamy *et al.,* synthesized a series of seven *N*1-(aryl thiocarbamoyl)-3-ar-l-5-(furan-2-yl)-pyrazoline derivatives and evaluated for their rMAOinhibitory activity. All the compounds were found to be selective towards rMAO-A, while compound having 3-methoxy phenyl thiocarbamoyl substitution at *N*1-position of the pyrazoline **45** (rMAO-A,K*i*= 175.90±11.80 nM, rMAO-B,K*i*= 460.450±29.900 nM) was found to be potent amongst the seven [57].

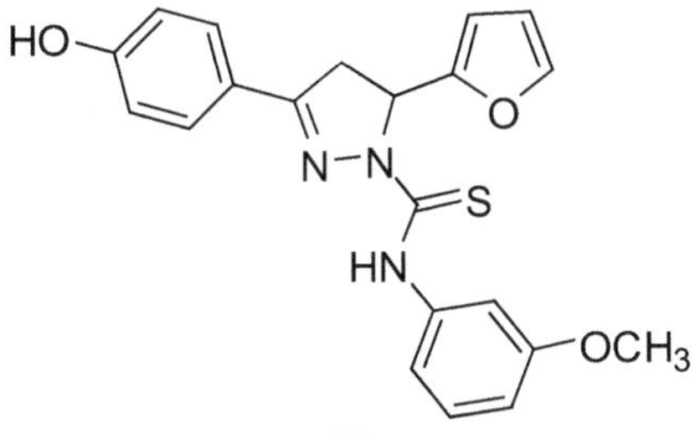

HO, N-N, S, HN, OCH_3, O

45

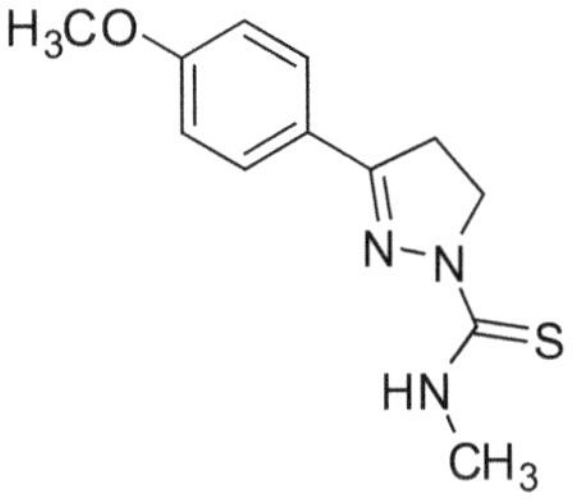

H_3CO, N-N, S, HN, CH_3

46

Maccioni *et al.,* evaluated a series of fifteen *N*1-thiocarbomoyl-3-aryl pyrazoline derivatives for their hMAO inhibitory activity. All fifteen compounds were found to be inactive against hMAO-A, while other seven compounds were found to be active against hMAO-B. Among the all one compound (**46**) contains 4-methoxy phenyl ring at 3rd position of pyrazoline (hMAO-B, IC_{50} =13.70 ± 0.95μM) was found to be more potent [58].

Fioravanti *et al.,* assessed the hMAO-B inhibitory activity of five novel prenylated pyrazoline *i.e., N1-* thiocarbomoyl - 3 -[(2'-hydroxy-4'-prenyloxy)-phenyl]-5-aryl-pyrazoline derivatives. Two compounds were found to be inactive against both the isoforms, while other three were active against only hMAO-B. Compound (**47**) having 4-phenyloxy phenyl substitution was found to be the potent (hMAO-B, pIC_{50} = 6.57) amongst the three actives [43].

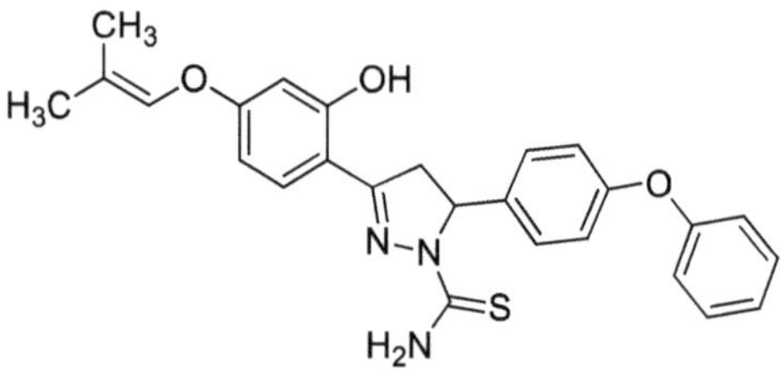

47 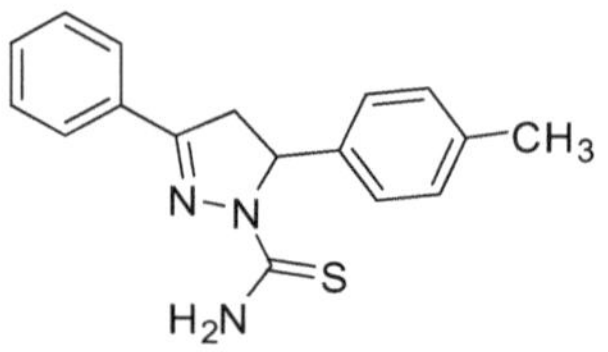 **48** 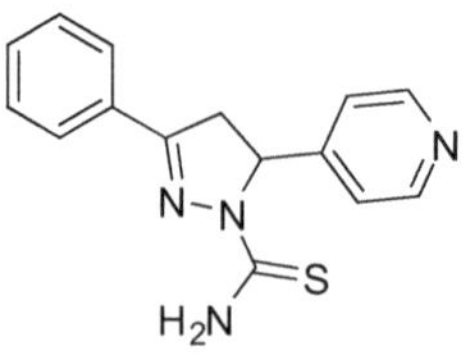 **49**

Jagrat *et al.,* reported the hMAO-inhibitory activity of three *N*1-thiocarbomoy--3,5-diaryl pyrazoline derivatives. Two compounds **48** (hMAO-A, IC_{50} =0.0333± 0.02μM, hMAO-B, IC_{50} =1.80 ± 0.11 μM), **49** (hMAO-A, IC_{50} =0.456 ± 0.02μM, hMAO-B, IC_{50} =4.00 ± 0.20 μM) were found to be selective towards hMAO-A, while the other one is non-selective. Both potency and selectivity were found to be poor [59].

A series of twelve *N*1-(phenylthiocarbomoyl)-3,5-diaryl pyrazoline derivatives were reported by Jagrat *et al.* The compounds were screened against hMAO-isoforms and all are found to be potent and selective inhibitors of hMAO-A. Compounds having 2-hydroxy phenyl substitution at 3rd position of the pyrazoline were found to be better than their 4-hydroxy phenyl counterparts. Compound (**50,** MAO-A, IC_{50}=0.10±0.01 μM, MAO-B, IC_{50}=979.00±41.00 μM) with 3-methoxy phenyl thiocarbamoyl substitution at 1*N*-position provided the most potent compound of the series [59].

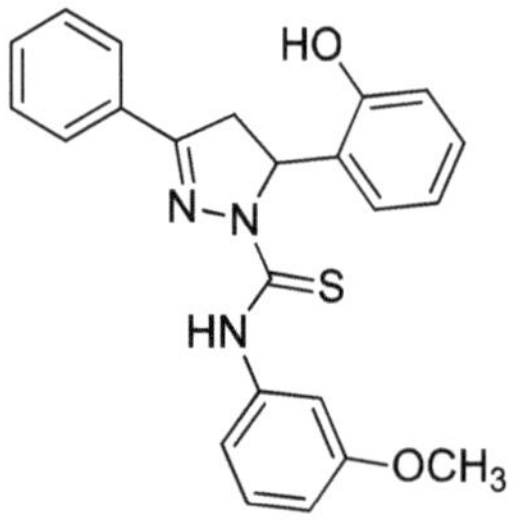

50 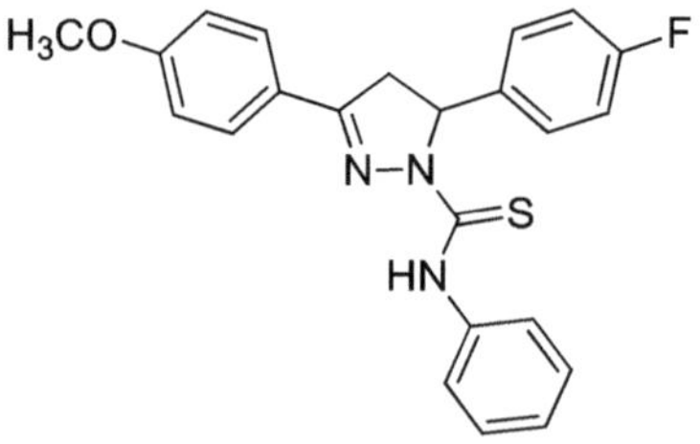 **51** 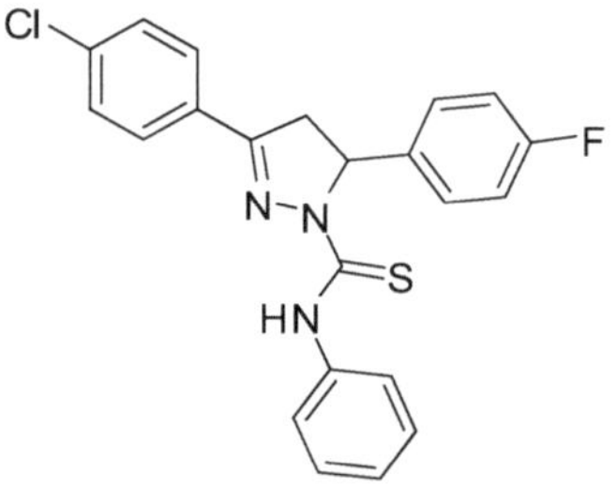 **52**

Senturk *et al.,* reported the hMAO-A inhibitory activity for a series of twelve *N*1-(alkyl/allyl thiocarbomoyl)-3-aryl-5-(4-fluorophenyl)-pyrazoline derivatives. They found that all compounds were potent and selective inhibitors of hMAO-A isoform. Selectivity Index was found to be low except for one compound **51** (MAO-A, IC_{50} = $1.0x10^{-3}$±$1.0x10^{-4}$ μM· MAO-B, IC_{50} = 2.15± 0.11 μM) that is having a methyl carbomoyl substitution at *N*I position and 4-methoxy phenyl substitution at 3rd position of the pyrazoline [60].

Four *N1*-(phenylthiocarbomoyl)-3,5-diaryl pyrazoline derivatives were reported by Senturk *et al.,* for their hMAO-isoform inhibitory activity. All the compounds were found to be potent and selective towards hMAO-A isoform. Compound **52** (MAO-A, IC_{50} = 0.21±0.01μM, MAO-B, IC_{50} = 0.70±0.05 μM) with 4-chloro phenyl substitution at 3rd position of the pyrazoline was found to be the most potent amongst the four derivatives [60].

N1, 3-Diaryl Pyrazolines

Chimenti *et al.,* reported the bovine brain mitochondrial MAO-isoform inhibitory activity of thirteen *N1*-phenyl, 3-aryl-pyrazoline derivatives. All were found to inhibit bMAO-A selectively. Compound **53** (bMAO-A, IC_{50} = $7.2x10^{-8}$ ± 0.11 μM, bMAO-B, IC_{50} = 4.0 x 10^{-5} ± 0.90 μM) having 2-hydroxy phenyl substitution at 3rd position of the pyrazoline ring was found to be potent among the series with best selectivity index [37].

Chimenti *et al.,* reported bovine brain mitochondrial MAO-isoform inhibitory activity of thirteen 1*N*,3-diaryl pyrazoline derivatives. All were found to inhibit bMAO-A selectively but were weaker both in potency and selectivity when compared with 3,5-diaryl counterparts [42].

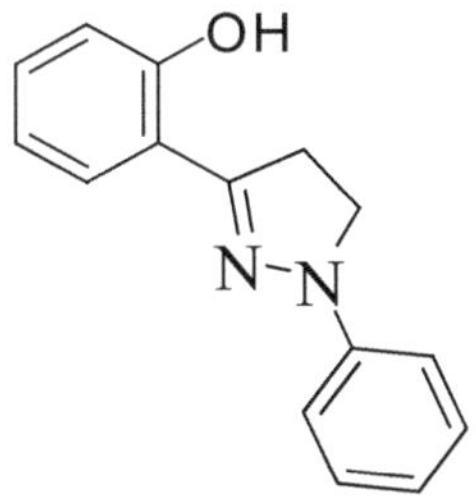

OH

N-N

53

N1-Acetyl-3-Aryl-Pyrazolines

Chimenti *et al.,* reported a series of fifteen novel *N1*-acetyl-3-aryl-pyrazoline derivatives with their inhibitory activity against bovine brain mitochondrial MAO-isoforms. All are found to be potent and selective against bMAO-A. Compounds having 4-chloro phenyl (**54**, bMAO-A, IC_{50} = $1.0x10^{-8}$ ± 0.04 μM, bMAO-B, IC_{50} = 1.0 x 10^{-4} ± 0.03 μM) and 4-bromo phenyl (**55**, bMAO-A, IC_{50} =

$1.0 \times 10^{-8} \pm 0.06$ μM, bMAO-B, $IC_{50} = 1.0 \times 10^{-4} \pm 0.05$ μM) at 3rd position of pyrazolines were found to be potent amongst the fifteen [37].

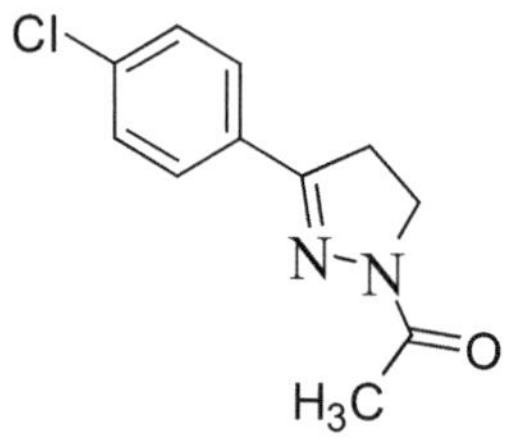

54 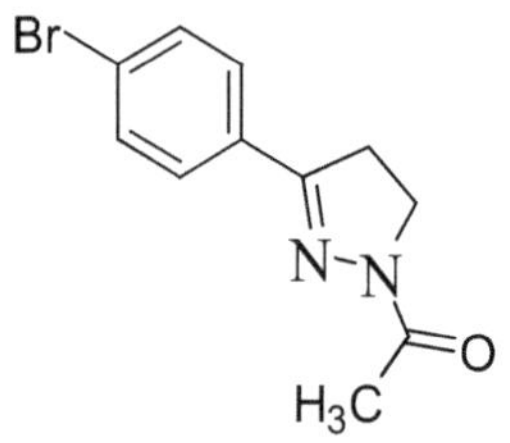 **55**

Chimenti *et al.*, have reported bovine brain mitochondrial MAO-isoform inhibitory activity of fifteen *N*1-acetyl-3-aryl pyrazoline derivatives. All were found to inhibit bMAO-A selectively but were weaker both in potency and selectivity when compared with 1*N*-acetyl-3,5-diaryl counterparts. Aryl substitution at 5th position of the pyrazoline seems to increase the potency as well as selectivity towards bMAO-A [42]

3-Aryl-5-Pyrrolyl-*N*1-Thiocarbomoyl Pyrazolines

Yabanoglu *et al.*, evaluated nine *N*1-(alkyl/allyl thiocarbamoyl)-3-aryl-5-(pyrol-2-yl)-pyrazoline derivatives for rat lung semicarbazide sensitive amine oxidase (SSAO) [61]. Later Goekhan *et al.*, evaluated the same compounds for their inhibitory activity on rat liver MAO-isoforms [62]. Compounds having 4-methyl phenyl substitution at 3rd position of pyrazoline were found to be non-selective, while those having 4-chloro phenyl were found to be selective towards rMAO-A and compound **56** [MAO-B, IC_{50}=58.55±4.27 μM (0min), MAO-B, IC_{50}=29.13±2.56 μM (60 min)] having 4-methoxy towards rMAO-B.

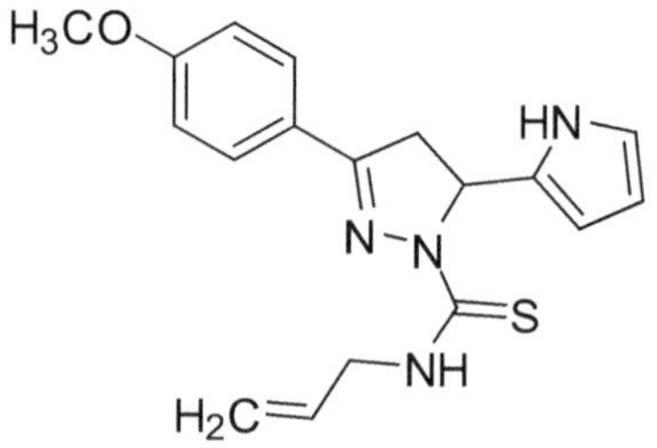

56

A series of three *N*1-(phenyl thiocarbamoyl)-3-aryl-5-(pyrrol-2-yl)-pyrazoline derivatives were screened for rat liver MAO-inhibitory activity by Yabanoglu *et al.* The one having 4-methyl phenyl substitution **57** [MAO-A, IC_{50}=323.19±29.90 μM at 0 min), MAO-A, IC_{50}= 300.18±28.13 μM at 60 min)] was found to be non-selective, while the other two having 4-chloro phenyl (**58**, MAO-A, IC_{50}= 98.22±8.13 μM, at 0 min) MAO-A, IC_{50}= 59.34±4.80 μM, at 60 min) and 4-methoxy phenyl (**59**, MAO-A, IC_{50}= 424.33±20.15 μM at 0 min), MAO-A, IC_{50}= 430.93±30.18 μM, at 60 min), were found to be selective towards rMAO-A and rMAO-B, respectively [62].

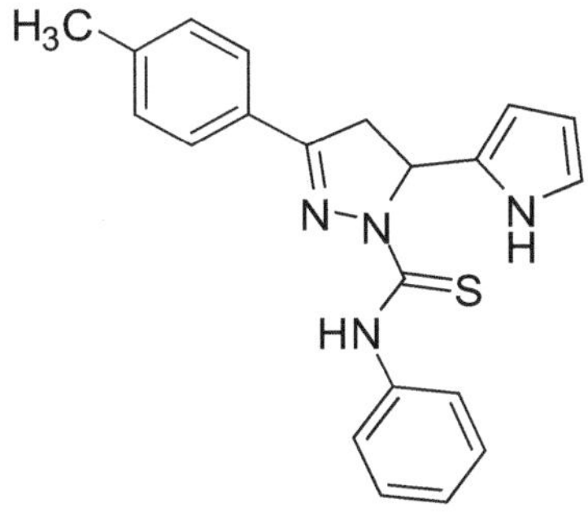

57 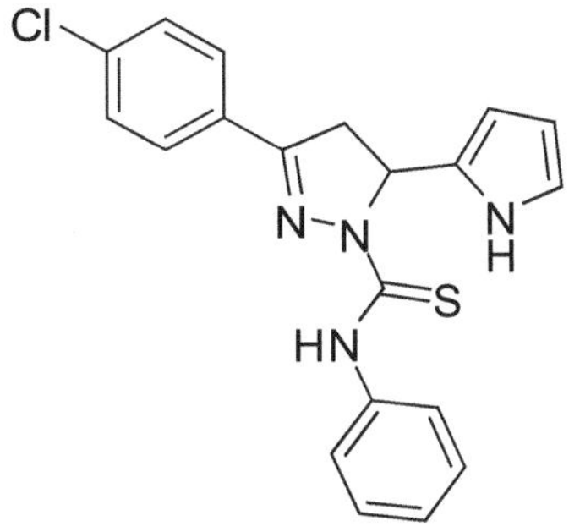 **58**

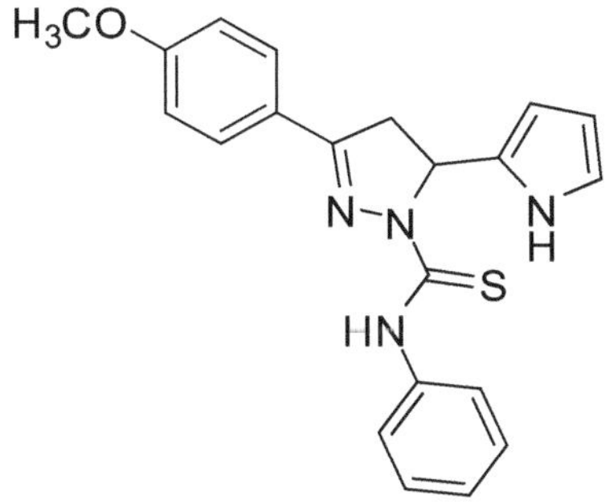

59 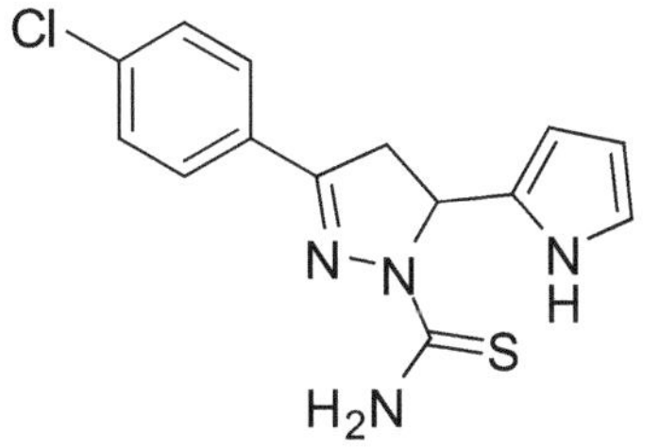 **60**

Chimenti *et al.,* reported the hMAO isoform inhibitory activity of *N*1-thiocarbamoyl-3-(4-chloro phenyl)-5-(pyrrol-2-yl)-pyrazoline. Compound **60** (MAO-A, IC_{50} = 50.14±4.96 μM,

MAO-B, IC_{50} = 29.38±2.87 μM) was found to be selective towards hMAO-B with low selectivity index of 1.7 [53].

3-Aryl-5-Aryl/Heteoaryl-*N1*-Guanyl Pyrazoline Derivatives

Goekhan-Kelekci *et al.,* introduced the quinzolinone ring in the 1*N*-position of pyrazoline nucleus. They prepared twelve compounds in which six were having either thiophenyl or furanyl ring at 5th position of pyrazoline while the other six were having phenyl ring. Compounds with phenyl ring at the 5th position of pyrazoline were found to be rat liver MAO-A selective while the others with heterocyclic system (thiophenyl/furanyl) were found to be selective towards rat liver MAO-B. Compounds having furanyl ring (**61**, MAO-A, IC_{50}=70.26±6.48 μM, 0min), MAO-A, IC_{50}=34.20±2.76 μM, 60 min) were better than their thiophenyl counterpart (**62**, MAO-A, IC_{50}=185.13±12.16 μM, 0min), MAO-A, IC_{50}=27.18±1.76 μM, 60 min) and the potent one seems to have 4-methoxy phenyl ring at 3rd position of pyrazoline in inhibiting MAO-B. In case of phenyl counterpart the one which having 3-chloro phenyl substitution at 5th position of pyrazoline (**63**, MAO-A, IC_{50}=0.90±0.07 μM, 0min) and MAO-A, IC_{50}=1.02±0.09 μM, 60 min) was found to be potent in inhibiting MAO-B [63].

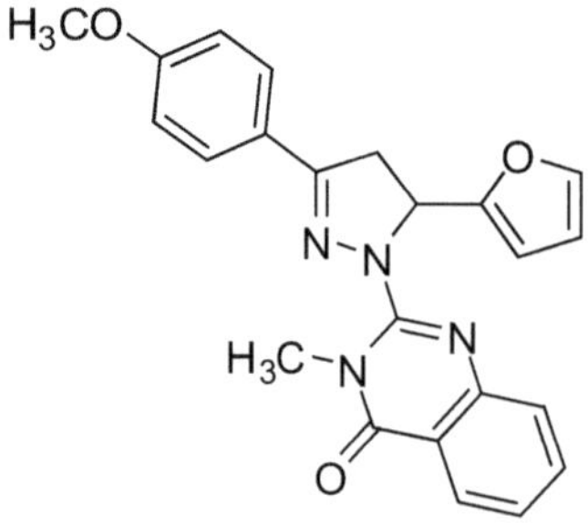

61 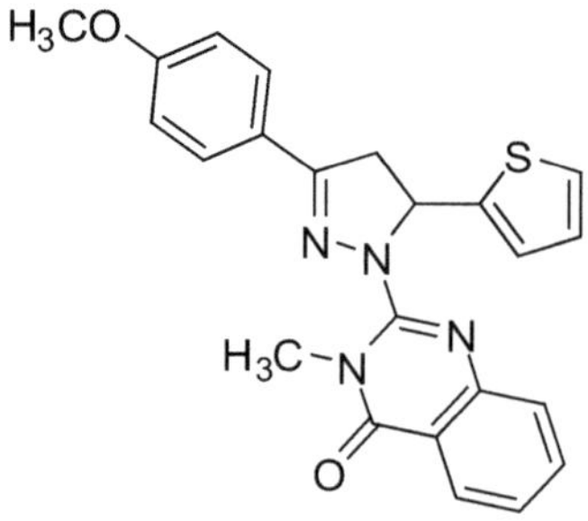 **62** 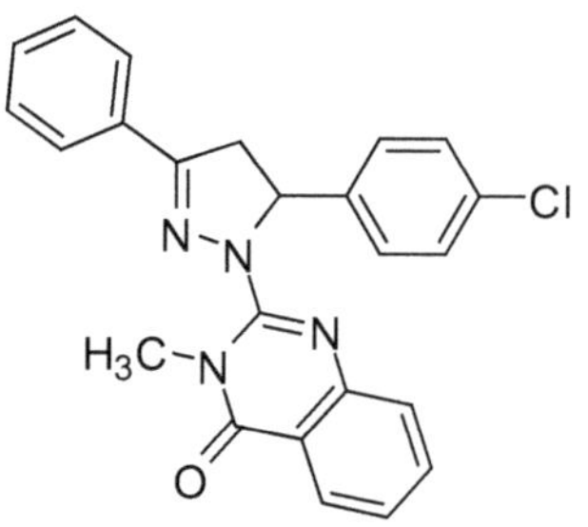 **63**

Sahoo *et al.,* tested the rat liver MAO inhibitory activity of two *N*1-(*N*-hydroxy amidinyl)-3-(2-hydroxy phenyl)-5-aryl pyrazoline derivatives **64** (MAO-A, K*i*= 15.66 μM, MAO-B, K*i*= 96.8 μM) and **65** (MAO-A, K*i*= 10.6 μM, MAO-B, K*i*= 210 μM) Both were found to be selective towards rat liver MAO-A but at the concentration K*i*> 10μM [48].

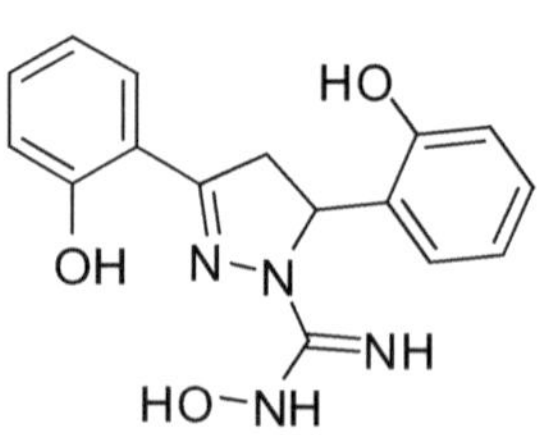

64 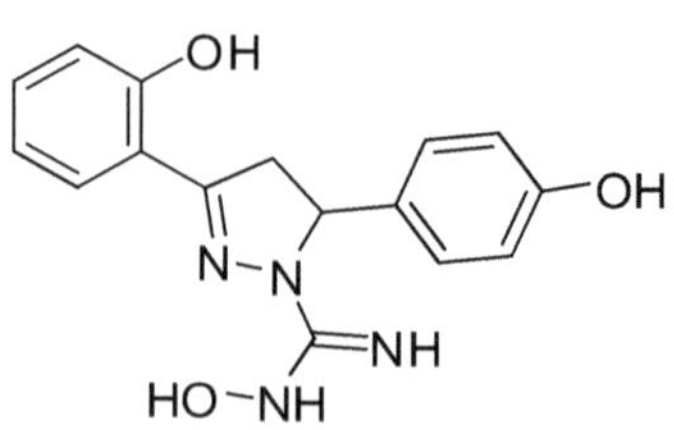 **65**

Jagrat *et al.* reported the synthesis and hMAO-inhibitory activity of three *N*1-amidinyl-3,5-diaryl pyrazoline derivatives **66** (hMAO-A, K*i*= 0.400 ± 0.02 μM, hMAO-B, K*i*= 4.11 ± 0.25 μM), **67** (hMAO-A,K*i*=0.670 ± 0.03 μM, hMAO-B,K*i*=4.80 ± 0.21 μM) and **68** (hMAO-A,K*i*= 0.150 ± 0.01 μM, hMAO-B,K*i*= 4.22 ± 0.19 μM) were found to be selective towards hMAO-A [59].

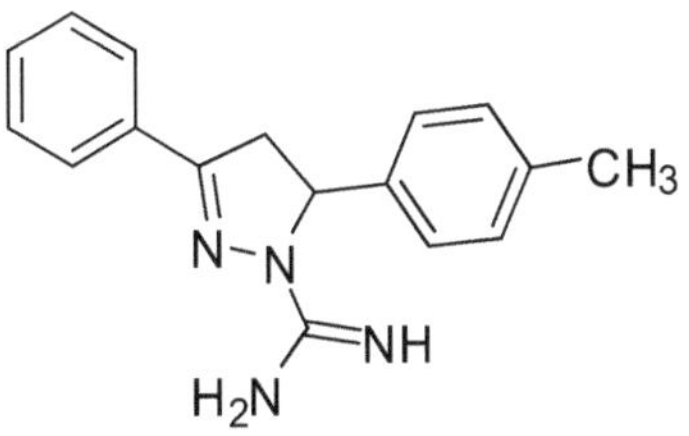

66 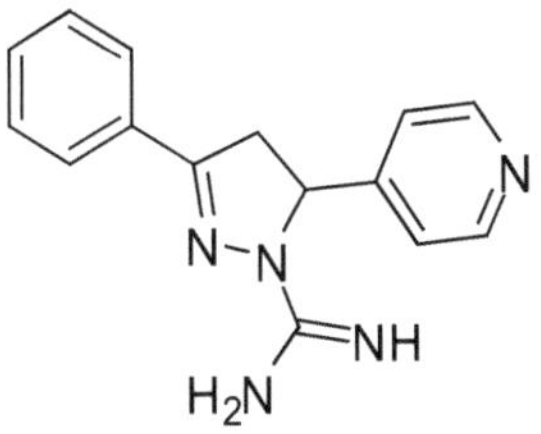 **67** 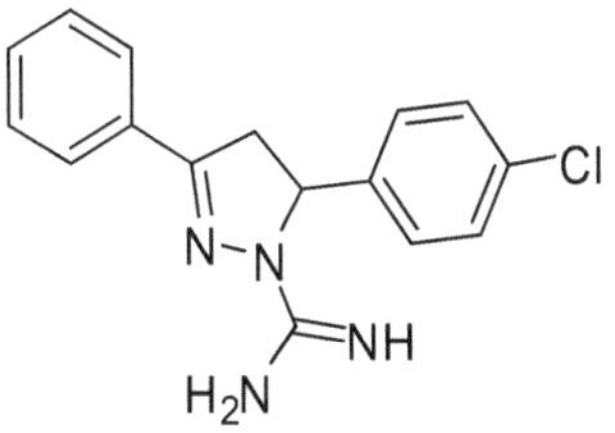 **68**

Hexahydroindazole Containing Pyrazolines

Gokhan *et al.,* reported fused pyrazoline derivatives and their rat liver MAO-isoform inhibitory activity. Increasing the bulkiness of the substitution at *N*1 position gradually shifted the selectivity from rMAO-B to rMAO-A. Furan-2-yl substitution at the 5th position of the pyrazoline was found to increase the potency towards rMAO-B when *N*1 substitutions were H, CH_3 and C_2H_5. On the other hand thiophen-2-yl at 5th position increased potency towards rMAO-A when *N*1 was having bulkier substitutions [64].

3, 5-Diary Pyrazolines

Sahoo *et al.,* reported the rat liver MAO-isoform inhibitory activity of two 3-(--hydroxy phenyl)-5-aryl pyrazoline derivatives. Compound having 2-hydroxy phenyl (**69**, MAO-B, K*i*= 0.78 μM, MAO-A, K*i*= 3.7 μM) and the other 4-hydroxy phenyl substitution at 5th position of the pyrazoline (**70**, MAO-B, K*i*= 0.60 μM, MAO-A, K*i*= 3.9 μM) were found to be equipotent and selective towards rat liver MAO-B [48].

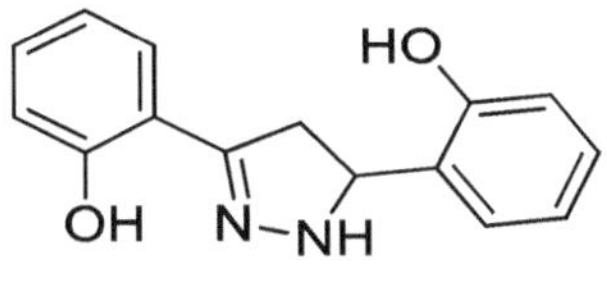

69 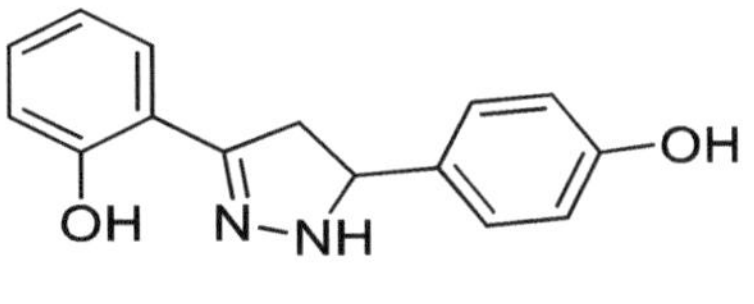 **70**

Mishra and Sasmal reported the design and synthesis of a series of ten novel 3-anthracenyl-5-aryl pyrazolines through High-throughput virtual screening of in-house generated library containing 18,000 molecules. The compounds were evaluated for their inhibitory activity against rat liver MAO-isoforms (rMAO) and human liver MAO-isoforms (hMAO). All the compounds were found to inhibit rMAO-B and hMAO-B selectively and are also competitive and reversible in nature. Amongst them compounds (**71**, hMAO-B, K_i= 0.31 nM, hMAO-A, K_i = 32.16 nM) and (**72**, hMAO-B, K_i= 1.70 nM, hMAO-A, K_i = 301.11 nM) were found to be potent and more than100-fold selective towards hMAO-B [65].

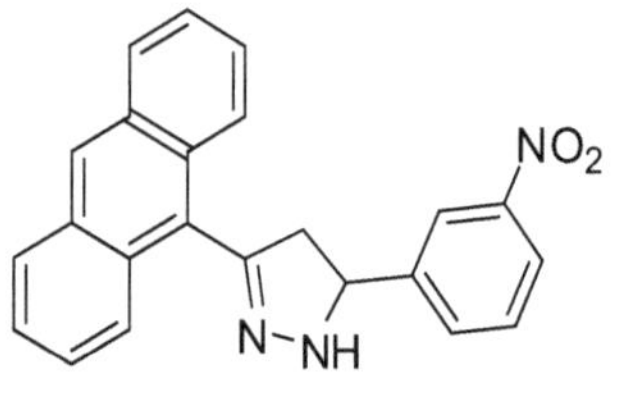

71 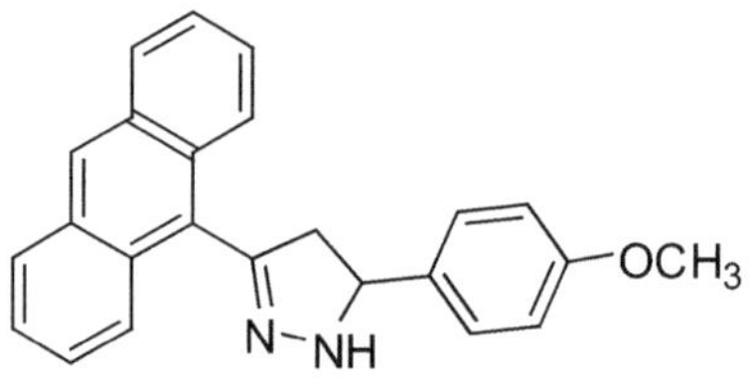 **72** 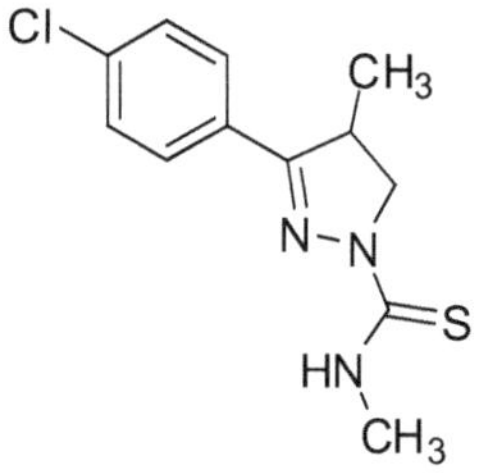 **73**

N1-Thiocarbomoyl-3-Aryl-4-Alkylpyrazoline Derivatives

A series of ten novel 1*N*-thiocarbomoyl-3-aryl-4-methyl pyrazolines were reported for their inhibitory activity by Maccioni *et al.* Seven compounds were inactive against both the isoforms, while three are active only against hMAO-B. Compound **73** (MAO-B, IC_{50} = 1.91 μM) having 4-chloro phenyl substitution was found to be potent amongst the three [58].

*N*1-Arylsulfonyl-3, 5-Diaryl- Pyrazolines

Sahoo *et al.,* synthesized four *N1*-(aryl sulfonyl)-3-(2-hydroxy phenyl)-5-aryl pyrazoline derivatives. All the four compounds were found to be potent and selective towards rat liver MAO-A. Compound with tosyl substitution at *N1* position **74** (MAO-A, K_i= 0.91 μM, MAO-B, K_i= 1550 μM), **75** (MAO-A, K_i= 0.68 μM, MAO-B, K_i= 700.2 μM) and compounds with 2-hydroxy phenyl substitution at 5th position of pyrazoline ring **76** (MAO-A, K_i= 0.36 μM, MAO-B, K_i= 620 μM), **77** (MAO-A, K_i= 0.60 μM, MAO-B, K_i= 285900 μM) were found to be potent [48].

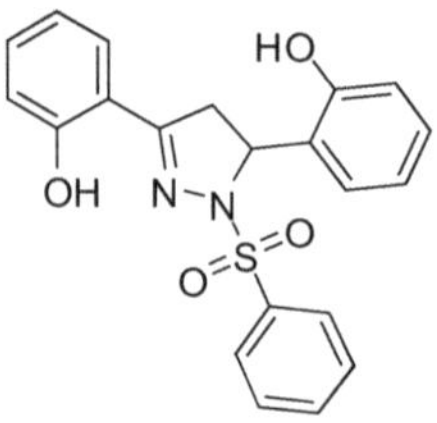

74 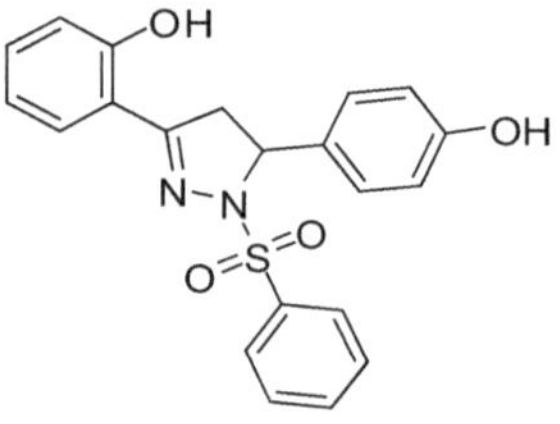 **75**

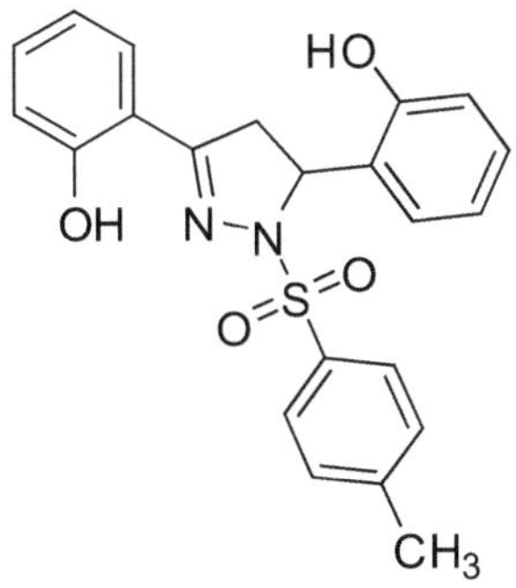

76 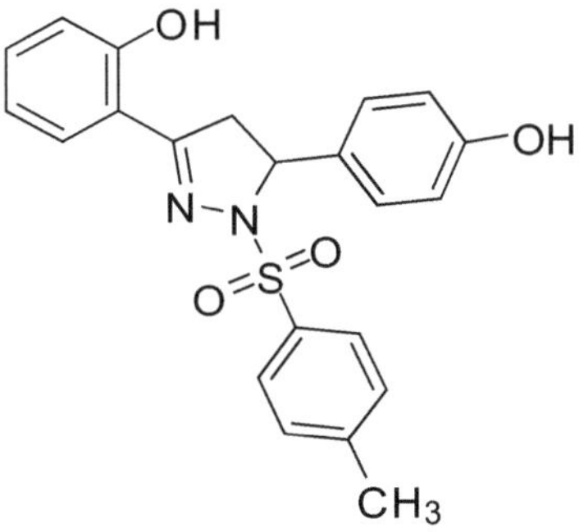 77

3-Pyrrolyl-5-Aryl-1*N*-Thiocarbomoyl Pyrazolines

Chimenti *et al.,* evaluated the hMAO inhibitory activity of a series of three 1*N*-thiocarbamoyl-3-(pyrrol-2-yl)-5-aryl-pyrazoline derivatives. All three compounds (**78**, **79** and **80**) were found to be inactive against both the isoforms at 100μM concentration [53].

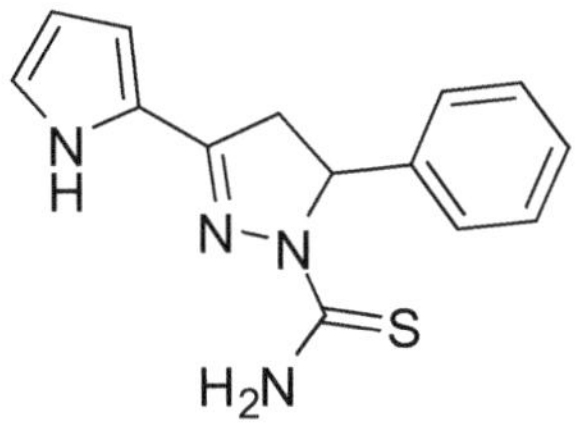

78 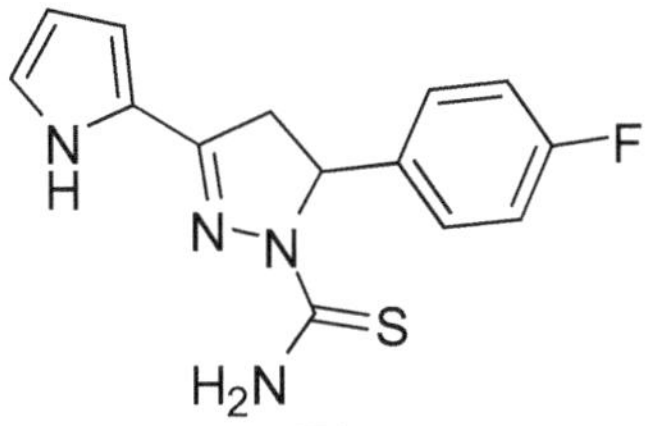 79 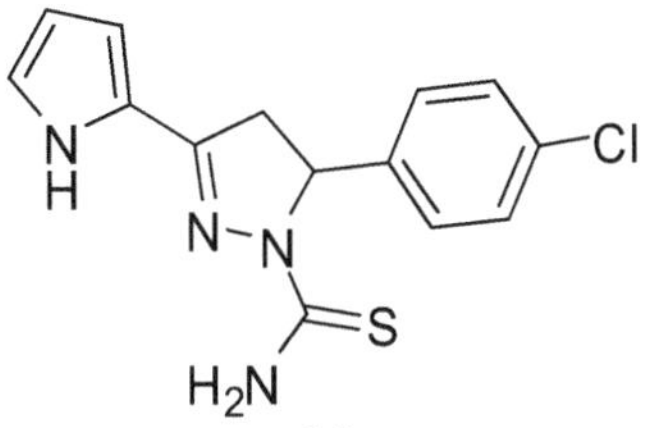 80

3-Furyl-5-Aryl-*N*1-Thiocarbomoyl Pyrazolines

Chimenti *et al.,* evaluated the hMAO inhibitory activity of two *N*1-thiocarbamoyl-3-(furan-2-yl)-5-aryl-pyrazoline derivatives. Both were found to be selective towards hMAO-B and one which is having 4-fluro phenyl substitution at 5th position of pyrazoline (**81**, hMAO-B, IC_{50} = 2.75±0.11 μM)was potent amongst the two [53].

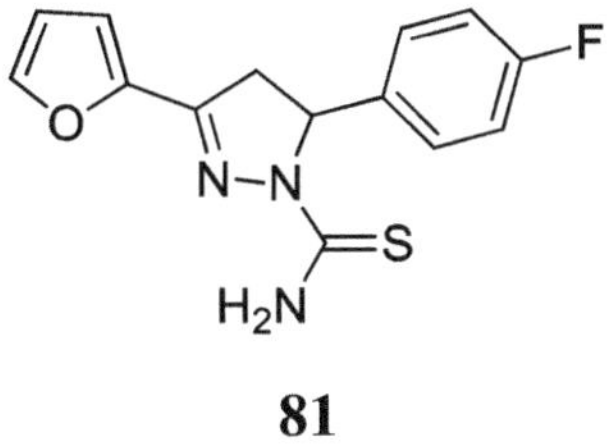

81

3, 5-Diaryl-*N*1-Carbomoyl Pyrazolines

A small series of four 1*N*-carbomoyl-3,5-diaryl-pyrazoline derivatives were synthesized and tested for their hMAO-inhibitory activity by Jagrat *et al.* Three compounds **82** (hMAO-A, K_i=0.490 ± 0.03 μM, hMAO-B, K_i=3.20 ± 0.18 μM), **83** (hMAO-A, K_i=7.00 ± 0.53 μM, hMAO-B, K_i=4.79 ± 0.24 μM), **84** (hMAO-A, K_i=0.980 ± 0.04 μM, hMAO-B, K_i=1.88 ± 0.09 μM) and **85** (hMAO-A, K_i=0.300 ± 0.02 μM, hMAO-B, K_i=1.66 ± 0.10 μM) were found to be selective towards hMAO-A, while the other one was selective towards hMAO-B. (selective hMAO-B compound was having pyridyl group at 5th position of pyrazolines) [59].

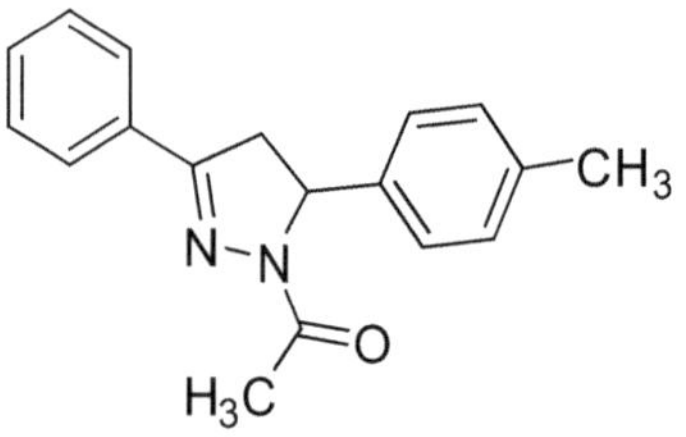

82 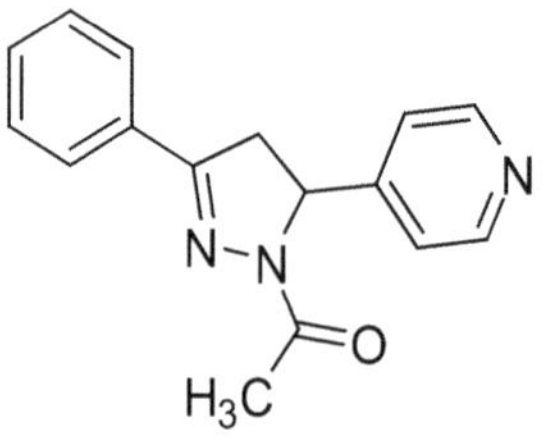 **83**

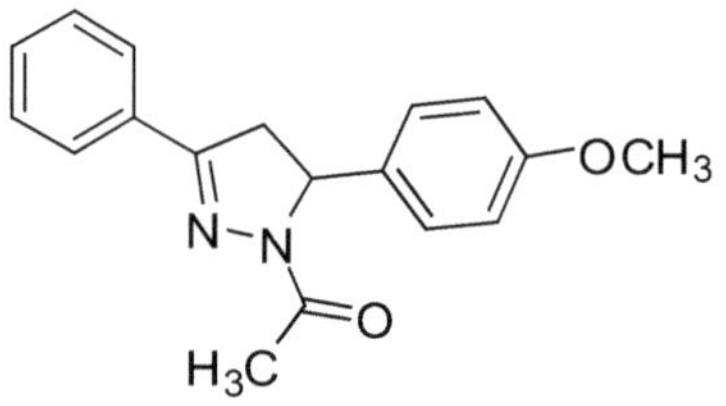

84 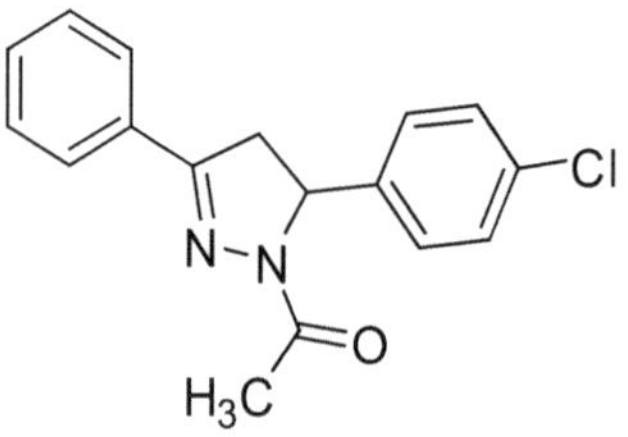 **85**

N-Alky-3,5-Diaryl Pyrazolines

Fioravanti *et al.,* reported hMAO inhibitory activity to a series of thirty 1*N*-methyl-3,5-diaryl-4,5-dihydro-1*H*-pyrazoles. Twenty-four compounds were found to be selective towards hMAO-A, while two compounds were non-selective and four did not showed any activity towards hMAO-isoforms. Compounds with unsubstituted phenyl ring at 3rd position of pyrazoline were found to be better than their 4-hydroxy phenyl and 2,4-dihydroxy phenyl counter parts. *N*1-methyl-3-phenyl, 5-(4-methyl phenyl) pyrazoline (**86**, hMAO-B, IC_{50} = 1.91 ± 0.06μM, hMAO-A, IC_{50} = 9.13 ± 0.52μM) was found to be the potent one amongst the three. Introduction of 4-hydroxy functional group on the phenyl group at 3rd position of pyrazoline reduces its potency, while introduction of 2, 4-dihydroxy totally abolishes its activity [66].

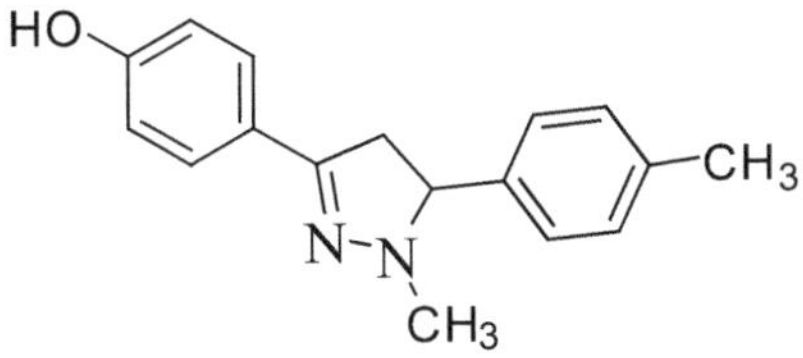

HO CH3 N-N CH3

86

3-Alkyl- 5-Aryl-*N*1-Carbomoyl Pyrazolines

Tong *et al.,* reported hMAO inhibitory activity for nine *N*1-acyl,3-methyl,5-aryl pyrazoline derivatives. All are found to be hMAO-A selective. Three compounds were inactive towards hMAO-B at 60 μM concentration [47]. Compound (**87,** IC_{50} = 2.00 μM) was found to be selective towards hMAO-A.

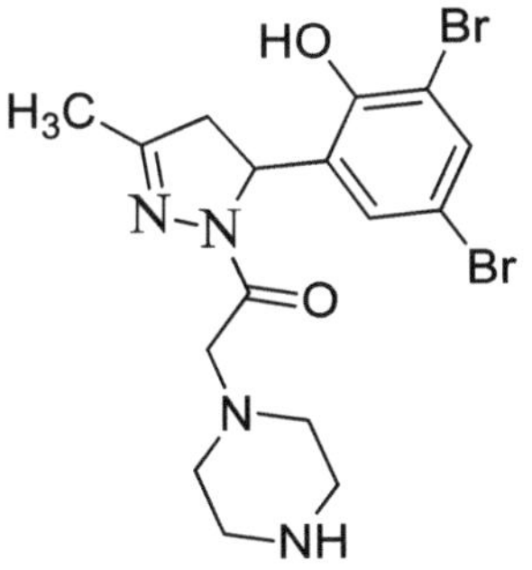

HO Br H3C N-N Br O N NH

87

*N*1-Ethyl And Phenyl Carbamate Derivatives Of Pyrazoline

Nayak *et al.,* investigated that phenyl carbamates (**88**, hMAO-A, Ki= 4.96± 0.21 nM) were shown better selectivity index (SI= 8.86x10-5) towards MAO-A, than ethyl carbamates (**89**, MAO-A, Ki=0.61± 0.03 μM) in *in vitro* human MAO enzyme assay [67]

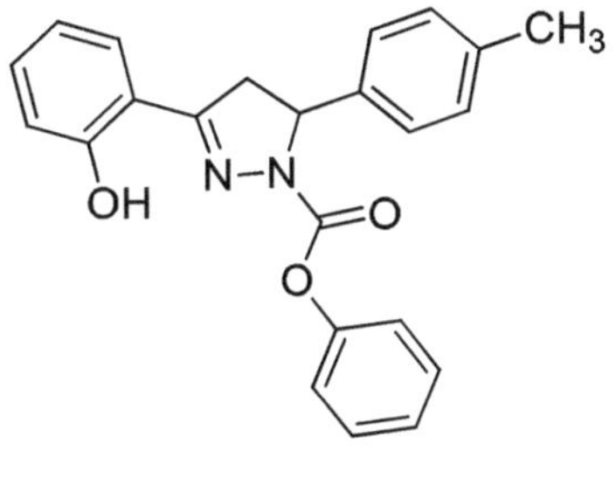

CH3 OH N-N O O

OCH3 OH N-N O O CH3

88 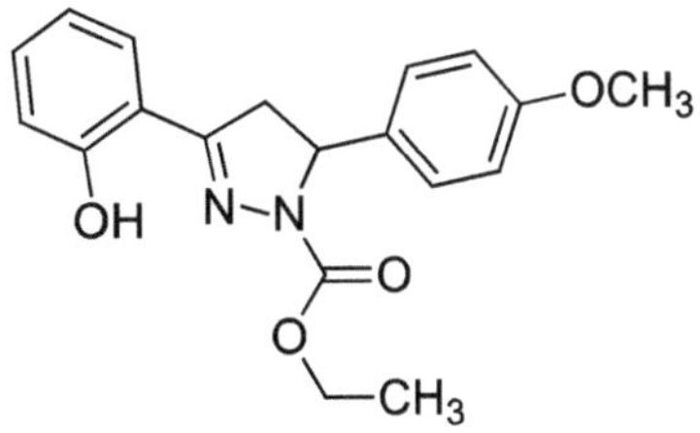 **89**

Curcumin-Based Pyrazolines Analogues

Nayak, *et al.,* designed curcumin based pyrazoline i.e aryl-α,β-unsaturated carbonyl portion of curcumin but by reversing the α, β-unsaturated carbonyl portion of the double bond (**90**, MAO-A, Ki= 0.06 ± 0.003 μM (SI= 1.02 × 10-5), MAO-B, Ki= 5900.00 ± 324.50 μM), (**91**, MAO-A, Ki= 5.02 ± 0.25 μM (SI= 14.343), MAO-B, Ki= ± 0.35 ± 0.02 μM) [68] and normal α, β-unsaturated carbonyl portion [69], and various substitution at *N*1 position of pyrazoline (**92**, MAO-A, Ki= 0.10±0.01 μM (SI=3.08x10^{-6}), MAO-B, Ki= 32500.00±1200.30 μM) and (**93**, MAO-A, Ki= 7.22±0.54 μM, (SI= 13.130, MAO-B, Ki= 0.55±0.03 μM). Compounds with no substitution at *N*1 position were selective towards hMAO-B and, compounds with bulkier substitution at *N*1 position were found to be selective against hMAO-A inhibitory activity.

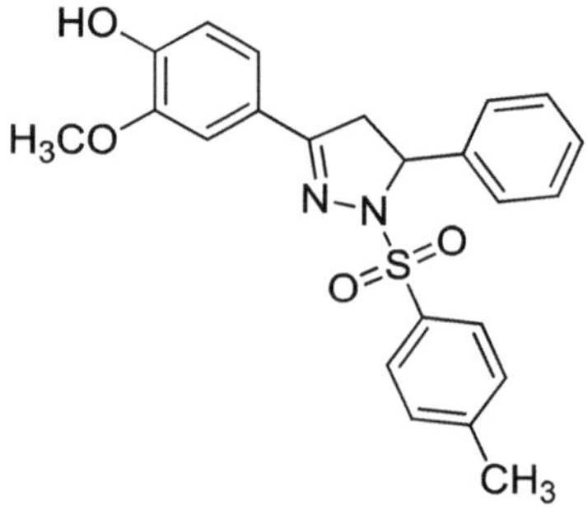

HO, H_3CO, N–N, O=S=O, CH_3

90

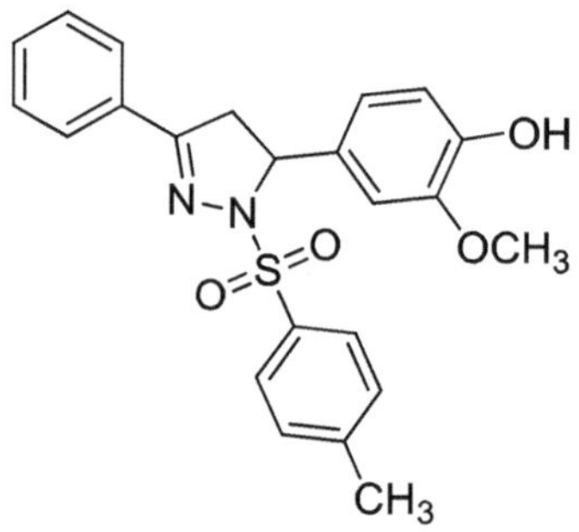

OH, N–N, O=S=O, OCH_3, CH_3

92

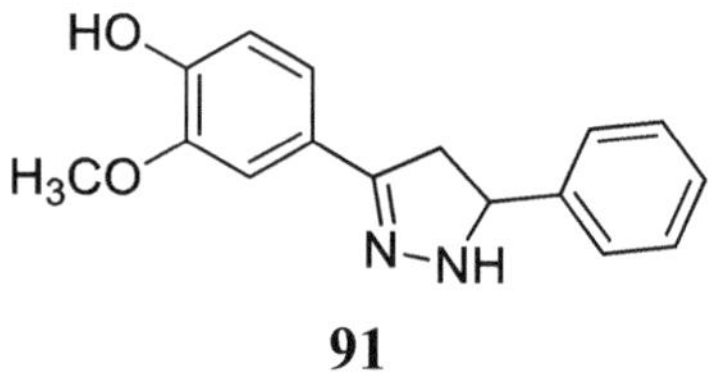

HO, H_3CO, N–NH

91

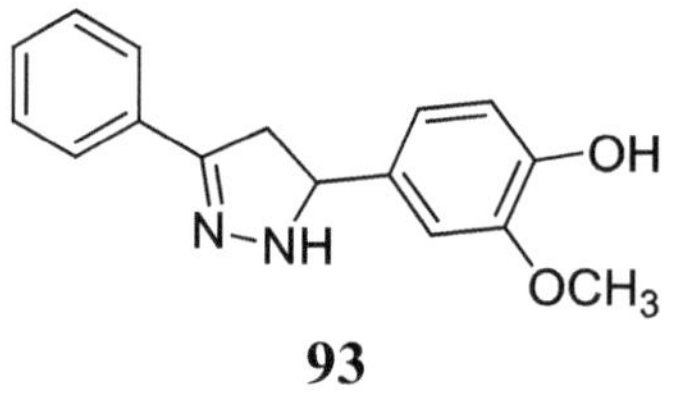

OH, N–NH, OCH_3

93

In continuation Nath *et al.,* designed a few novel curcumin based pyrazoline by reversing the α, β-unsaturated carbonyl portion position of the double bond, interestingly with *p*-chloro at ring B at C5 and *p*-hydroxy substitution on phenyl ring at C3 (**94**, MAO-A, Ki= 0.080 ± 0.009μM (SI= 1751.25), MAO-B, Ki= 140.10 ± 12.00 μM) these scaffolds shifted the selectivity toward hMAO-A [70], with no cytotoxicity (in HepG2 cell), and good permeability through blood brain barrier to reach biological targets located in Central Nervous system.

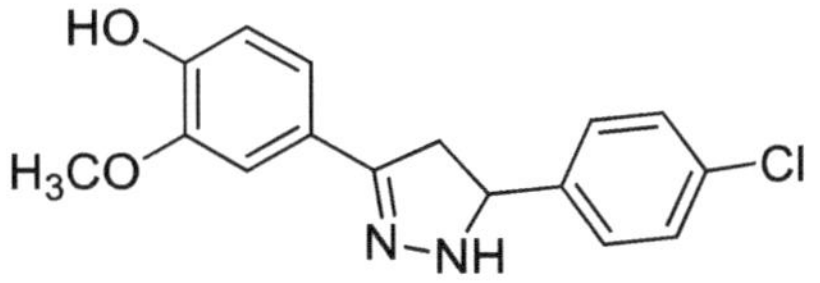

HO
H_3CO
N-NH
Cl

94

*N*1-2-Oxoethyl Benzofuran-2(3H)-One, 5-Dihydro-1*H*-Pyrazolines

Goksen, *et al*., reported the synthesized, absolute configuration using vibrational circular dichroism, and also suggested compound (**95**, R-isomer: MAO-A (Ki $=0.85 \times 10^{-3} \pm 0.05 \times 10^{-3}$ μM, SI= 2.35×10^{-5}), S- isomer: MAO-A (Ki=0.184 ± 0.007 and SI=0.001), R enantiomer was potent and a selective towards Mao-A than S isomer in *in vitro* [71].

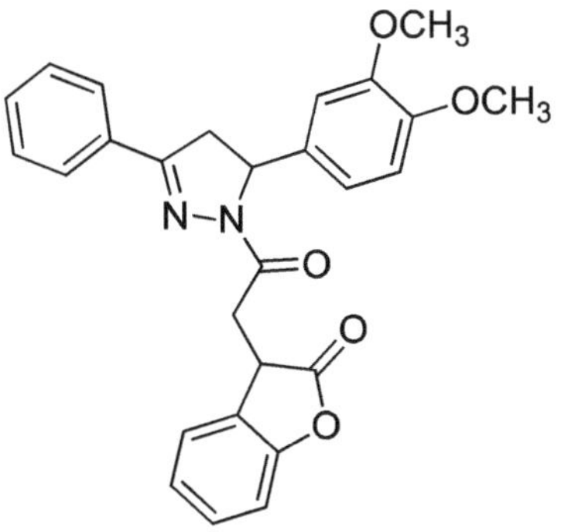

OCH_3
OCH_3
N-N
O
O
O

95

5-(Anthracen-9-Yl)-3-(3-Nitrophenyl)-4,5-Dihydro-1H-Pyrazole

Mishra and Sasmal reported modulation of brain amines and dopaminergic behavior by a novel, reversible and selective MAO-B inhibitor [72], studied the effect of brain amines upon acute and chronic administration of a potent, reversible and selective inhibitor of hMAO-B identified by them. It was found that there was a significant increase in striatal dopamine level upon chronic administration of the selective hMAO-B inhibitor. They also observed that there was no hypertensive crisis upon co-administration of tyramine.

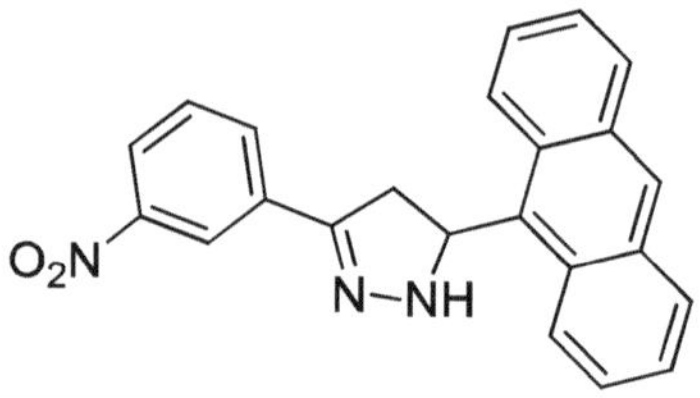

O_2N N–NH

96

ANTIDEPRESSANT ACTIVITIES OF PYRAZOLINES

MAO-A is involved in the metabolism of serotonin, adrenaline and noradrenaline. As a consequence of prolonged excessive activity of these enzymes the level of these neurotransmitters decreases in brain leading to the onset and progression of depression. The level can be restored by the administration of MAO-inhibitors and thus they find their potential utility in the treatment of depression.

N1-Thiocarbomoyl-3,5-Diaryl Pyrazolines

Bilgin *et al.,* carried out the antidepressant activity (Porsolt's behavioural despair test" on Swiss-Webster mice) of some *N*1-thiocarbamoyl-3,5-diphen-l-2-pyrazolines (**97**). They found that these derivatives were having activity equivalent to or higher than that of pargyline and tranylcypromine. Most of the active ligands were having the methoxy, methyl and chloro substitutent's at 4th positions of phenyl rings were shown the good antidepressant activity [73].

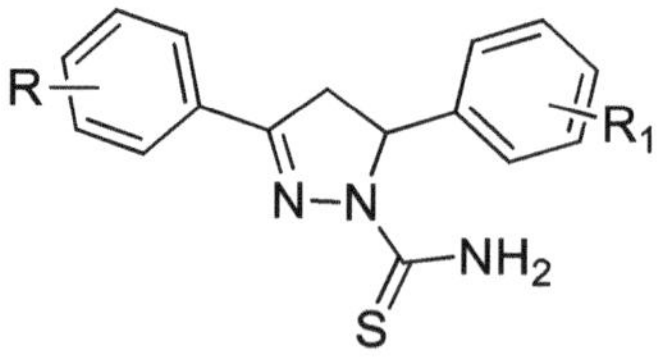

R R_1 N–N NH_2 S

97

3, 5-Diaryl, *N*1-Benzenesulfonyl Pyrazoline

Tripathi, *et al.,* reported a series of 3, 5-diaryl, with 4-nitrobenzenesulfonyl chloride, among all compounds with thiophene at ring B (**98**, Duration of immobility's (DOIs) in FST (s) (Mean ± SD): 51.00 ± 7.48, DOIs in TST (s) (Mean ± SD): 82.50 ± 13.16) exhibited highest antidepressant activity by Porsolt's behavioral despair or forced swim test (FST) and Tail suspension test (TST) in mice [74].

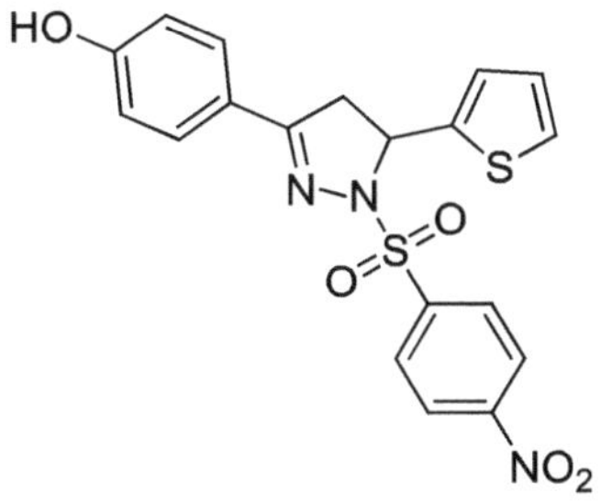

98 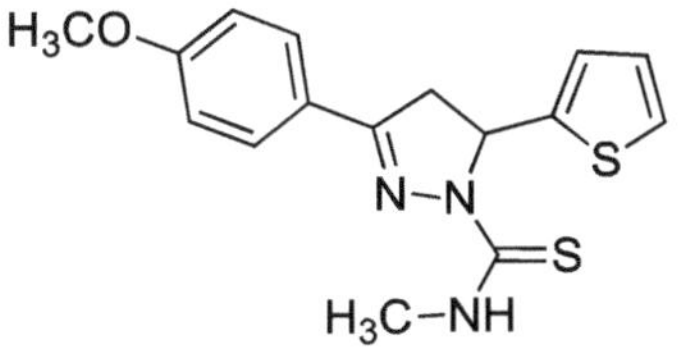 **99** 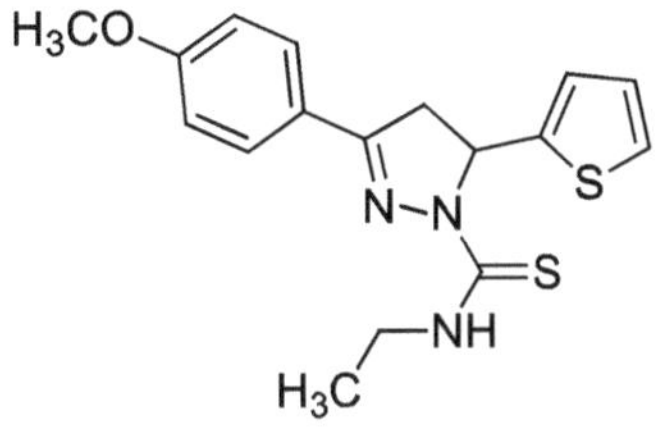 **100**

Gokhan, *et al.,* reported the antidepressant activity of a few *N*1-substituted thiocarbamoyl-3-phenyl-5-thienyl-2-pyrazolines (**99**, DOIs: Mean ± SEM =177.4 ± 12.38) and (**100**, DOIs: Mean ± SEM =175.4 ± 12.27) along with MAO inhibitory activity, but they were found to be less potent when compared with compounds having phenyl substitution at 5th position. The effects of the compounds on anxiety and depression were evaluated by using the Porsolt's forced swimming test and plus-maze respectively on Swiss-Webster mice [54].

Ozdemir, *et al.*, synthesized a few 3-(2-thienyl) pyrazoline derivatives and investigated for their antidepressant activities [Porsolt's behavioral despair test (forced swimming)] on albino mice. Among them compounds, *N*-methyl-3-5-di(thiophen-2-yl)-4,5-dihydro-1*H*-pyrazole-1-carbothioamide (**101**, DOIs=43± 15.3) and phenyl-3,5-di(thiophen-2-yl)-4,5-dihydro-1*H*-pyrazole-1-carbothio amide (**102**, DOIs= 48±18.9) showed significant antidepressant activity [75].

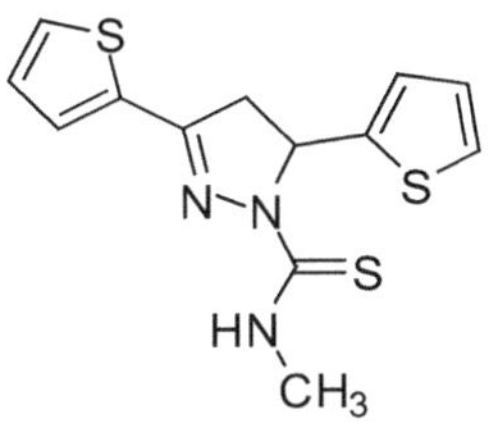

101 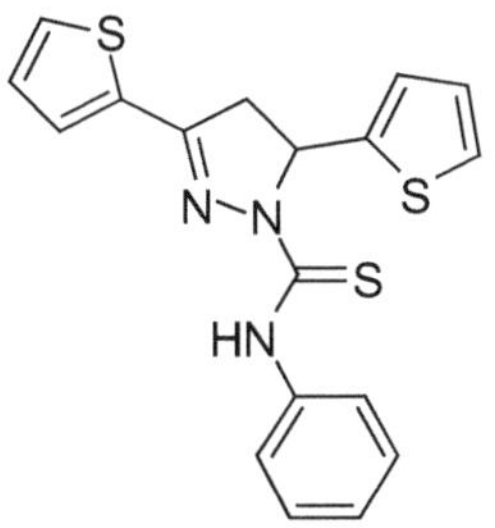 **102** 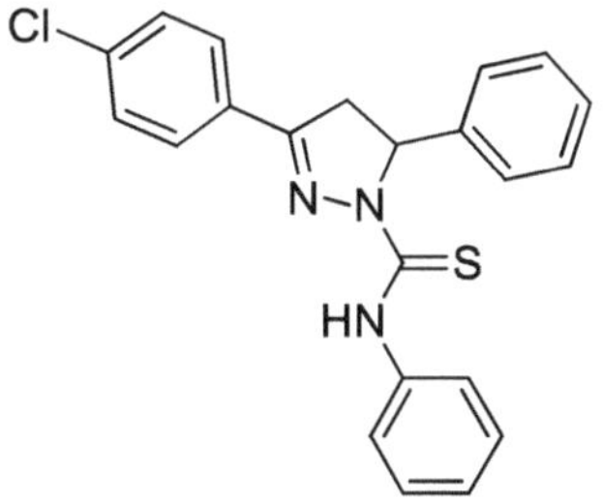 **103**

Siddique *et al.,* evaluated antidepressant activity of the 3,5-diaryl-4,5-dihy-ro-pyrazole-1-carbothioic acid phenylamides. Compound (**103**, DOIs: Mean ± SEM =113±19) was found to have significant antidepressant activity at 25mg/kg dose using Imipramine sulphate as standard drug [76].

1, 3, 5-Triaryl Pyrazolines

Bilgin *et al.,* investigated the antidepressant activity of 1,3,5-triphenyl-2-pyrazolines by Porsolt's behavioural despair Test" using Swiss-Webster mice. They found that bromide substitution on phenyl ring at 5th position enhanced the antidepressant activity [77].

Palaska *et al.,* screened a series of new 1,3,5-triaryl-2-pyrazoline derivatives for their antidepressant activities by the "porsolt's behavioral despair test" model using Swiss-Webster mice. It was found that 1-phenyl-3-(4 methylphenyl)-5-(3-4-dimethoxyphenyl)-2-pyrazoline (**104**, DOIs=2.08±3.6) and 1-phenyl-3-(4-methylphenyl)-5-(2-chloro-3,4-dimethoxyphenyl)-2-pyrazoline (**105**, DOIs= 24.5±4.3) were showed significant antidepressant activity. Methyl substitution on the phenyl ring at 3rd position enhances the antidepressant activity and replacement by halogens decreases the activity [78].

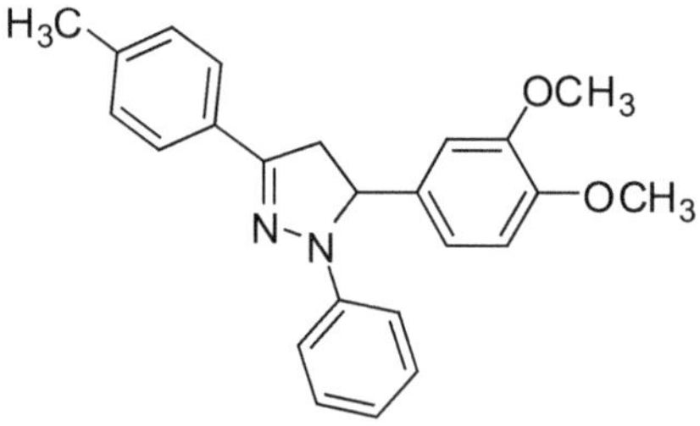

104 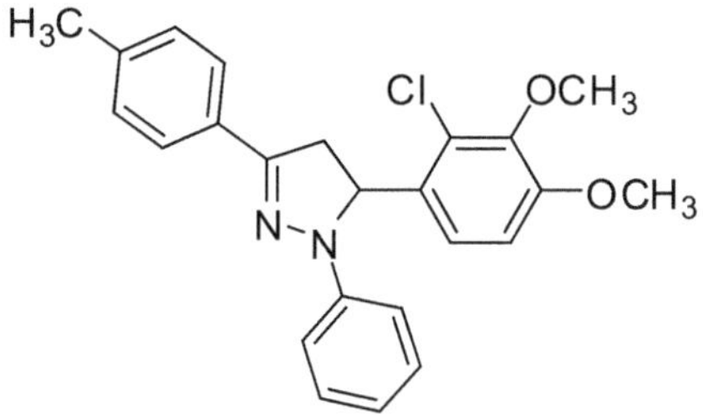 **105**

Prasad *et al.,* evaluated the antidepressant activity of 1,3,5-triaryl-2-pyrazolines by using "Porsolt's behavioral test" on Swiss-webster mice. They found that 4-(1,3-diphenyl-4,5-dihydro-1*H*-pyrazol-5-yl)-N,N-dimethylaniline (**106**, DOIs= 22.95±4.21) reduced the immobility times at a dose of 100 mg kg^{-1}. They also reported that the presence of electron releasing groups such as methoxy, dimethylamino and hydroxyl on either of phenyl ring on 3rd and 5th position is essential for enhancement of the antidepressant activity [79].

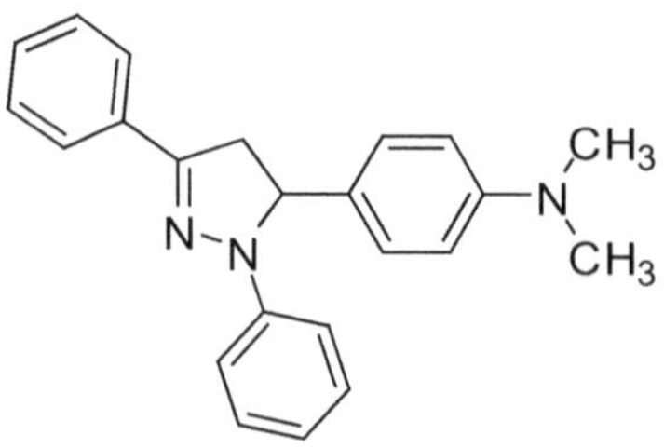

106 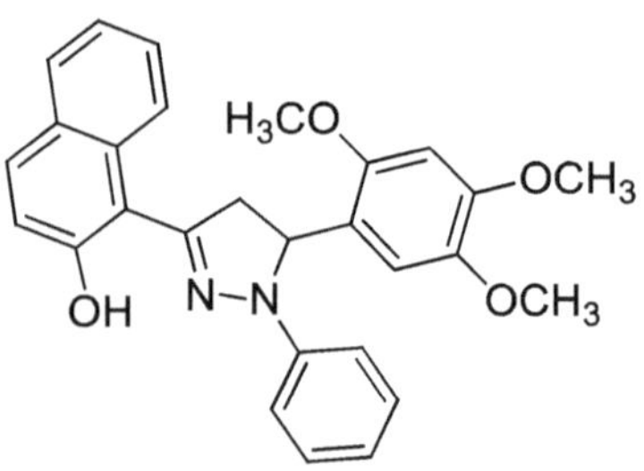 **107**

Prasad *et al.*, evaluated the antidepressant activity (Porsolt's behavioral test" on Swiss-webster mice) of 3-(3"-coumarinyl)-1,5-diphenyl-2-pyrazolines and 3-(2--hydroxy naphthalen-1"-yl)-1,5-diphenyl-2-pyrazolines. They observed that 2-pyrazolines derived from 3-acetyl coumarin showed greater potency when compared with the one's derived from 2-hydroxy-1-acetonaphthone (**107**, DOIs=22.80 ± 4.19). They also found that the substitution on rings at 3rd and 5th position with electron releasing groups enhanced the antidepressant activity [80].

Patil *et al.,* investigated the antidepressant activity of 1,3,5-triaryl-2-pyrazoline derivatives by using forced swim test on mice. They found that the 1,5-dipheny--3-(4-methoxyphenyl)-2-pyrazoline (**108**, DOIs=8 .0 ± 1.30) showed maximum antidepressant activity comparable with Imipramine, a standard drug used in the study. Electron releasing groups like methoxy functional group on phenyl ring at 3rd position was found to increase the antidepressant activity. Replacement of electron releasing group with electron withdrawing group found to decreases the activity [81].

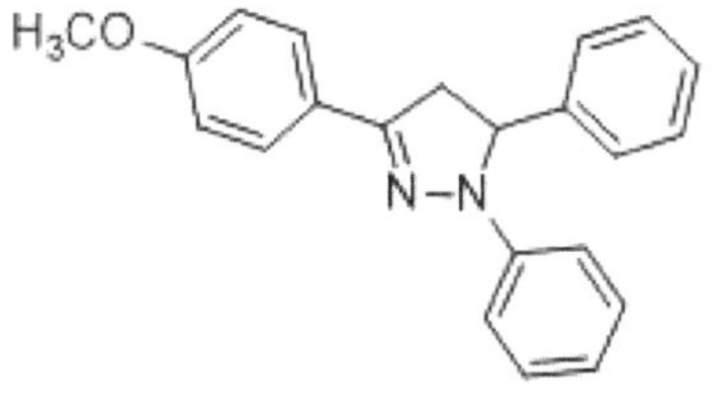

108 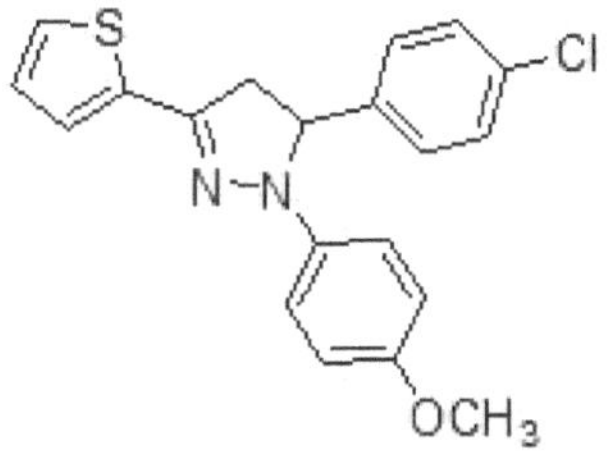 **109**

Das *et al.,* reported the antidepressant activity of *N*1-substituted/unsubstituted 5-(4-chlorophenyl)-3-(2-thienyl)pyrazolines by using Porsolt's behavioral despair (forced swimming) test in mice [82]. Compound **109** (DOIs: Mean ± SEM=71 ± 5.3) exhibited good activity profile against depression.

3, 5-Diaryl Pyrazolines

Palaska *et al.,* carried out the antidepressant activity of 3,5-diaryl-2-pyrazolines by the "Porsolt's behavioral despair test" on Swiss-Webster mice, and found that 3-(4-methoxyphenyl)-5-(2-chloro-3,4-dimethoxyphenyl)-2-pyrazoline (**110**, DOIs =24.5±5.4) and 3-(4-Methoxy phenyl)-5-(3,4-dimethoxyphenyl)-2-pyrazoline (**111**, DOIs= 25.2±5.8) reduced 41.94-48.62% immobility times at 100 mg kg^{-1} dose level. They also found that 4-chloro and 4-methoxy substituents on the Phenyl ring at 3rd position the pyrazoline ring increased the antidepressant activity, while replacement of these groups by -Br and $-CH_3$ substituents decreased activity [83].

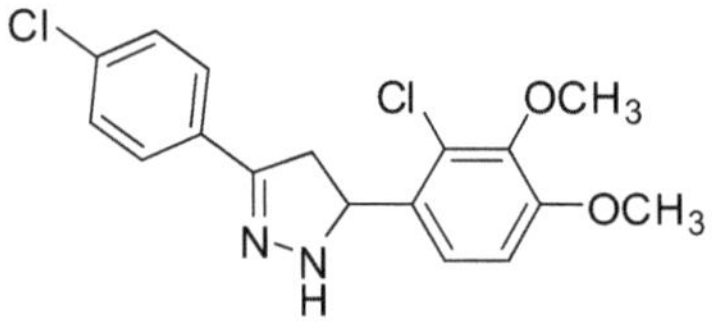

110 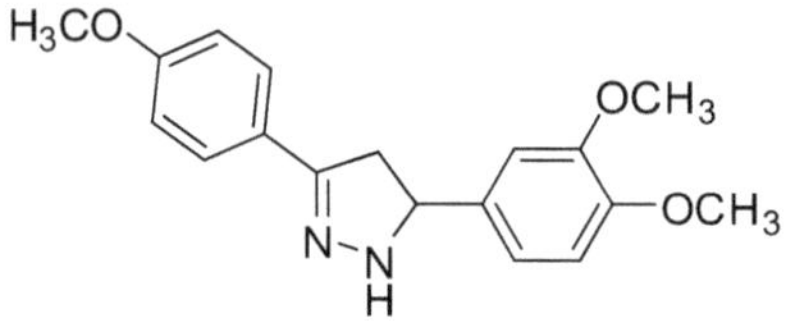 **111** 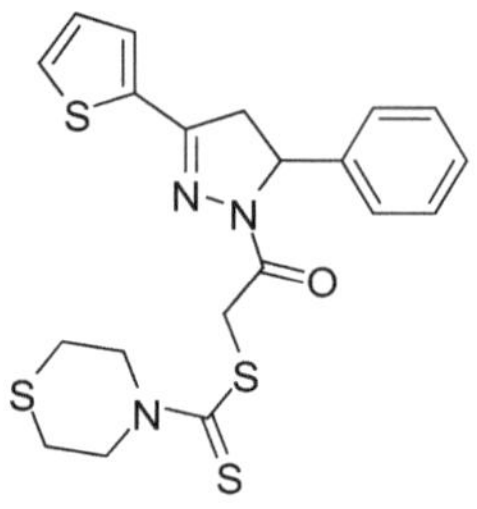 **112**

N1-Acyl-3, 5-Diaryl Pyrazolines

Gok *et al.,* investigated the antidepressant like activity of new 1-[(*N*,*N*-disubstituted thiocarbamoylthio)acetyl]- 3-(2-thienyl)-5-aryl-2-pyrazolines by using the forced-swim test on mice. 2-oxo-2-(5-phenyl-3-(thiophen-2-yl)-4, 5-dihydro-1*H*-pyrazol-1-yl)ethylthio morpholine-4-carbodithioate (**112**, DOIs: Mean ± SEM=84 ± 15) was found to be more effective than the standard drug clorpramine and tranylcypromine. They also concluded that the presence of dithiocarbamate moiety on pyrazoline is essential for the antidepressant activity [84].

CHIRAL SEPARATION AND COMPUTATIONAL STUDIES OF PYRAZOLINES

The 5th carbon of pyrazoline is chiral in nature and two isomers are possible (Fig. **3**). Very few researchers separated the individual enantiomers (R-and S-) by using various separation techniques to understand the effect of chirality that determines the potency and selectivity of the isomers (R- and S-) on MAO-inhibition. The computational studies of reported inhibitors were carried out by different groups (Table **3**), they were proposed that most of the ligand-receptor interactions were have the π-π stacking, hydrophobic, hydrogen bonding, *etc.*

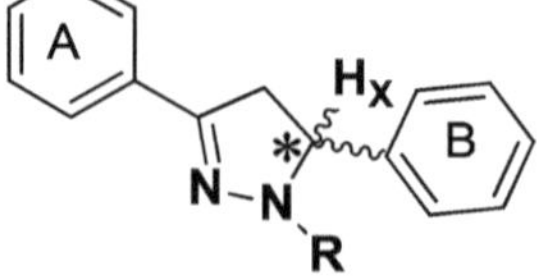

Fig. (3). General structure of pyrazoline ring with chiral proton (Hx) system at 5C carbon of pyrazoline.

Cirilli *et al.,* were the first to develop a semi preparative chiral chromatographic method for the separation of individual enantiomers (**113** and **114**). Chiracel OD column of semi preparative scale was used to achieve the separation of three compounds. X-ray crystal structure for one compound was solved to assign the configuration of chiral carbon of pure enantiomer [41]. The inhibitory activity of the (+)-(R)-enantiomer of was found to be 1.5–3.0 times more potent than (+)-(S- -form toward both MAO isoform.

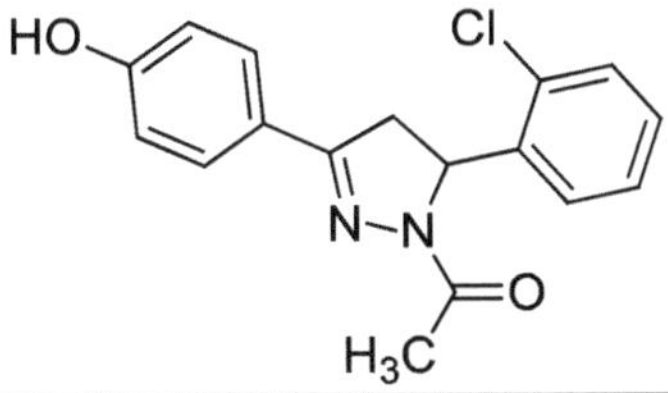

113	IC_{50} (Mean±SD)		SI[a]
	MAO-A	MAO-B	
Racemic (±)	$8.6x10^{-9} \pm 0.4$	$8.7x10^{-5} \pm 0.4$	10,116
(-)-(S)	$4.8x10^{-9} \pm 0.4$	$6.5x10^{-5} \pm 0.3$	13,542
(+)-(R)	$3.0x10^{-9} \pm 0.5$	$2.0x10^{-5} \pm 0.6$	6,666

Data represent mean values of at least of three separate experiments. [a]SI = IC_{50} (MAO-B)/IC_{50} (MAO-A).

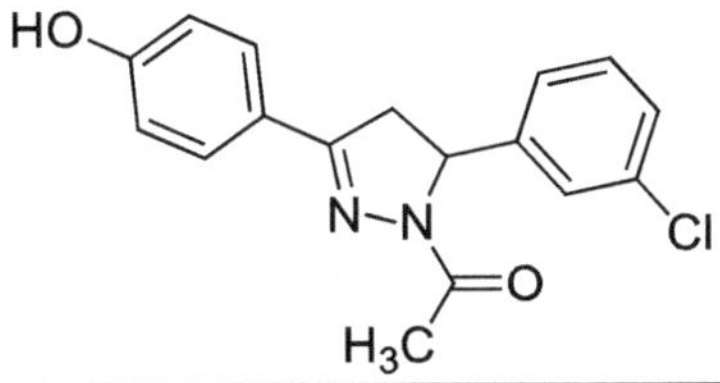

114	IC_{50} (Mean ± SD)		SI[a]
	MAO-A	MAO-B	
Racemic(±)	$1.0x10^{-8} \pm 0.3$	$2.3x10^{-5} \pm 0.2$	2,300
(-)-(S)	$6.0\ x10^{-9} \pm 0.8$	$2.2x10^{-5} \pm 0.8$	3,666
(+)-(R)	$3.0x10^{-9} \pm 0.2$	$1.0x10^{-5} \pm 0.4$	3,333

Data represent mean values of at least of three separate experiments. [a]SI= IC_{50} (MAO-B)/IC_{50} (MAO-A).

Chimenti *et al.,* selected two compounds (**115** and **116**) with best selectivity index amongst the twelve compounds and separated the enantiomers of both by using analytical and the semi preparative scale by enantioselective HPLC on a chiral

Chiralcel OD column packed with cellulose carbamate derivative/silica gel. The separated individual enantiomers were evaluated for their potency and selective inhibitory activity on MAO-isoforms [40]. All the compounds with (-)- were found to be potent, and selective towards MAO-A than (+)-enantiomer.

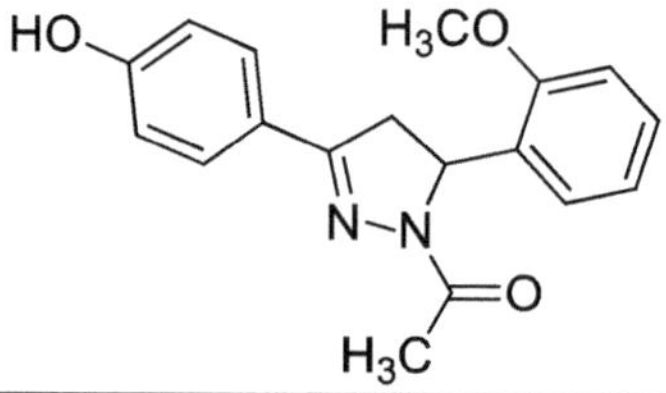

115	K_i MAO-A	K_i MAO-B	SI[b]
Racemic	$9.0x10^{-9}$± 0.010	$7.6x10^{-4}$± 0.02	84444
(-)-(S)	$2.0x10^{-9}$± 0.015	$3.3x10^{-4}$± 0.05	165000
(+)-(R)	$6.0x10^{-9}$± 0.020	$1.0x10^{-3}$± 0.03	166666

[a]Data represent mean values of at least of three separate experiments. [b]SI= IC_{50} ± MAO-B)/IC_{50} ± MAO-A).

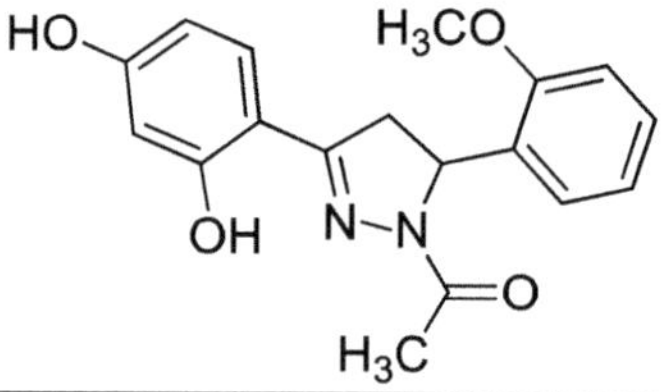

116	K_iMAO-A	K_i MAO-B	SI[b]
Racemic (±)	$8.0x10^{-9}$± 0.050	$6.0x10^{-4}$± 0.04	75000
(-)-(S)	$4.0x10^{-9}$± 0.016	$3.2x10^{-4}$± 0.04	80000
(+)-(R)	$7.0x10^{-9}$± 0.020	$2.7x10^{-4}$± 0.07	38571

[a]Data represent mean values of at least of three separate experiments. [b]SI= IC_{50} ± MAO-B)/IC_{50} ± MAO-A).

Chimenti *et al.,* synthesized a series of 1-thiocarbamoyl-3, 5-diaryl-4, 5-dihydr--(1*H*)-pyrazole derivatives and investigated for their MAO-isoform inhibitory activity. Then they separated the potent compounds (**117** and **118**) on analytical and semi preparative scale by enantioselective HPLC on an amylose phenylcarbamate based chiral stationary phase (CSP) [51]. Reported the selectivity of the (-)- (*S*)-**1** enantiomer were found to be more potent than (-)-(*S*)-**4** enantiomer against both MAO-isoforms

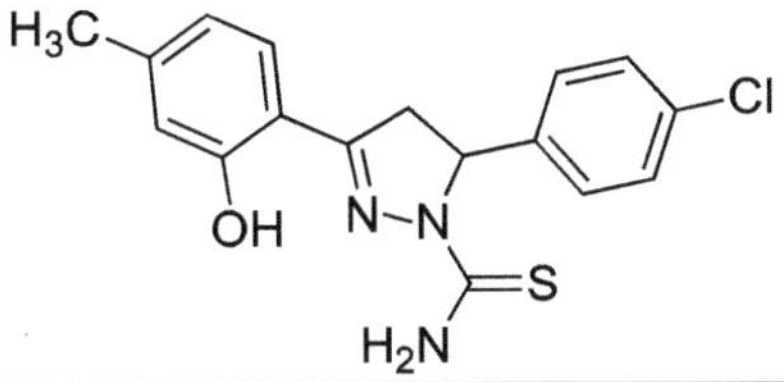

117	K_i M (±SD)		[b]SIB/A	[c]SIA/B
	MAO-A	MAO-B		
Racemic(±)	$3.1x10^{-8}$± 0.05	$1.5x10^{-9}$± 0.02	0.05	20.70
(-)-(S)	$5.0x10^{-8}$± 0.02	$1.0x10^{-9}$± 0.01	0.02	50.00
(+)-(R)	$1.3x10^{-8}$± 0.04	$2.7x10^{-9}$± 0.07	0.20	4.80

[a]Data represent mean values of at least of three separate experiments. [b]SI= K_i(MAO-B)/K_i(MAO-A). [c]SI= K_i(MAO-A)/K_i(MAO-B)

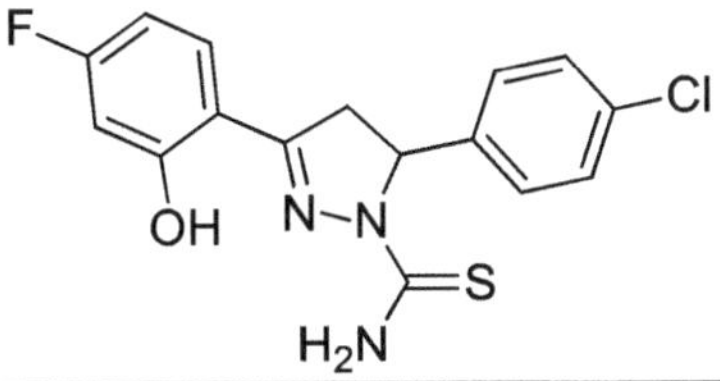

118	K_i M (±SD)		[b]SIB/A	[c]SIA/B
	MAO-A	MAO-B		
Racemic(±)	$6.0x10^{-9}$± 0.03	$1.0x10^{-6}$± 0.04	166.00	0.006
(-)-(S)	$5.0x10^{-9}$± 0.04	$2.4x10^{-6}$± 0.04	480.00	0.002
(+)-(R)	$1.2x10^{-8}$± 0.02	$1.4x10^{-6}$± 0.05	116.00	0.008

[a]Data represent mean values of at least of three separate experiments. [b]SI= K_i(MAO-B)/K_i(MAO-A). [c]SI= K_i(MAO-A)/K_i(MAO-B)

Molecular docking studies has been widely employed to understand the interaction of inhibitors with the MAO-isoforms at molecular level. Few groups also performed molecular dynamics studies to get much better picture on molecular level interaction (Table **3**). Summarizes the experimental model of proteins (PDB) used and software tools employed to carry out the simulation studies.

Table 3. Computational studies available on pyrazolines as MAO inhibitors.

PDB Used		Software Used	Reference
MAO-A (PDB ID)	MAO-B (PDB ID)		
-	IGOS	Glide, MOLLINE	Manna *et al.*, [39]
105W	IGOS	Macromodel v7.2, Glide and Schrodinger LLC	Chimenti *et al.*, [51]
2BXR	IGOS	Macromodel v7.2 Maestro, MOLLINE	Chimenti *et al.*, [42]
2BXR	IGOS	Maestro-Glide	Chimenti *et al.*, [37]
2BXR	2BYB	AutoDock-4.0	Jayaprakash *et al.*, [56]
2BXR	IGOS	Macromodel v7.2, MOLLINE	Chimenti *et al.*, [45]
2BXS	1S3E	AutoDock-4.01	Goekhan *et al.*, [63]
2Z5X	2V60	Maestro GUI, AutoDock Vina	Fioravanti *et al.*, [43]
2Z5X	2BK3	AutoDock Vina	Maccioni *et al.*, [58]
2BXR	2BYB	AutoDock-4.0	Karuppasamy *et al.*, [57]
2BXR	2BYB	AutoDock-4.0	Sahoo *et al.*, [48]
2BXR	2BYB	AutoDock-4.0	Jagrat *et al.*, [59]
2BXR	2BYB	AutoDock-4.0	Mishra, *et al.*, [65]
2BXR	-	Schrodinger-Maestro	Das *et al.*, [82]
2Z5X	2BK3	Molecular Operating Environment	Senturk *et al.*, [60]
2BXR	2BYB	AutoDock-4.2	Nayak, *et al.*, [67, 69, 70, 85]
2Z5X	-	AutoDock-4.2, GPU Molecular dynamics (version of Amber 14)	C. Nath, *et al.*, [70]
2Z5X	2V5Z	AutoDock 4.2.6	Goksen, *et al.*, [71]
2Z5X	-	Schrödinger, LLC(Version 6.5)	Tripathi, *et al.*, [74]
2Z5X	4A79	AutoDock 4.2	Guglielmi, *et al.*, [44]

SUMMARY AND CONCLUSION

In this chapter we reviewed the MAO-inhibitory activity and antidepressant activity of 4, 5-dihydro-1*H*-pyrazole. Pyrazolines are also having the proficiency of binding to MAO enzyme and its isoforms reversibly. Both substitution and stereochemistry plays a crucial role in determining the potency and selectivity of the compounds towards MAO isoforms. Smaller biaryl substituted pyrazolines were found to inhibit MAO-B selectively, while bulkier triaryl substituted derivatives inhibit MAO-A selectively. Studies with single enantiomer of 1*N*-acetyl and 1*N*-thiocarbomoyl derivatives, invariably proven that *S*-isomer has improved potency and best selectivity towards MAO-A isoform. While similar studies are not available for all the compounds, simulation studies were reported by few researchers. In most of them *S*-isomer seems to show better affinity towards MAO-A isoform in comparison with its *R*-counterpart. As literature on pyrazoline derivatives is growing and X-ray crystal structure of human MAO isoforms in complex with inhibitors is also available, medicinal chemists of these days are well equipped to design newer derivatives. With modern tools, one can expect that the optimized candidates with pyrazoline scaffold may enter in to clinical studies in coming days.

CONSENT FOR PUBLICATION

Not applicable.

CONFLICT OF INTEREST

The authors declare no conflict of interest, financial or otherwise.

ACKNOWLEDGEMENTS

Author was thankful to Department of Pharmaceutical Sciences and Technology, Birla Institute of Technology for providing financial support as a prestigious Institute Fellowship.

REFERENCES

[1] Thase ME, Trivedi MH, Rush AJ. MAOIs in the contemporary treatment of depression. Neuropsychopharmacology 1995; 12(3): 185-219. [http://dx.doi.org/10.1016/0893-133X(94)00058-8] [PMID: 7612154]

[2] Bortolato M, Chen K, Shih JC. Monoamine oxidase inactivation: from pathophysiology to therapeutics. Adv Drug Deliv Rev 2008; 60(13-14): 1527-33. [http://dx.doi.org/10.1016/j.addr.2008.06.002] [PMID: 18652859]

[3] Anderson MC, Hasan F, McCrodden JM, Tipton KF. Monoamine oxidase inhibitors and the cheese effect. Neurochem Res 1993; 18(11): 1145-9. [http://dx.doi.org/10.1007/BF00978365] [PMID: 8255365]

[4] Youdim MBH, Weinstock M. Therapeutic applications of selective and non-selective inhibitors of monoamine oxidase A and B that do not cause significant tyramine potentiation. Neurotoxicology 2004; 25(1-2): 243-50. [http://dx.doi.org/10.1016/S0161-813X(03)00103-7] [PMID: 14697899]

[5] Dowson JH. MAO Inhibitors in Mental Disease: Their Current Status BT - Monoamine Oxidase Enzymes: Review and Overview. Vienna: Springer Vienna 1987; pp. 121-38.

[6] Ebadi M, Brown-Borg H, Ren J, Sharma S, Shavali S. Therapeutic efficacy of selegiline in neurodegenerative disorders and neurological diseases. Curr Drug Targets 1513-29.

[7] Youdim MBH, Bar Am O, Yogev-Falach M, *et al.* Rasagiline: neurodegeneration, neuroprotection, and mitochondrial permeability transition. J Neurosci Res 2005; 79(1-2): 172-9. [http://dx.doi.org/10.1002/jnr.20350] [PMID: 15573406]

[8] Collins GGS, Sandler M, Williams ED, Youdim MBH. Multiple forms of human brain mitochondrial monoamine oxidase. Nature 1970; 225(5235): 817-20.

[http://dx.doi.org/10.1038/225817a0] [PMID: 5415111]

[9] Tipton KF, Boyce S, O'Sullivan J, Davey GP, Healy J. Monoamine oxidases: certainties and uncertainties. Curr Med Chem 2004; 11(15): 1965-82.
[http://dx.doi.org/10.2174/0929867043364810] [PMID: 15279561]

[10] Slotkin TA. Mary Bernheim and the discovery of monoamine oxidase. Brain Res Bull 1999; 50(5-6): 373.
[http://dx.doi.org/10.1016/S0361-9230(99)00110-0] [PMID: 10643441]

[11] Bach AW, Lan NC, Johnson DL, *et al.* cDNA cloning of human liver monoamine oxidase A and B: molecular basis of differences in enzymatic properties. Proc Natl Acad Sci USA 1988; 85(13): 4934-8.
[http://dx.doi.org/10.1073/pnas.85.13.4934] [PMID: 3387449]

[12] Youdim MBH, Collins GGS, Sandler M, Bevan Jones AB, Pare CMB, Nicholson WJ. Human brain monoamine oxidase: multiple forms and selective inhibitors. Nature 1972; 236(5344): 225-8.
[http://dx.doi.org/10.1038/236225b0] [PMID: 4553640]

[13] Thorpe LW, Westlund KN, Kochersperger LM, Abell CW, Denney RM. Immunocytochemical localization of monoamine oxidases A and B in human peripheral tissues and brain. J Histochem Cytochem 1987; 35(1): 23-32.
[http://dx.doi.org/10.1177/35.1.3025289] [PMID: 3025289]

[14] Muller CP, Jacobs B. Handbook of the Behavioral Neurobiology of Serotonin. Academic Press 2009; 21.

[15] Yanez M, Fernando Padin J, Alberto Arranz-Tagarro J, Camina M, Laguna R. history and therapeutic use of mao-a inhibitors: a historical perspective of mao-a inhibitors as antidepressant drug. Curr. Top Med. Chem.2012; 12(20): 2275-82.

[16] Foye WO, Lemke TL, Williams DA. Foye's Principles of Medicinal Chemistry. Lippincott Williams & Wilkins 2008.

[17] Lavian G, Finberg JP, Youdim MB. The advent of a new generation of monoamine oxidase inhibitor antidepressants: pharmacologic studies with moclobemide and brofaromine. Clin Neuropharmacol 1993; 16 (Suppl. 2): S1-7.
[PMID: 8313392]

[18] Da Prada M, Keller HH, Kettler R. Comparison of the new MAO-A inhibitors moclobemide, brofaromine and toloxatone with tranylcypromine in an animal experiment: significance for clinical practice. Psychiatr Prax 1989; 16 (Suppl. 1): 18-24.
[PMID: 2587673]

[19] Youdim MBH, Bakhle YS. Monoamine oxidase: isoforms and inhibitors in Parkinson's disease and depressive illness. Br J Pharmacol 2006; 147(S1) (Suppl. 1): S287-96.
[http://dx.doi.org/10.1038/sj.bjp.0706464] [PMID: 16402116]

[20] Mayersohn M, Guentert TW. Clinical pharmacokinetics of the monoamine oxidase-A inhibitor moclobemide. Clin Pharmacokinet 1995; 29(5): 292-332.
[http://dx.doi.org/10.2165/00003088-199529050-00002] [PMID: 8582117]

[21] Raaflaub J, Haefelfinger P, Trautmann KH. Single-dose pharmacokinetics of the MAO-inhibitor moclobemide in man. Arzneimittelforschung 1984; 34(1): 80-2.
[PMID: 6538424]

[22] Nair NPV, Ahmed SK, Kin NM. Biochemistry and pharmacology of reversible inhibitors of MAO-A agents: focus on moclobemide. J Psychiatry Neurosci 1993; 18(5): 214-25.
[PMID: 7905288]

[23] Barrett JS, Szego P, Rohatagi S, *et al.* Absorption and presystemic metabolism of selegiline hydrochloride at different regions in the gastrointestinal tract in healthy males. Pharm Res 1996; 13(10): 1535-40.
[http://dx.doi.org/10.1023/A:1016035730754] [PMID: 8899847]

[24] Laine K, Anttila M, Helminen A, Karnani H, Huupponen R. Dose linearity study of selegiline pharmacokinetics after oral administration: evidence for strong drug interaction with female sex steroids. Br J Clin Pharmacol 1999; 47(3): 249-54. [http://dx.doi.org/10.1046/j.1365-2125.1999.00891.x] [PMID: 10215747]

[25] Khalil NA, Ahmed EM, El-Nassan HB, Ahmed OK, Al-Abd AM. Synthesis and biological evaluation of novel pyrazoline derivatives as anti-inflammatory and antioxidant agents. Arch Pharm Res 2012; 35(6): 995-1002. [http://dx.doi.org/10.1007/s12272-012-0606-9] [PMID: 22870808]

[26] Azarifar D, Shaebanzadeh M. Synthesis and characterization of new 3, 5-dinaphthyl substituted 2-pyrazolines and study of their antimicrobial activity. Molecules 2002; 7(12): 885-95. [http://dx.doi.org/10.3390/71200885]

[27] Ali MA, Yar MS, Kumar M, Pandian GS. Synthesis and antitubercular activity of substituted novel pyrazoline derivatives. Nat Prod Res 2007; 21(7): 575-9. [http://dx.doi.org/10.1080/14786410701369367] [PMID: 17613813]

[28] Puig-Basagoiti F, Tilgner M, Forshey BM, *et al.* Triaryl pyrazoline compound inhibits flavivirus RNA replication. Antimicrob Agents Chemother 2006; 50(4): 1320-9. [http://dx.doi.org/10.1128/AAC.50.4.1320-1329.2006] [PMID: 16569847]

[29] Kawazura H, Takahashi Y, Shiga Y, Shimada F, Ohto N, Tamura A. Cerebroprotective effects of a novel pyrazoline derivative, MS-153, on focal ischemia in rats. Jpn J Pharmacol 1997; 73(4): 317-24. [http://dx.doi.org/10.1254/jjp.73.317] [PMID: 9165368]

[30] Amir M, Kumar H, Khan SA. Synthesis and pharmacological evaluation of pyrazoline derivatives as new anti-inflammatory and analgesic agents 2008; 18: 918-22.

[31] Havrylyuk D, Zimenkovsky B, Vasylenko O, Zaprutko L, Gzella A, Lesyk R. Synthesis of novel thiazolone-based compounds containing pyrazoline moiety and evaluation of their anticancer activity. Eur J Med Chem 2009; 44(4): 1396-404. [http://dx.doi.org/10.1016/j.ejmech.2008.09.032] [PMID: 19000643]

[32] Ozdemir Z, Kandilci HB, Gümüşel B, Caliş U, Bilgin AA. Synthesis and studies on antidepressant and anticonvulsant activities of some 3-(2-furyl)-pyrazoline derivatives. Eur J Med Chem 2007; 42(3): 373-9. [http://dx.doi.org/10.1016/j.ejmech.2006.09.006] [PMID: 17069933]

[33] Secci D, Bolasco A, Chimenti P, Carradori S. The state of the art of pyrazole derivatives as monoamine oxidase inhibitors and antidepressant/anticonvulsant agents. Curr Med Chem 2011; 18(33): 5114-44. [http://dx.doi.org/10.2174/092986711797636090] [PMID: 22050759]

[34] Marella A, Ali MR, Alam MT, *et al.* Pyrazolines: a biological review. Mini Rev Med Chem 2013; 13(6): 921-31. [http://dx.doi.org/10.2174/1389557511313060012] [PMID: 23544604]

[35] Parmar SS, Pandey BR, Dwivedi C, Harbison RD. Anticonvulsant activity and monoamine oxidase inhibitory properties of 1,3,5-trisubstituted pyrazolines. J Pharm Sci 1974; 63(7): 1152-5. [http://dx.doi.org/10.1002/jps.2600630730] [PMID: 4850598]

[36] Manna F, Chimenti F, Bolasco A, *et al.* Inhibitory effect of 1,3,5-triphenyl-4,5-dihydro-(1H)-pyrazole derivatives on activity of amine oxidases. J Enzyme Inhib 1998; 13(3): 207-16. [http://dx.doi.org/10.3109/14756369809028341] [PMID: 9629538]

[37] Chimenti F, Bolasco A, Manna F, *et al.* Synthesis, biological evaluation and 3D-QSAR of 1,3,5-trisubstituted-4,5-dihydro-(1H)-pyrazole derivatives as potent and highly selective monoamine oxidase A inhibitors. Curr Med Chem 2006; 13(12): 1411-28. [http://dx.doi.org/10.2174/092986706776872907] [PMID: 16719786]

[38] Manna F, Chimenti F, Bolasco A, *et al.* Selective inhibition of FAD and copper-dependent amine

oxidases by N-acetyl pyrazole derivatives. Inflamm Res 2001; 50(2) (Suppl. 2): S128-9. [PMID: 11411587]

[39] Manna F, Chimenti F, Bolasco A, *et al.* Inhibition of amine oxidases activity by 1-acetyl-3,5-diphe-yl-4,5-dihydro-(1H)-pyrazole derivatives. Bioorg Med Chem Lett 2002; 12(24): 3629-33. [http://dx.doi.org/10.1016/S0960-894X(02)00699-6] [PMID: 12443791]

[40] Chimenti F, Bolasco A, Manna F, *et al.* Synthesis and selective inhibitory activity of 1-acetyl-3, 5-diphenyl-4, 5-dihydro-(1 h)-pyrazole derivatives against monoamine oxidase. 2004; 20071-74.

[41] Cirilli R, Ferretti R, Gallinella B, *et al.* Enantiomers of C(5)-chiral 1-acetyl-3,5-diphenyl-4,5-di-ydro-(1H)-pyrazole derivatives: Analytical and semipreparative HPLC separation, chiroptical properties, absolute configuration, and inhibitory activity against monoamine oxidase. Chirality 2004; 16(9): 625-36. [http://dx.doi.org/10.1002/chir.20085] [PMID: 15382204]

[42] Chimenti F, Bolasco A, Manna F, *et al.* Synthesis and molecular modelling of novel substituted-4,--dihydro-(1H)-pyrazole derivatives as potent and highly selective monoamine oxidase-A inhibitors. Chem Biol Drug Des 2006; 67(3): 206-14. [http://dx.doi.org/10.1111/j.1747-0285.2006.00367.x] [PMID: 16611214]

[43] Fioravanti R, Bolasco A, Manna F, *et al.* Synthesis and molecular modelling studies of prenylated pyrazolines as MAO-B inhibitors. Bioorg Med Chem Lett 2010; 20(22): 6479-82. [http://dx.doi.org/10.1016/j.bmcl.2010.09.061] [PMID: 20934874]

[44] Guglielmi P, Carradori S, Poli G, *et al.* Design, synthesis, docking studies and monoamine oxidase inhibition of a small library of 1-acetyl- and 1-thiocarbamoyl-3,5-diphenyl-4,5-dihydr--(1H)-pyrazoles. Molecules 2019; 24(3): 484. [http://dx.doi.org/10.3390/molecules24030484] [PMID: 30700029]

[45] Chimenti F, Fioravanti R, Bolasco A, *et al.* Synthesis, molecular modeling studies and selective inhibitory activity against MAO of N1-propanoyl-3,5-diphenyl-4,5-dihydro-(1H)-pyrazole derivatives. Eur J Med Chem 2008; 43(10): 2262-7. [http://dx.doi.org/10.1016/j.ejmech.2007.12.026] [PMID: 18281126]

[46] Salgin-Gökşen U, Yabanoğlu-Çiftçi S, Ercan A, Yelekçi K, Uçar G, Gökhan-Kelekçi N. Evaluation of selective human MAO inhibitory activities of some novel pyrazoline derivatives. J Neural Transm (Vienna) 2013; 120(6): 863-73. [http://dx.doi.org/10.1007/s00702-013-0980-6] [PMID: 23361656]

[47] Tong X, Chen R, Zhang T-T, Han Y, Tang W-J, Liu X-H. Design and synthesis of novel 2-pyrazolin--1-ethanone derivatives as selective MAO inhibitors. Bioorg Med Chem 2015; 23(3): 515-25. [http://dx.doi.org/10.1016/j.bmc.2014.12.010] [PMID: 25541201]

[48] Sahoo A, Yabanoglu S, Sinha BN, Ucar G, Basu A, Jayaprakash V. Towards development of selective and reversible pyrazoline based MAO-inhibitors: Synthesis, biological evaluation and docking studies. Bioorg Med Chem Lett 2010; 20(1): 132-6. [http://dx.doi.org/10.1016/j.bmcl.2009.11.015] [PMID: 19945874]

[49] Evranos-Aksöz B, Yabanoğlu-Çiftçi S, Uçar G, Yelekçi K, Ertan R. Synthesis of some novel hydrazone and 2-pyrazoline derivatives: monoamine oxidase inhibitory activities and docking studies. Bioorg Med Chem Lett 2014; 24(15): 3278-84. [http://dx.doi.org/10.1016/j.bmcl.2014.06.015] [PMID: 24986657]

[50] Evranos-Aksöz B, Baysal İ, Yabanoğlu-Çiftçi S, *et al.* Synthesis and screening of human monoamine oxidase-a inhibitor effect of new 2-pyrazoline and hydrazone derivatives. Arch Pharm (Weinheim) 2015; 348(10): 743-56. [http://dx.doi.org/10.1002/ardp.201500212] [PMID: 26293971]

[51] Chimenti F, Maccioni E, Secci D, *et al.* Synthesis, molecular modeling studies, and selective inhibitory activity against monoamine oxidase of 1-thiocarbamoyl-3,5-diaryl-4,5-dihydro-(1H)-pyrazole derivatives. J Med Chem 2005; 48(23): 7113-22.

[http://dx.doi.org/10.1021/jm040903t] [PMID: 16279769]

[52] Palaska E, Aydin F, Uçar G, Erol D. Synthesis and monoamine oxidase inhibitory activities of 1-thiocarbamoyl-3,5-diphenyl-4,5-dihydro-1H-pyrazole derivatives. Arch Pharm (Weinheim) 2008; 341(4): 209-15.
[http://dx.doi.org/10.1002/ardp.200700159] [PMID: 18266289]

[53] Chimenti F, Carradori S, Secci D, *et al.* Synthesis and inhibitory activity against human monoamine oxidase of N1-thiocarbamoyl-3,5-di(hetero)aryl-4,5-dihydro-(1H)-pyrazole derivatives. Eur J Med Chem 2010; 45(2): 800-4.
[http://dx.doi.org/10.1016/j.ejmech.2009.11.003] [PMID: 19926363]

[54] Gökhan N, Yeşilada A, Uçar G, Erol K, Bilgin AA. 1-N-substituted thiocarbamoyl-3-pheny--5-thienyl-2-pyrazolines: synthesis and evaluation as MAO inhibitors. Arch Pharm (Weinheim) 2003; 336(8): 362-71.
[http://dx.doi.org/10.1002/ardp.200300732] [PMID: 14502756]

[55] Ucar G, Gokhan N, Yesilada A, Yabanoglu S, Bilgin AA. Interaction of Some 1-N-Substituted Thiocarbamoyl-3-Phenyl-5-Thienyl-2-Pyrazolines with Rat Liver Semicarbazide-Sensitive Amine Oxidase (SSAO). Hacettepe Univ J Fac Pharm 2005; 25(1): 23-4.

[56] Jayaprakash V, Sinha BN, Ucar G, Ercan A. Pyrazoline-based mycobactin analogues as MAO-inhibitors. Bioorg Med Chem Lett 2008; 18(24): 6362-8.
[http://dx.doi.org/10.1016/j.bmcl.2008.10.084] [PMID: 18980841]

[57] Karuppasamy M, Mahapatra M, Yabanoglu S, *et al.* Development of selective and reversible pyrazoline based MAO-A inhibitors: Synthesis, biological evaluation and docking studies. Bioorg Med Chem 2010; 18(5): 1875-81.
[http://dx.doi.org/10.1016/j.bmc.2010.01.043] [PMID: 20149663]

[58] Maccioni E, Alcaro S, Orallo F, *et al.* Synthesis of new 3-aryl-4,5-dihydropyrazole-1-carbothioamide derivatives. An investigation on their ability to inhibit monoamine oxidase. Eur J Med Chem 2010; 45(10): 4490-8.
[http://dx.doi.org/10.1016/j.ejmech.2010.07.009] [PMID: 20702005]

[59] Jagrat M, Behera J, Yabanoglu S, *et al.* Pyrazoline based MAO inhibitors: synthesis, biological evaluation and SAR studies. Bioorg Med Chem Lett 2011; 21(14): 4296-300.
[http://dx.doi.org/10.1016/j.bmcl.2011.05.057] [PMID: 21680183]

[60] Sentürk K, Tan OU, Ciftçi SY, Uçar G, Palaska E. Synthesis and evaluation of human monoamine oxidase inhibitory activities of some 3,5-diaryl-N-substituted-4,5-dihydro-1H-pyrazole-1-carbothioamide derivatives. Arch Pharm (Weinheim) 2012; 345(9): 695-702.
[http://dx.doi.org/10.1002/ardp.201100448] [PMID: 22674756]

[61] Yabanoglu S, Ucar G, Gokhan N, Salgin U, Yesilada A, Bilgin AA. Interaction of rat lung SSAO with the novel 1-N-substituted thiocarbamoyl-3-substituted phenyl-5-(2-pyrolyl)-2-pyrazoline derivatives. J Neural Transm (Vienna) 2007; 114(6): 769-73.
[http://dx.doi.org/10.1007/s00702-007-0686-8] [PMID: 17385065]

[62] Gökhan-Kelekçi N, Yabanoğlu S, Küpeli E, *et al.* A new therapeutic approach in Alzheimer disease: some novel pyrazole derivatives as dual MAO-B inhibitors and antiinflammatory analgesics. Bioorg Med Chem 2007; 15(17): 5775-86.
[http://dx.doi.org/10.1016/j.bmc.2007.06.004] [PMID: 17611112]

[63] Gökhan-Kelekçi N, Koyunoğlu S, Yabanoğlu S, *et al.* New pyrazoline bearing 4(3H)-quinazolinone inhibitors of monoamine oxidase: synthesis, biological evaluation, and structural determinants of MAO-A and MAO-B selectivity. Bioorg Med Chem 2009; 17(2): 675-89.
[http://dx.doi.org/10.1016/j.bmc.2008.11.068] [PMID: 19091581]

[64] Gökhan-Kelekçi N, Simşek OO, Ercan A, *et al.* Synthesis and molecular modeling of some novel hexahydroindazole derivatives as potent monoamine oxidase inhibitors. Bioorg Med Chem 2009; 17(18): 6761-72.

[http://dx.doi.org/10.1016/j.bmc.2009.07.033] [PMID: 19682910]

[65] Mishra N, Sasmal D. Development of selective and reversible pyrazoline based MAO-B inhibitors: virtual screening, synthesis and biological evaluation. Bioorg Med Chem Lett 2011; 21(7): 1969-73. [http://dx.doi.org/10.1016/j.bmcl.2011.02.030] [PMID: 21377879]

[66] Fioravanti R, Desideri N, Biava M, Proietti Monaco L, Grammatica L, Yáñez M. Design, synthesis, and *in vitro* hMAO-B inhibitory evaluation of some 1-methyl-3,5-diphenyl-4,5-dihydro-1H-pyrazoles. Bioorg Med Chem Lett 2013; 23(18): 5128-30. [http://dx.doi.org/10.1016/j.bmcl.2013.07.035] [PMID: 23927971]

[67] Vishnu Nayak B, Ciftci-Yabanoglu S, Jadav SS, *et al.* Monoamine oxidase inhibitory activity of 3,5-biaryl-4,5-dihydro-1H-pyrazole-1-carboxylate derivatives. Eur J Med Chem 2013; 69: 762-7. [http://dx.doi.org/10.1016/j.ejmech.2013.09.010] [PMID: 24099995]

[68] Badavath VN, Baysal İ, Ucar G, Sinha BN, Jayaprakash V. Monoamine oxidase inhibitory activity of novel pyrazoline analogues: curcumin based design and synthesis. ACS Med Chem Lett 2015; 7(1): 56-61. [http://dx.doi.org/10.1021/acsmedchemlett.5b00326] [PMID: 26819666]

[69] Badavath VN, Ucar G, Sinha BN, Mondal SK, Jayaprakash V. Monoamine oxidase inhibitory activity of novel pyrazoline analogues: curcumin based design and synthesis-II. ChemistrySelect 2016; 1(18): 5879-84. [http://dx.doi.org/10.1002/slct.201600914]

[70] Nath C, Badavath VN, Thakur A, *et al.* Curcumin-based pyrazoline analogues as selective inhibitors of human monoamine oxidase A. MedChemComm 2018; 9(7): 1164-71. [http://dx.doi.org/10.1039/C8MD00196K] [PMID: 30109004]

[71] Goksen US, Sarigul S, Bultinck P, *et al.* Absolute configuration and biological profile of pyrazoline enantiomers as MAO inhibitory activity. Chirality 2019; 31(1): 21-33. [http://dx.doi.org/10.1002/chir.23027] [PMID: 30468523]

[72] Mishra N, Sasmal D. Modulations of brain amines and dopaminergic behavior by a novel, reversible and selective MAO-B inhibitor. Brain Res 2012; 1470: 45-51. [http://dx.doi.org/10.1016/j.brainres.2012.06.037] [PMID: 22765918]

[73] Bilgin AA, Palaska E, Sunal R. Studies on the synthesis and antidepressant activity of some 1-thiocarbamoyl-3,5-diphenyl-2-pyrazolines. Arzneimittelforschung 1993; 43(10): 1041-4. [PMID: 8267665]

[74] Tripathi AC, Upadhyay S, Paliwal S, Saraf SK. Derivatives of 4, 5-dihydro (1h) pyrazoles as possible mao-a inhibitors in depression and anxiety disorders: synthesis, biological evaluation and molecular modeling studies. Med Chem Res 2018; 27: 1485-503. [http://dx.doi.org/10.1007/s00044-018-2167-z]

[75] Ozdemir Z, Kandilci HB, Gumusel B, Calis U, Bilgin AA. Synthesis and studies on antidepressant and anticonvulsant activities of some 3-(2-thienyl)pyrazoline derivatives. Arch Pharm (Weinheim) 2008; 341(11): 701-7. [http://dx.doi.org/10.1002/ardp.200800068] [PMID: 18816586]

[76] Siddiqui N, Alam P, Ahsan W. Design, synthesis, and *in-vivo* pharmacological screening of N,3-(substituted diphenyl)-5-phenyl-1*H*-pyrazoline-1-carbothioamide derivatives. Arch Pharm (Weinheim) 2009; 342(3): 173-81. [http://dx.doi.org/10.1002/ardp.200800130] [PMID: 19194967]

[77] Bilgin AA, Palaska E, Sunal R, Gümüşel B. Some 1,3,5-triphenyl-2-pyrazolines with antidepressant activities. Pharmazie 1994; 49(1): 67-9. [PMID: 8140135]

[78] Palaska E, Erol D, Demirdamar R. Synthesis and Antidepressant Activities of Some 1, 3, 5-Tripheny--2-Pyrazolines. Eur J Med Chem 1996; 31(1): 43-7.

[http://dx.doi.org/10.1016/S0223-5234(96)80005-5]

[79] Rajendra Prasad Y, Lakshmana Rao A, Prasoona L, Murali K, Ravi Kumar P. Synthesis and antidepressant activity of some 1, 3, 5-triphenyl-2-pyrazolines and 3-(2″-hydroxy naphthalen-1′--yl)-1,5-diphenyl-2-pyrazolines. Bioorg Med Chem Lett 2005; 15(22): 5030-4. [http://dx.doi.org/10.1016/j.bmcl.2005.08.040] [PMID: 16168645]

[80] Prasad YR, Kumar PR, Deepti CA, Ramana MV. Synthesis and Antidepressant Activity of Some 3-(3"-Coumarinyl)-1, 5-Diphenyl-2-Pyrazolines and 3-(2"-Hydroxy Naphthalen-1"-Yl)-1, 5-Diphenyl-2-Pyrazolines. Asian J Chem 2007; 19(6): 4790.

[81] Patil PO, Belsare DP, Kosalge SB, Fursule RA. Microwave assisted synthesis and antidepressant activity of some 1,3,5-triphenyl-2-pyrazolines. Int J Chem Sci 2008; 6(2): 717-25.

[82] Das N, Dash B, Dhanawat M, Shrivastava SK. Design, synthesis, preliminary pharmacological evaluation, and docking studies of pyrazoline derivatives. Chem Pap 2012; 66: 67-74. [http://dx.doi.org/10.2478/s11696-011-0106-2]

[83] Palaska E, Aytemir M, Uzbay IT, Erol D. Synthesis and antidepressant activities of some 3,5-diphenyl-2-pyrazolines. Eur J Med Chem 2001; 36(6): 539-43. [http://dx.doi.org/10.1016/S0223-5234(01)01243-0] [PMID: 11525844]

[84] Gok S, Demet MM, Ozdemir A, Turan-Zitouni G. Evaluation of antidepressant-like effect of 2-pyrazoline derivatives. Med Chem Res 2010; 19(1): 94-101. [http://dx.doi.org/10.1007/s00044-009-9176-x]

[85] Badavath VN, Sinha BN, Jayaprakash V. Design, *in-silico* docking and predictive adme properties of novel pyrazoline derivatives with selective human mao inhibitory activity. Int J Pharm Pharm Sci 2015; 7(12): 277-82.

CHAPTER 4

Flavonoids Antagonize Effects of Alcohol in Cultured Hippocampal Neurons: A Drug Discovery Study

Eduard Korkotian[1,2,*], **Menahem Segal**[1], **Alena Botalova**[2] and **Tatyana Bombela**[3]

[1] *Department of Neurobiology, The Weizmann Institute of Science, Rehovot, Israel*

[2] *Department of Immunology, Perm State University, Perm, Russia*

[3] *Department of Pharmacognosy, Perm State Pharmaceutical Academy, Perm, Russia*

Abstract: Alcohol dependence is one of the top priority public health problems on a global scale. The costs of medical treatments of patients with alcohol dependence, a decrease in labor productivity, an increased risk of developing somatic and mental disorders, and early mortality are all consequences of acute and chronic alcohol abuse. The brain is one of the main targets of alcohol intoxication. Extensive neurobiological studies have revealed a number of synaptic and extra-synaptic mechanisms, affected by alcohol. A primary target of it is GABAergic transmission. Nevertheless, the exciting and disinhibiting actions of alcohol at the system and cellular levels have not been satisfactorily elucidated. It remains unclear whether effects of ethanol are highly complex, manifested only at the level of entire brain or concerns also individual cells, their subcellular structures, organelles, ion channels and receptors. With this approach, small, cultured neural networks that are isolated from the rest of the brain are of particular interest. A serious problem of modern pharmaceuticals is the lack of drugs that have a therapeutic effect on alcohol toxicity of the brain and nervous system, despite the abundance of so-called "traditional medicines". Substances obtained from some herbs containing a mixture of biologically active substances that exhibit a wide range of properties are of particular interest. Among them - flavonoids, which are polyphenols of plant origin and often reveal a sign of sedative, neuroprotective, antidepressant properties, and may improve cognitive function. The aims of our study is to reveal the mechanisms of various concentrations of ethanol, as well as its chronic effects on the functional properties of neurons in small neural networks such as the primary neuronal culture of the rat hippocampus. We have also performed a complex neuropharmacology screening and the study of flavonoids, extracted from *Scrophulariaceae* plant family, which is known in the traditional medicine for its anti-alcohol properties.

[*] **Corresponding author Eduard Korkotian:** Department of Neurobiology, The Weizmann Institute of Science, Rehovot, Israel; Department of Immunology, Perm State University, Perm, Russia; E-mail: eduard.korkotian@weizmann.ac.il

Atta-ur-Rehman and M. Iqbal Choudhary (Eds.)

Keywords: Calcium Imaging, Electrophysiology, Ethanol, Flavonoids, Hippocampal Culture, Inhibition, SK-channels.

INTRODUCTION

Alcohol dependence is a top priority public health hazard on a global scale. According to WHO [1], excessive alcohol consumption is among the leading causes of morbidity and premature death in many countries where the purchase of alcohol is not regulated legislatively, having a serious impact on the quality and duration of human life. The costs of medical treatment of patients with alcohol dependence, a decrease in labor productivity, an increased risk of developing somatic and mental disorders, and early mortality are all consequences of acute and chronic alcohol abuse.

The brain is a major target of alcohol intoxication. The potential costs associated with brain damage produced by alcohol are enormous. In 7-10% of the population of developed countries, alcohol dependence is diagnosed; of which 9% have clinical brain damage. It is shown that the brain retains the dysfunctions accumulated in the past, even if alcohol toxicity is discontinued [2]. It is shown that along with chronic alcohol consumption, the spatial memory, which is stored in the hippocampus and is responsible for forming memories of the location in space, combined with information about related events, deteriorates [3, 4]. Perhaps therefore the strong alcohol intoxication is accompanied by a poor memorization of the events, including those related to movement in space. Thus, studies related to hippocampus, can make a valuable contribution to understanding the mechanisms of ethanol (EtOH).

It should be noted that the concentration of alcohol in the blood, after its consumption in any form of alcoholic beverages, reaches values of 0.5-1 ppm (0.05-0.1%) in a case of light and easy form of drunkness, 2-3 ppm (0.2-0.3%) in a case of average levels of drunkenness and about 4-5 ppm (0.4-0.5%) with a very strong intoxication. A further increase in the volume of alcohol in the blood is considered with a life hazard [5].

According to the modern view, the main cause of death in acute alcohol intoxication is its depressive effect on cellular activity in the vital breathing center of the medulla oblongata, which leads to an arrest of breathing and subsequent coma. However, the specific level of achievement of this condition depends on a whole range of factors, such as the dynamics of alcohol intake and the individual tolerance of the organism to its accumulation and effects. The limiting dose of alcohol in the blood in different patients can fluctuate in the range from 0.5 to 0.8% and even higher [6, 7].

At the same time, the correlation between the level of alcohol in the blood and in the brain is not that unambiguous. In particular, it was found that the concentrations of EtOH in the brain during the first 5-15 minutes after its intake exceed those of the blood by 1.5 times, and in a case of rapid intake - by 3 times [8]. Thus, physiological, life-compatible concentrations of EtOH in the brain can reach 1.5-2%, but hardly exceed 2.5%, and the concentration of EtOH above 3%, used in some *in vitro* experiments, when a complete inhibition of neuronal activity is observed, cannot be recognized as physiologically relevant [9, 10]. Thus, despite the arbitrary nature of the study of alcohol intoxication *in vitro*, there is a very good correlation between *in vitro* alcohol levels, at which a strong decline in neuronal activity begins and the attainment of concentrations incompatible with life in the brain *in vivo*.

Extensive neurobiological studies have revealed a number of synaptic and extra-synaptic mechanisms, affected by alcohol. It interacts with lipids and thereby influences the viscosity of cell membranes [11]. The molecular targets of acute (short-term) effects of alcohol in the brain have been suggested [12 - 15], including potassium channels [16, 17], glutamate and GABA [18, 19] receptors as well as synaptic scaffold proteins [20, 21].

The primary target of ethanol is likely to be GABAergic transmission: either directly, by affecting synaptic and extra-synaptic GABA receptors, or by the involvement of neurosteroids [22 - 29]. However, the exciting or disinhibiting effects of alcohol at the structural and cellular levels have not been satisfactorily elucidated. Similarly, the stimulating and disinhibiting effect of alcohol on the psyche have not yet received a clear mechanistic explanation [30, 31].

Particularly, it remains unclear whether effects of EtOH in humans are manifested only at the level of specific brain structures or the entire nervous system, or concerns also individual cells, their subcellular structures, organelles, ion channels and receptors. With this approach, small, cultured neural networks that are isolated from the rest of the brain are of particular interest. Such a testing model system can demonstrate the effect of different pharmacological substances on the local activity, without the involvement of concomitant effects of incoming afferents from external structures or blood supply of the tested region of interest.

Besides all the above, the mechanism of chronic (long-term) effect of alcohol on neurons remains unclear as well. Using a dissociated culture of central neurons, a diversity of conflicting morphological and chemical consequences of chronic exposure to EtOH was found. On one hand, they include neuronal death [32], a decrease in the density of dendritic spines and their degree of maturity [20], but on the other hand - an increase in the size of dendritic spines associated with an increase in the density of NMDA receptor clusters [33]. The variety of effects may depend on different concentrations of alcohol, duration of exposure and age at the onset of chronic use, as well as on differences in growth conditions and the source of the test tissue (dissociated culture versus slice-culture). In addition, virtually no studies have combined observations on changes in the activity of neurons with their morphological modifications. This question is especially important to determine whether the effects of chronic effects of EtOH are primary or secondary. Additionally, few studies have documented the effects of chronic EtOH on the electrical activity of nerve tissue [34, 35], in contrast to its acute effects (*e.g.* [36, 37]).

The age of the cultured cells is another important factor for the effect of EtOH, as the local network may be at different stages of development after plating. A certain analogue of this experimental approach is the testing of animals of different ages in the context of the influence of pharmacological substances. It should be noted that the life span of cultured neurons is limited to about six to ten weeks. For this reason, a direct comparison of cultures is possible with fairly young animals, up to the age of two months. There are almost no publications in which the effect of EtOH on the primary culture of different ages is investigated. In animal studies, it has been shown that there is a significant correlation between the chronic effect of EtOH on the brain with the age of the animal [38 - 40]. In particular, it was found that in younger animal's behavioral tests show more pronounced locomotor activity with EtOH and a less pronounced sedative effect than in adult animals [38, 40]. Chronic exposure to EtOH causes an increase in anxiety in both young and mature animals [40]. Little is known about the specific effects of alcohol on children and adolescents compared to adults [41].

Despite intensive studies on possible molecular mechanisms and the entire spectrum of behavioral effects, there is limited information on the effects of agonists and antagonists of EtOH in specific target cells. Cultured neurons should demonstrate the effect of a pharmacological substance on local network activity, without the involvement of incoming afferentation, blood supply or other complicating conditions.

Therefore, the study of the mechanisms of action of EtOH on local neural networks remains incomplete until the issue of pharmacological counteraction of the effects of alcohol on intercellular and synaptic activity is examined. In this respect, it should be noted that a serious problem of modern pharmaceutics is the lack of drugs that have a therapeutic effect on alcohol toxicity, despite the abundance of so-called "traditional medicine", which in some way can alleviate the complex symptoms associated with alcohol poisoning. At the moment, drugs of chemical origin used for the treatment of chronic alcohol intoxication, such as benzodiazepines, naltrexone, acamprosate, show mixed results in clinical trials. Therefore, it is reasonable that substances obtained from some herbs used in ethnoscience practice and containing a mixture of biologically active substances are of particular interest [42]. Among them - flavonoids, which are polyphenols of plant origin and often reveal a range of sedative, neuroprotective, antidepressant properties, and may improve cognitive function [43 - 45]. In the case study [46], flavonoids have been shown to eliminate the intoxicating effect of alcohol in the brain. Anthocyanins, which also belong to the flavonoid group, protect hippocampal neurons from apoptosis caused by ethanol [47]. Cyanidin-3-glucoside prevents the inhibition of neurite growth caused by ethanol [48]. Isoflavones of the plant extract of *Pueraria montana* roots (kudzu) reduce alcohol intoxication in clinical trials [49]. Thus, studies of biologically active substances from the group of flavonoids as potential drugs for the treatment of alcohol dependence are promising.

EFFECTS OF ALCOHOL IN CULTURED NEURONS: AN OVERVIEW

In clinical studies, the use of alcohol by humans is associated with both stimulating and depressing effects. The first phases of intoxication affect personal control, disrupting the basic braking mechanisms that usually serve to suppress inappropriate behavior, provoke disinhibition and impulsiveness. Then the inhibitory effects begin, and finally the sedative effects develop [50]. Interestingly, at the prevalence of stimulating effects on the sedative, the risk of alcohol intake increases, and vice versa [51]. It is reasonable to assume that these two phases can involve different synaptic pathways in the brain, acting on different receptors.

Have molecular targets been found for the excitatory and inhibitory effects of alcohol in neuronal culture? Below is the summary of what is currently known about the acute and chronic effects of EtOH on the spontaneous activity of the neural network, as well as on the morphology of cultured neurons.

Acute Effects

Mechanisms of Acute Effect of Ethanol on Excitatory and Inhibitory Neurons

After the first discovery that EtOH acts as an agonist in GABAergic synapses, the exact mechanisms underlying the physiological effects of both acute and chronic exposure to EtOH are still being investigated.

The potentiation of GABAergic synaptic inhibition by EtOH occurs at both pre- and postsynaptic locations. Postsynaptic action arises as a result of potentiation of $GABA_A$ or other anion-related receptors/channels. It is hypothesized that acute exposure to EtOH increases the function of Cys-loop ligand-gated ion channel superfamily which includes $GABA_A$ receptors, nicotinic acetylcholine (nAChR), serotonin (5-HT3) receptors, glycine (GlyR) and several others [52 - 54]. However, inhibition of nAChR and $GABA_A$ receptors have also been reported [54 - 57]. The simplest action of EtOH is observed when it affects the probability of channel opening. Particularly, already moderate concentrations of EtOH are able to increase the channel opening duration [58]. Alternatively, it can increase the affinity of receptor to the natural agonist [59, 60]. This potentiation by EtOH typically affects the synaptic receptors, but their extrasynaptic pool may also be influenced, particularly taking into consideration that extrasynaptic effect may require some lower doses of alcohol [61 - 64] due to easier access. Thus, EtOH increases the amplitude or duration of inhibitory postsynaptic currents [61, 63].

Inhibitory effect of ethanol may also be expressed in other way, by affecting the amount of neurotransmitter release from presynaptic vesicles. The effect of synaptic inhibition may be enhanced if more GABA is accumulated or the probability of release is higher in this case [65]. Thus, GABAergic synaptic transduction has been shown to rise in the presence of alcohol in different areas of the brain, including the hippocampus [22, 56, 61, 63, 66]. As can be seen, both the probability of GABA release and the agonistic effect of postsynaptic channels/receptors may be proposed as the main source of inhibitory effects of EtOH. Therefore, an important issue is the particular parameter of inhibitory postsynaptic currents to be modified by EtOH: the frequency of events recorded, which suggests the presynaptic mechanism or the amplitude of potentials, most probably involving the postsynaptic modifications. This problem is still debated in literature even though more researchers suggest the presynaptic effect as the main reason of chronic effect of EtOH on the dynamics of synaptic transduction, particularly in hippocampus and some other brain areas [22, 56, 66]. Still, an argument that inhibitory effects of EtOH are quickly washed out after alcohol withdrawal and for this reason they should be more likely attributed to the presynaptic ones is doubtful, as presynaptic effects are also often reversed.

However, some studies suggest that EtOH is unable to demonstrate any significant effect on spontaneous GABAergic synaptic activity in cultured neurons of the hippocampus, and therefore the verdict on the role of GABA in the effect of EtOH is not final. Thus, acute EtOH did not alter the frequency of mIPSC in the hippocampal and cortical neurons, and the acute exposure to EtOH only slightly increased the duration of mIPSC in hippocampal neurons, while did not change the kinetics of mIPSC in cortical neurons [23].

Other studies indicate that the interaction between EtOH and presynaptic activity of $GABA_B$ autoreceptors regulates the sensitivity of GABAergic synapses to EtOH [22].

The effect of EtOH on glutamate neurotransmission has been studied, showing that EtOH has an inhibitory effect on glutamate receptors [67]. Synaptic responses mediated by NMDAR are also reduced by EtOH [68, 69]. Arancio's group could not find an effect of acute EtOH on mEPSC amplitudes, while they found suppression of mEPSC frequency. This effect was recorded 15-20 minutes after the onset of exposure to EtOH, the time required for activation of endocannabinoid receptors [37].

The variety of effects of EtOH indicates that different types of cells can react differently to a low concentration of EtOH, as indicated in another study conducted with cultured cortical neurons [70]. These effects may be age-dependent and slow to develop [71].

Calcium-dependent Potassium Channels Mediate Excitatory Effects of Ethanol

Control of cell excitability is essential for neurons as it affects the probability and speed of cellular responses as well as the overall responsiveness. These processes are foremost dependent on potassium outward currents, which are particularly mediated by calcium-dependent potassium channels of small (SK) and high conductivity (BK, MaxiK). SK and BK channels are of interest as possible pharmacological targets for the action of EtOH [36].

The selective and concentration-dependent amplification of ion currents are mediated by high conductance, voltage and Ca^{2+} -dependent K^+ channels in response to a short exposure (1-2 minutes) to physiological concentrations (10-100 mM) of EtOH, on the neurohypophysis nerve terminals of the rat [72, 73]. Some other studies also support the functional interactions between EtOH at physiological concentrations and BK channels [74 - 76]. However, some studies show that EtOH at physiologically relevant concentrations not only leads to potentiation of the BK channel current, but also can lead to refractivity or inhibition of BK channel current [76, 77]. The final effect depends on many factors, including the intracellular calcium level, the isoform of Slo1 (protein forming BK channel), the composition of the BK beta subunit, the posttranslational modification of the BK proteins, the lipid microenvironment of the channel, and the route of administration of EtOH [77, 78].

Fewer studies address the interaction of EtOH with SK channels. When an action potential develops, Na^+ and calcium ions enter the cell, which activate the SK channels. This, in turn, leads to an increased release of K^+ ions from the cell, repolarization, and allows for a new discharge. Discovery of SK channels helps to understand the facilitation of the cell repolarization stage, during which the initial resting membrane potential is restored creating conditions for a rapid postsynaptic response [79, 80]. In a few studies, the SK channel has been proposed as a potential target for the action of EtOH. It was shown that the excitatory effect of low concentrations of EtOH is due to direct participation of SK channels of dopaminergic neurons in the ventral tegmental [81]. Additionally, EtOH increased the spontaneous activity of dopaminergic neurons [82]. Participation of SK channels in the increased activity of neurons in nucleus accumbens and alcohol seeking during abstinence have also been found [83]. Studies by Mulholland *et al.* show changes in SK-channel expression and function after chronic exposure to EtOH (75 mM for 7-9 days) in the CA1 region of hippocampus. This exposure resulted in a decrease in apamin-sensitive SK currents and suppression of SK-channel expression [84]. Thus, Ca^{2+} -activated K^+ -channel is an evolving field for research, which is of particular importance for understanding the molecular mechanism of the excitatory action of EtOH.

Chronic Effects

Chronic alcohol abuse, due to its severe social and medical consequences, have been carefully studied in recent years at the behavioral and molecular levels.

Chronic alcohol consumption can cause addiction and physical dependence [85]. Cessation of alcohol consumption after its prolonged leads to an increase in neuronal excitability and may be manifested by anxiety, irritability, and even convulsion [86, 87]. As with many long-term treatments related to GABAergic system, chronic exposure to EtOH may lead to insensitivity to some important pharmacological means of treatment, such as sedative, anxiolytic and similar effects [88, 89].

Chronic use of EtOH may differentially change the gene expression of different $GABA_A$ subunits in different regions of the brain. For example, chronic administration of EtOH reduced the levels of the delta subunit of $GABA_A$ receptors in rat cerebellum and hippocampus. And in contrast to this, cerebral cortex in regard to the protein levels stayed unchanged [90]. Modifications of $GABA_A$ receptor gene expression depend on the location and time. For example, the chronic EtOH modified the level of the alfa 4 subunit of $GABA_A$ in the hippocampus after 40 days, but not at the earlier stages of treatment [91]. Data suggest that the chronic effect of EtOH differently changes the expression of

$GABA_A$ receptor in the hippocampus and in other areas of the brain and these changes are dependent on the persistence of exposure to EtOH [92].

In an early study, Olsen and Spigelman [93] developed chronic intermittent ethanol (CIE) exposure mode, in which rats received EtOH at a dose of 5 to 6 g/kg (60 times in 120 days) with alternating intoxication and withdrawal stages, or with intermittent addition of EtOH directly to the neuronal culture. After cessation of procedures a convulsive activity could be detected [93].

In different study, immunocytochemistry and patch-clamp techniques were used to study directly the effect of the CIE protocol on rat hippocampal GABAergic synapses. A large increase in alpha4 and gamma2 $GABA_A$ subunits and decrease in alpha1 and delta subunits were found in the hippocampal homogenates after implementation of CIE protocol in animals and after removal of EtOH during two days [94]. Chronic effects of EtOH led to mutual changes in alpha1 and alpha4 subunits [95].

The mentioned [94] study reports significant decreases in the amplitude and half-decay of TTX-resistant miniature inhibitory postsynaptic currents (mIPSCs), recorded from pyramidal neurons of CA1 hippocampal region treated with CIE protocol [94]. These may be associated with the changes in the expression of alpha1 and alpha4 $GABA_A$ subunits along with reduction in the frequency of mIPSC. It should be underlined that these data suggest both presynaptic and a postsynaptic decrease in GABAergic transmission in the hippocampus of rats treated using CIE protocol.

However, in a later study, the chronic EtOH did not change the frequency of mIPSCs in the hippocampal and cortical neurons, while there was only temporary decrease in the decay time of mIPSC in cortical neurons and no change in kinetics of mIPSC in hippocampal neurons [23].

Release of GABA may be altered through presynaptic mechanisms. Thus, decrease in the probability of GABA release following chronic consumption of EtOH was detected in dentate gyrus [96] and in CA1 region [94] of hippocampus. These effects may be understood and explained as a peculiar compensation for the enhanced GABA release in a case of acute consumption of EtOH. Another outcome of the increased release of GABA in CA1 region *in vivo* is the decrease of $GABA_B$ receptor activity [97]. As mentioned above, reduced GABAergic transmission in different regions of the brain in the presence of chronic alcohol may include both presynaptic and postsynaptic mechanisms. Thus, neuromodulatory, circumstantial (even humoral) and direct effects of chronic EtOH may be proposed as possible integrative effects of alcohol on GABA release and transmission. In one case, decline of overall inhibition and some activation will be expected while the other possibility is associated with long-term depression of activity following EtOH withdrawal [98].

Collectively, these studies show that GABAergic synapses undergo complex changes after the chronic exposure to EtOH, which, for the most part, will lead to a decrease in the inhibitory tone. These data also suggest that long-term exposure to EtOH results in both pre-and postsynaptic changes, and these changes may vary between different areas of the brain, eg, in hippocampus, cerebral cortex or in the amygdala [68].

The chronic exposure to EtOH involves many neuroadaptive changes in the CNS, including glutamatergic synaptic transmission. Induction of long-term potentiation (LTP) in CA1 region of hippocampus by tetanic stimulation of Schaffer's collaterals was completely blocked in hippocampal slices exposed to alcohol. LTP remained blocked 1 day after removal of EtOH, indicating that the neuroadaptive changes caused by alcohol were not easily reversible. Partial reduction in LTP was observed 5 days after removal of EtOH [56, 99].

Quite inconclusive reports of the effect of EtOH on the morphology of dendritic spines has been reported. Enlarged spine volume was associated with an increase in NMDA receptor clusters [33], while in another study a decrease in spine density was reported [20].

Increased levels of extracellular glutamate may enhance NMDA function. But in contrast to this hippocampal and amygdalar LTP is highly suppressed by chronic EtOH [99 - 102]. However, it is still unknown which factors are involved in the disruption of LTP production in LTP, but the downregulation of the NMDA receptors expression levels following its excessive activation can serve as a plausible explanation.

Molecular Mechanisms of Alcohol-modified Neuronal Activity in Culture

Acute Effects of Ethanol

Spontaneous Network Activity in Hippocampal Neuronal Culture: Calcium Imaging

Stable background neuronal activity is an important precondition for further examination of the effects of EtOH. Fig. (**1A**) provides recordings from three cultured hippocampal neurons loaded with Fluo-4 (AM). Each trace coded in red, blue and green represents a region of interest drawn around soma of the given neuron. Calcium transients ("events") represent electrical bursts in the neurons, recorded as the change in Fluo-4 fluorescence and expressed in arbitrary units.

For further analysis, arbitrary units have been transformed into ΔF/F units where F is the basal fluorescence and ΔF is the net fluorescence change. Same cells were imaged during 40 minutes. Example images taken at the beginning and in 10, 30 and 40 minutes are shown on panel A. Fig. (**1B**) represents the averaged activity from many cells and no statistically significant change in the number of calcium events can be seen. On 1C averaged, normalized single events of the same cell, taken at time points of 0, 10, 30 and 40 min are compared. Results reveal no significant differences in the dynamics of events: neither in their rise nor in decay time course.

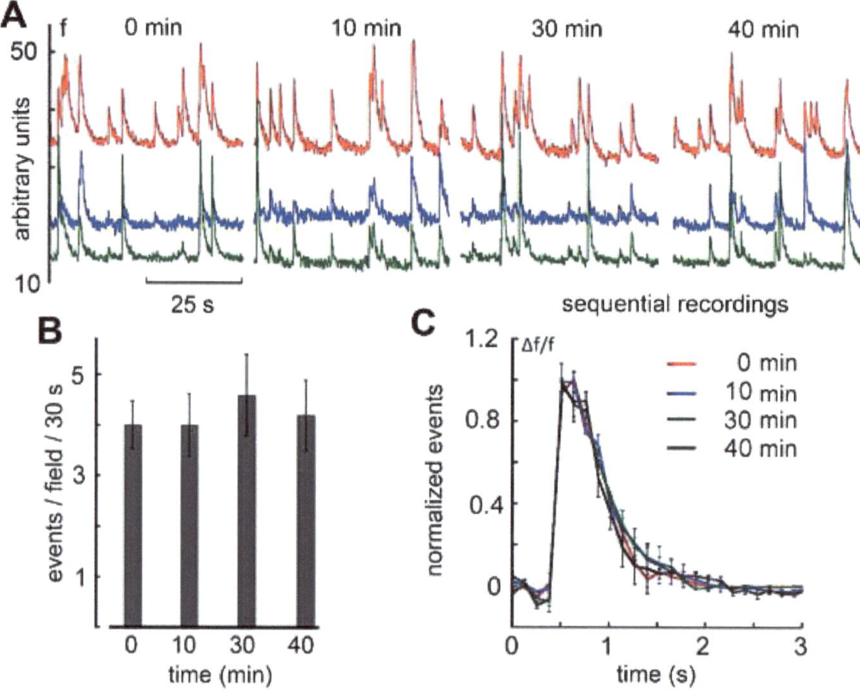

Fig. (1). Stable network activity in cultured hippocampal neurons over 40 minutes of recording. (Modified from [9]). For overview of primary hippocampal culture preparation and calcium imaging see [103 - 106].

We then tested the effect of a range of EtOH concentrations on spontaneous neuronal activity in hippocampal cultures of same type and age. Fig. (**2A**) shows a representative field of recording with several cells, three of which have been marked as ROIs using red, green and blue lines. Left panel shows the basal calcium level and the middle panel represents the peak of calcium event ("spike") showing elevated fluorescence levels.

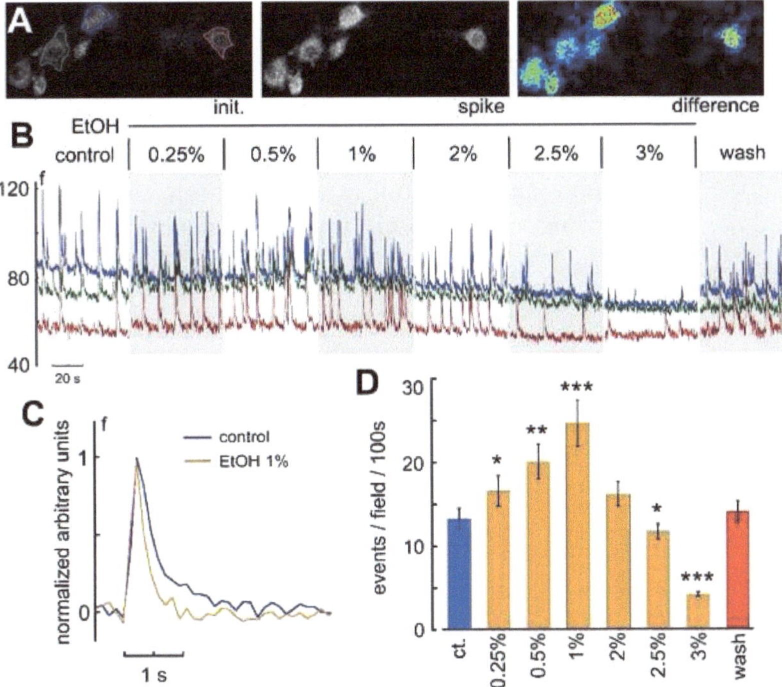

Fig. (2). Low ethanol facilitates and high ethanol suppresses network activity in hippocampal culture. A. sample illustration of several neurons in the field of view. B. continuous record of activity of the neurons exposed to increasing concentrations of EtOH. C. Averaged time course of the rise and decay of the calcium response. D. Mean number of events. (Modified from [9]). (Also, see [103]).

The lowest concentrations (0.25%, 0.5%, and 1%, equivalent to 40, 80, and 160 mM, respectively) caused an increase in the discharge rate of the neurons. This increase was accompanied by the shortening of duration of representative calcium events, as shown on panel C. Surprisingly, higher concentrations of EtOH, 2, 2.5 and 3% (corresponding to 320, 400 and 480 mM), caused a significant decrease in the discharge rate, up to the almost complete cessation of activity. After washout of EtOH, a gradual return to the basal level of discharges was observed. This suggests that a short (5-10 minutes) exposure to even high concentrations of EtOH does not cause a toxic effect on neuronal activity. Fig. (**2D**) summarizes results, obtained from 5 cover glasses with 34 cells in total. An 85.5% increase in the bursting rate, from 13.15 ± 1.12 to 24.4 ± 2.4 events per 100 seconds was recorded in 1% EtOH compared to control ($p < 0.001$). The minimum dosage of the EtOH, still able to provide a statistically significant increase in the activity rate was about 0.09% (≤15 mM, $p < 0.05$). In 3% EtOH the activity was reduced to 4.13 ± 0.11, a 68.6% decrease, compared to the control level ($p < 0.001$) (taken from [9]).

A conspicuous effect of EtOH was the shortening of calcium transients (Fig. **3**). This change could be due to the acceleration of the decay time of discharges (1/2 decay = 0.442 ± 0.065 seconds in the control, to 0.319 ± 0.041 in the presence of 0.5% EtOH, p <0.001) as shown in Fig. (**3**), where all spikes of a given cell indicates were averaged at control (blue) and 0.5% EtOH (red). But the same figure evidences that such acceleration remains about the same also in the presence of 3% alcohol (brown trace), which in fact reduces the rate of activity.

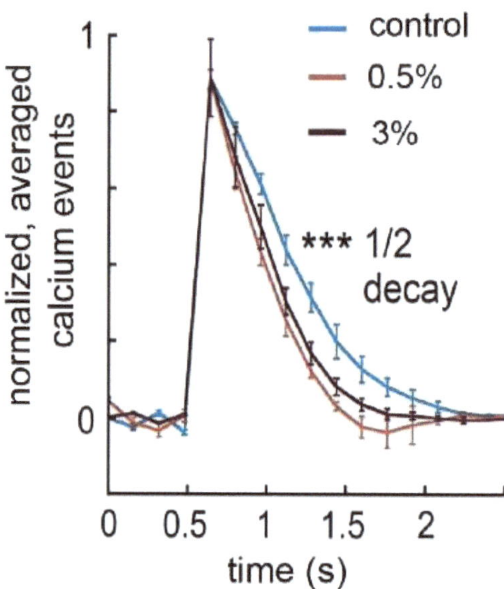

Fig. (3). Both low and high ethanol accelerate the time course of half decay in averaged calcium events, compared to control condition. (Modified from [9]).

This observation suggests that either acceleration of spike decay is not related to the change in the rate of activity, or that another, independent factor suppresses the activity following high alcohol despite the facilitation seen with lower EtOH.

Thus, low concentrations of EtOH (0.25-1%) cause an increase in the spontaneous activity of neurons compared to the control activity, while higher concentrations (2-3%) inhibit the activity. Additionally, all acute EtOH effects are non-toxic and reversible after wash.

Electrophysiological Effects of Acute Ethanol in Hippocampal Culture

Possible synaptic targets of EtOH were studied using patch-clamp technique, on 11 neurons (one cell per cover glass), obtained in three different dissections. The recordings were done in the presence of TTX to block action potentials, and bicuculline to suppress the possible effects of EtOH on inhibitory synapses.

Under standard conditions, the basal activity level was recorded for two minutes, followed by 0.5% EtOH (recorded for 2 minutes) and 3% EtOH (recorded for another two minutes). The resistance in the pipette was stable throughout the recording period. The average size of mEPSC did not differ significantly in the three recording conditions [see 9 for details] (Fig. **4A** and Fig. **B**). The mEPSC rate was variable among the three recording conditions, but in most cases the frequency of mEPSCs increased after exposure to EtOH (panel D). Individual changes between the recording conditions in EtOH versus control were analyzed and significant growth was observed (panel E). It is interesting to note that the rise time of mEPSCs was significantly faster during exposure to both concentrations of EtOH than in control (panel F).

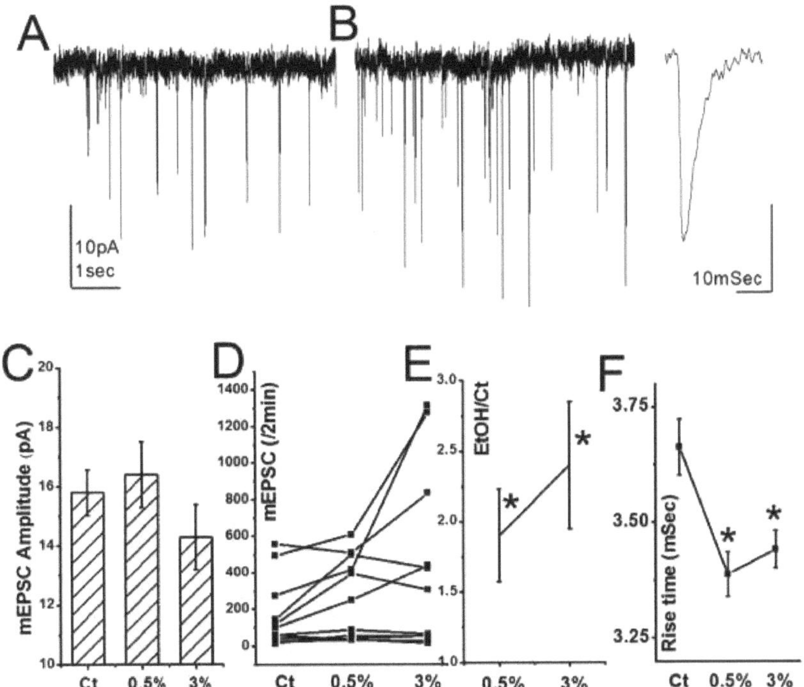

Fig. (4). Electrophysiological effects of EtOH in patch-clamped cultured hippocampal neurons. (Modified from [9]).

These experiments show that EtOH can have both a presynaptic locus of action (expressed in an increase in the mEPSC frequency) and a postsynaptic locus, expressed in change of the kinetics of mEPSC.

Acute Effect of Ethanol on $GABA_A$ Receptors

Possible involvement of GABAergic neurotransmission in the effect of facilitation mediated by low concentrations of EtOH or in suppression, induced by its high concentrations was tested [9]. First, cultures were exposed to low EtOH, which resulted in a typical increase in activity, followed by 3% EtOH, which suppressed the activity (not shown). Ethanol was then washed and cultures were perfused with 10 μM bicuculline, a $GABA_A$ receptor antagonist. Bicuculline caused a 1.5-2-fold increase in the amplitude and a noticeable increase in the duration (Fig. **5**, two left panels), associated with prolonged electrical bursts.

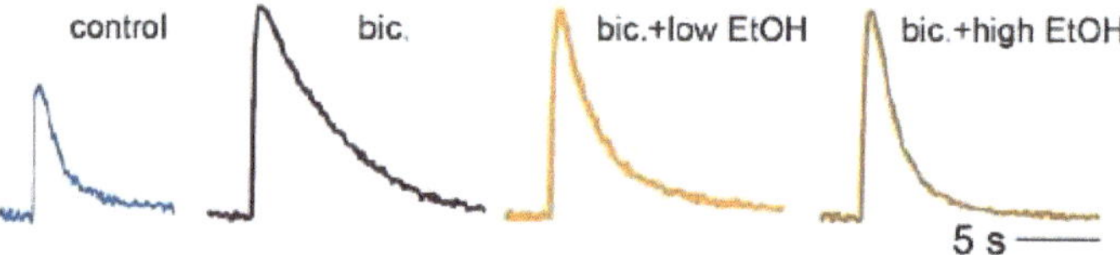

Fig. (5). Representative calcium transients recorded from the same cell in control, after 10μM bicuculline and with addition of low and high concentrations of EtOH. (Modified from [9]).

A typical large calcium transient recorded in the presence of bicuculline is shown in Fig. (**6**). Top panel represents the resting condition and the middle panel is taken at the peak of spike. Lower panel shows the net response coded in spectrum range.

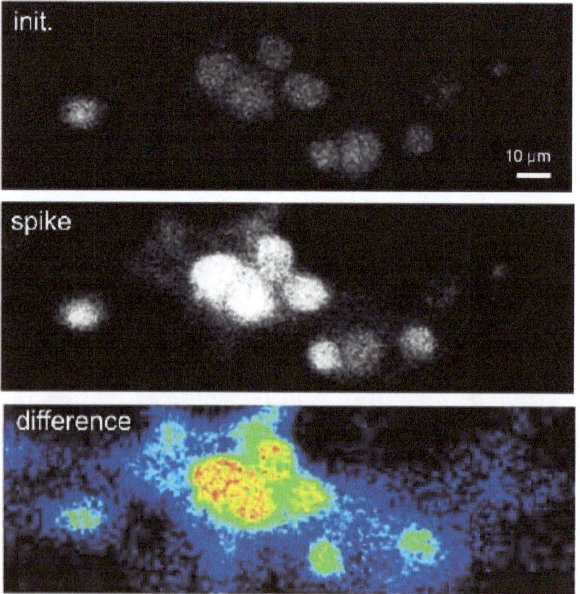

Fig. (6). Calcium transient in the presence of 10 μM bicuculline. (Also, see [103]).

In the presence of bicuculline, 0.5% EtOH was still able to increase significantly the discharge frequency: from 9.2 ± 1.04 in control and 10.8 ± 0.88 in bicuculline to 16.9 ± 1.17, p <0.001) (Figs. **7A** and **B**). Accordingly, the amplitude of calcium events, related to the size of electric bursts rose as well (Figs. **7A** and **C**).

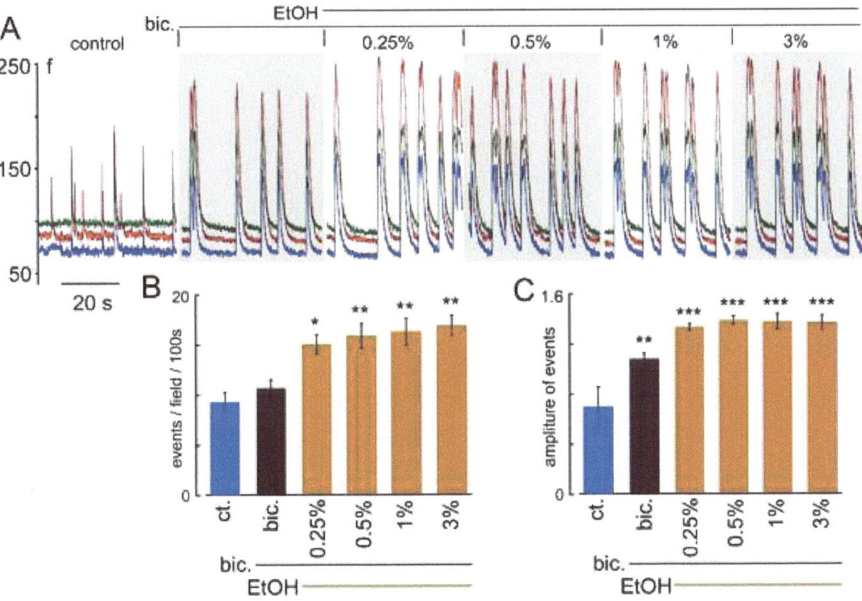

Fig. (7). Low and high ethanol increase the amplitude and frequency of calcium events in the presence of 10μM bicuculline, a $GABA_A$ receptor blocked. (Modified from [107]).

It is important to note that the high level of EtOH (3%) was no longer able to suppress spontaneous neuronal activity, which remained almost unchanged following the increasing concentrations of alcohol (Fig. 7). Still, the durations of typical calcium events were decreased due to a reduction in the decay time (Fig. **5**, right panels).

These results suggest that the high concentration of EtOH facilitates the GABAergic effects in the culture by either selectively activating the GABAergic neurons or (most likely) by acting as a GABA receptor co-agonist. Nevertheless, the facilitation seen after exposure to low concentrations of EtOH does not include GABAergic neurotransmission and is not blocked by bicuculline.

Ethanol Acts via SK Channels

Earlier studies suggest that EtOH may affect potassium channels of predominantly low conductivity (SK channels) [36, 84, 108]. We investigated the role of SK channels in the action of EtOH on neuronal activity, using a selective SK channel antagonist, apamin. Exposure to low concentration of apamin (40 nM) caused a significant but temporary (about two fold) increase in the discharge rate during first 3-5 minutes of exposure (Fig. **8**), as well as an increase in the average duration of discharges (Fig. **9**, blue *vs* dark blue trace) and their amplitude (Fig. **10**, left panel, 8 experiments, 51 neurons).

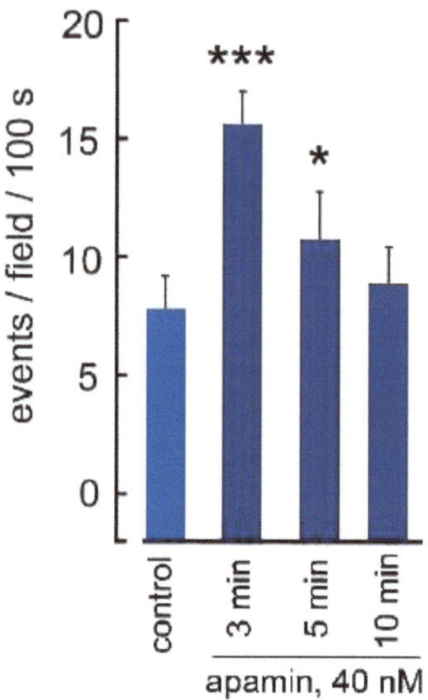

Fig. (8). Temporary increase of cell spontaneous activity by 40 nM apamin.

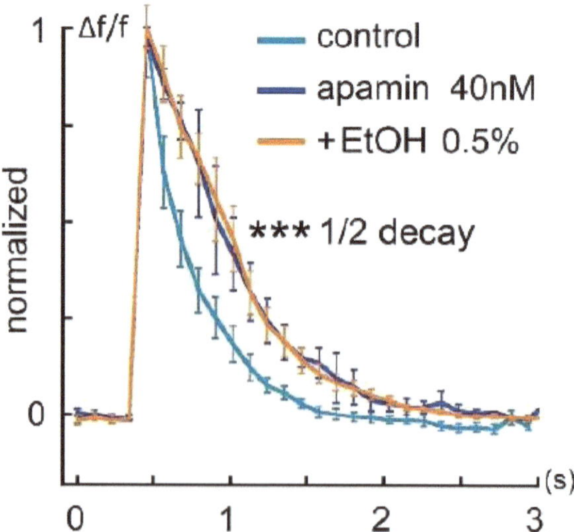

Fig. (9). Averaged time courses of calcium events of the same representative cell in control, in the presence of 40nM apamin and after addition of 0.5% alcohol. (Modified from [9]).

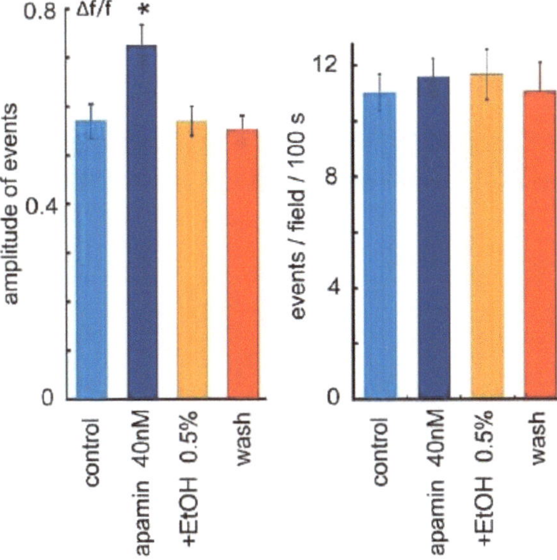

Fig. (10). Apamin slightly increases the averaged amplitude of calcium events but suppresses the facilitation of neuronal spontaneous activity induced by 0.5% alcohol (EtOH). (Modified from [9]).

However, in the presence of apamin, low concentrations of EtOH (0.25-0.5%) no longer caused an increase in neuronal activity (Fig. **10**, right panel, from [9]), G, and were also unable to reduce the slower decay of the averaged events shown in Fig. (**9**), orange trace.

In contrast, high concentrations of EtOH still suppressed the background cell activity level to zero (not shown), which indicates that this effect is not mediated by the action of SK channels. Washing away the substances caused a complete recovery of activity (Fig. **10**).

To verify that the interaction between apamin and EtOH was not due to the consecutive use of substances, EtOH was first used in another series of experiments to provide a typical steady increase in the discharge rate. Then, apamin was applied and it blocked the increase in the discharge rate. In addition, apamin caused an increase in the size and duration of discharges.

This experimental protocol, where apamin is applied in the presence of low ETOH concentrations, is summarized in Fig. (**11**). Panel A of the figure demonstrates the increased amplitude of typical calcium event, recorded in the presence of 40 nM apamin. Traces of neurons marked on A using red, green and blue are shown on the panel B. As in the previous experiments, 0.25 and 0.5% EtOH gradually increase the activity, while addition of 20 and 40 nM of apamin in the presence of 0.55 EtOH decreased the rate of spontaneous events to the basal level. Moreover, further application of additional portion of alcohol (0.25%) could not anymore change the activity rate. Representative calcium transient time course of the same cell, taken at control (blue), in Fig. (**11**).

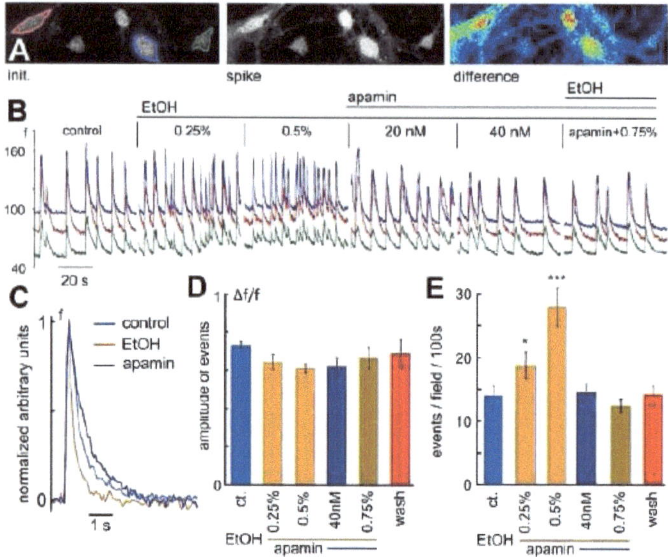

Fig. (11). Apamin (at 20 and 40 nM) abolish the facilitation of cell activity induced by EtOH. (Modified from [107]).

presence of EtOH and then – apamin are shown on panel C. While EtOH accelerates the decay time, further application of apamin elongates the time course slightly above the control level.

Panels D and E represent averaged amplitude (D) and the number of events per 100 s (E) of several experiments. Washout of the drugs could recover the initial parameters of spontaneous activity.

These experiments show that, regardless of the order of applications, apamin blocked the increase in burst rate caused by low EtOH, while maintaining a steady effect of its own expressed in the change in the size and decay of discharges.

The effects of apamin and EtOH in a joint application were studied in the presence of a $GABA_A$ - receptor antagonist, bicuculline, in order to identify possible interactions between apamin and the GABAergic system. As shown above (Figs. **6** and **7**), bicuculline caused a significant increase in the discharge size, which is associated with a marked prolongation of the discharge duration. In addition, the presence of bicuculline did not affect the facilitation effect of the EtOH on activity rate (Figs. **7A** & **B** and Fig. **12**, orange column).

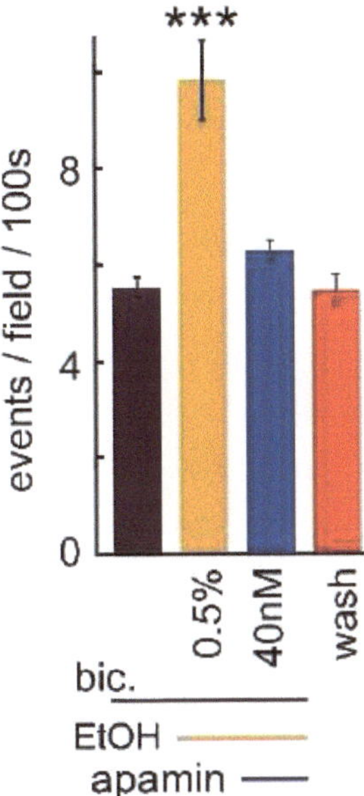

Fig. (12). Blocking effect of apamin on the facilitation, induced by 0.5% ethanol in the presence of 10 μM bicuculline.

Following the addition of 40 nM apamin, the discharge frequency decreased significantly (Fig. **12**), dark blue column), while washout of all the substances recovered the initial activity state. These results indicate that while bicuculin and apamin may have a joint effect on the duration of single discharges (as shown on Figs. **5** and **9**), most probably due to the activation of various synaptic and channel properties, they are distinguished by their ability to block both the facilitative and inhibitive effects of EtOH.

Finally, if the effects of EtOH are mediated by the activation of SK channels, it is important to compare the effects of EtOH with the SK channel agonist - 1-EBIO (1-ethyl-1,3-dihydro-2H-benzimidazol-2-one). At high concentrations (200 μM) [84], 1-EBIO caused a marked suppression of spontaneous activity, which results from activating potassium channels (Fig. **13A**, from [9]).

Importantly, much lower concentrations of 1-EBIO (200-500 nM) led to an increase in the discharge rate by 51.2% and slight decrease in the amplitude of events (Figs. **13A** & **B**). This was associated with acceleration of the half-decay of the averaged bursts: the opposite effect to that caused by apamin, and similarly to the effect of low concentrations of EtOH (panels C&D). The combined use of low concentrations of EtOH and 1-EBIO lead to their synergistic action and caused either amplification or termination of any of them, since both substances at high concentrations suppress spontaneous neuronal activity. These 1-EBIO effects could be completely recovered by 40 nM apamin (dark blue columns on A&B and dark blue trace on C), [from 9].

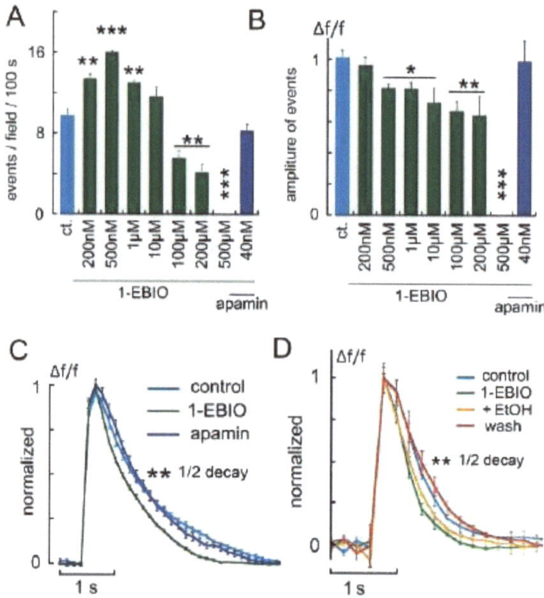

Fig. (13). Low concentrations of 1-EBIO (200-500 nM) act similarly to low doses of EtOH (0.25-1%) and the effect can be blocked by apamin (40 nM). (Modified from [9]).

Chronic Ethanol AFFECTS Spontaneous Activity in Hippocampal Culture

As it was shown on Fig. (**2**) for acute effect of EtOH, its typical effect on the level of spontaneous activity of cultured neurons depends on the concentration, so that the lower, 0.5 to 1% ones increase the activity and the higher, around 3% suppress it. This effect is seen in a case of short application of each concentration during several minutes and the washout almost immediately recovers the initial level of activity. It means that the "brief" and "long" wash look about the same (Fig. **14**, left).

On the right panel, the initial conditions are the same and effects of EtOH look similar, including the 3% EtOH applied for 5 hours. Nevertheless, the initial part of wash, after chronic exposure to EtOH looks very different, revealing an increase in the level of activity far above the control level. Only continuous wash during next 30 minutes restores the initial activity.

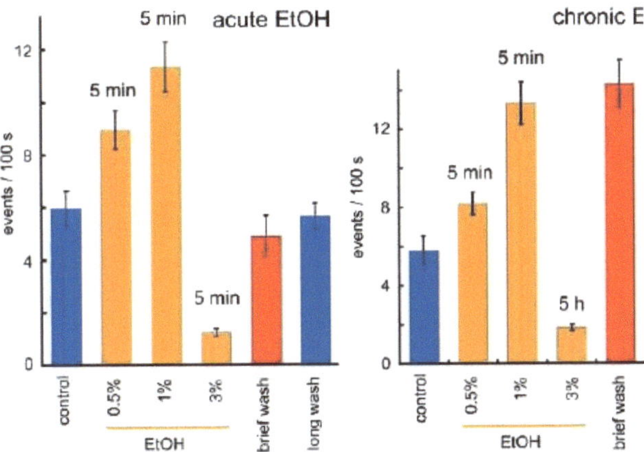

Fig. (14). Effects of brief (5 min) and long (5 hours) application of 3% ethanol (EtOH) and two stages of its wash: "brief" and "long". (Modified from [10]).

This effect is shown on Fig. (**15**), where activity two cells in the presence of 3% EtOH during 5 hours, is compared to the level, observed during brief wash for same neurons.

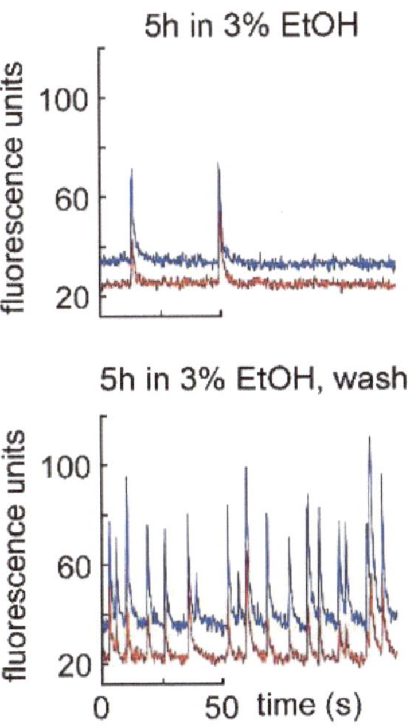

Fig. (15). Calcium transients of two cells in 3% ethanol (EtOH) during 5 hours of application and following brief wash. (Modified from [10]).

In order to clarify whether this chronic effect is limited to the high dose of EtOH, we performed the same experiment with 1% EtOH, applied for periods of 5 and 12 hours (Fig. **16** left and right panels, respectively). However, even in this case, the washout of EtOH increased the activity. Summary of these two experiments are shown on Fig. (**17**), although facilitative effect on cell activity after 12 hours of incubation was less pronounced.

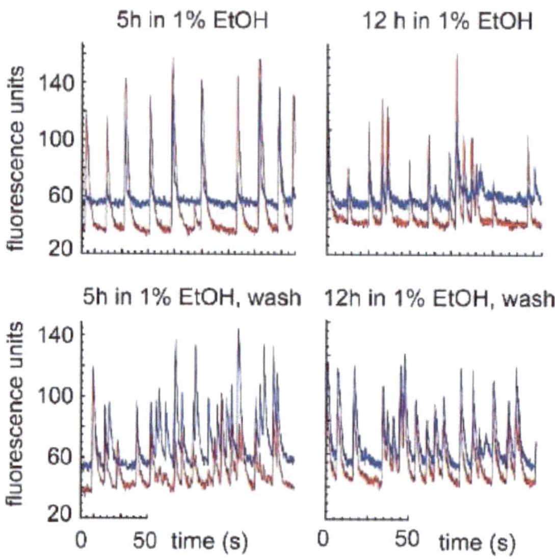

Fig. (16). Calcium transients of two cells in 1% ethanol (EtOH) during 5 hours (left) and 12 hours (right) of application and following wash (Modified from [10]).

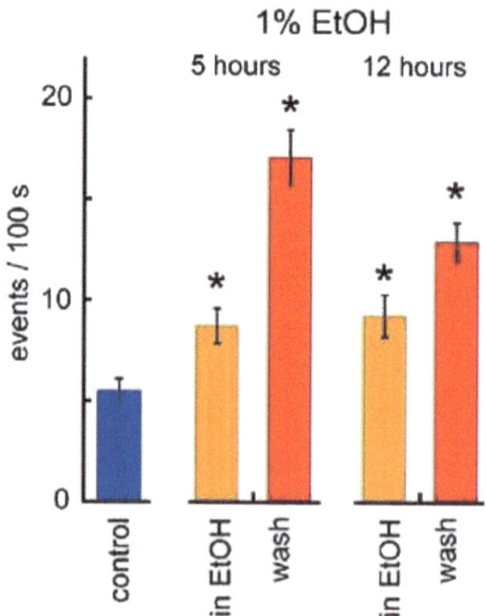

Fig. (17). Chronic effect of EtOH applied for 5 and 15 hours, measured after its washout [10].

Although relatively short chronic applications of 1% EtOH: for 5 and 12 hours still increased the rate of bursts, even to the much lower levels than in acute experiments, the longer incubation with 1% EtOH was not facilitative any longer. Fig. (**18A**) shows the reduced activity following 1-day incubation and even more pronouncedly reduction – in 5 days (B).

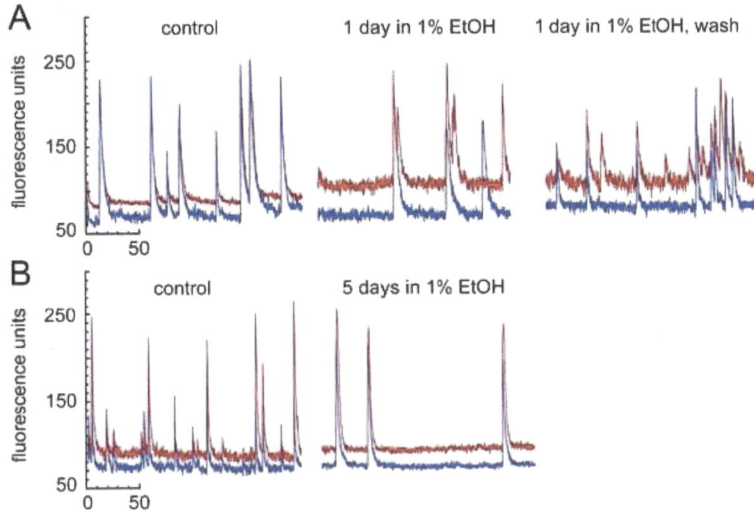

Fig. (18). Chronic application of 1% ethanol (EtOH) for 1 (A) and 5 (B) days. (Modified from [10]).

Washout of EtOH after its chronic 1, 2 and 5 days exposure was also shifted to more inhibitory state. This magnitude of this shift depends on two factors: the EtOH concentration and the time course of exposure. This, 0.5% EtOH is less inhibitory that 1 and 3%, and 5 days of action is more inhibitory that 1 and 2 days. These results are summarized on Fig. (**19**).

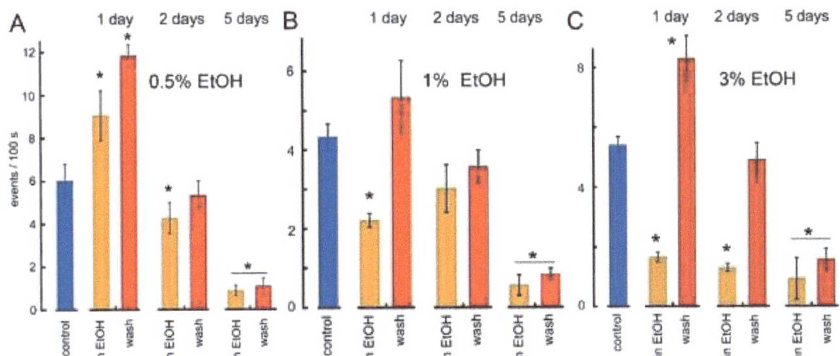

Fig. (19). Chronic exposure to 0.5, 1 and 3% ethanol (EtOH) for 1, 2 and 5 days, followed by washout. (Modified from [10]).

If the presence of 0.5% EtOH for 1 day facilitated the activity similarly to its acute exposure, 1% and 3% EtOH suppressed it. Still, in all 3 cases the wash leads to an overshoot of activity. Two days of exposure demonstrate a transitional effect, not changing much the initial activity levels neither during the incubation, not after removal of a substance. Interestingly, a significant suppression of activity seen in the presence of 3% EtOH if followed by its recovery during the wash. Finally, 5 days of EtOH exposure brought activity to very low, almost zero values with no recovery seen after washout of the drug.

It must be indicated that these long exposures to the drug did not lead to cell toxicity or neuronal death at least for several days after the exposure.

In the present series of acute experiments, we have shown that the inhibitory effects of high, 2-3% EtOH are due to enhancement of inhibition in culture and therefore can be abolished by 10 μM of $GABA_A$ receptor blocker, bicuculline (Fig. **7**). Moreover, when overall activity in hippocampal culture is influenced by low concentrations of TTX, which reduces the excitatory glutamatergic more than GABAergic tone, the inhibitory effects of alcohol could be detected already at the low concentrations (data not shown). Therefore, a similar experiment was performed with chronic, 5-day exposure to 1% EtOH with introduction of bicuculline after extensive wash of alcohol.

(Figs. **20** and **21**) show that cell activity is persistently reduced after long-term exposure of 1% EtOH, while addition of bicuculline could restore activity. A similar effect could be seen with lower doses of EtOH as well as with higher amount used for only 2 days (data not shown). We conclude that non-toxic inhibitory effect of EtOH is directed to GABAergic activity.

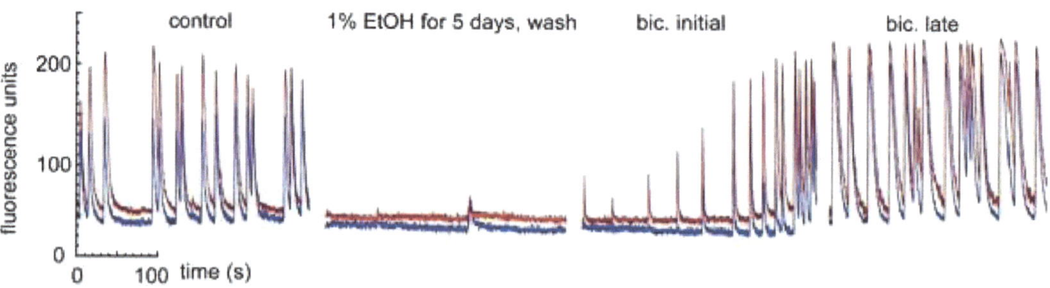

Fig. (20). Bicuculline (bic) is able to restore activity reduced by chronic ethanol (EtOH).

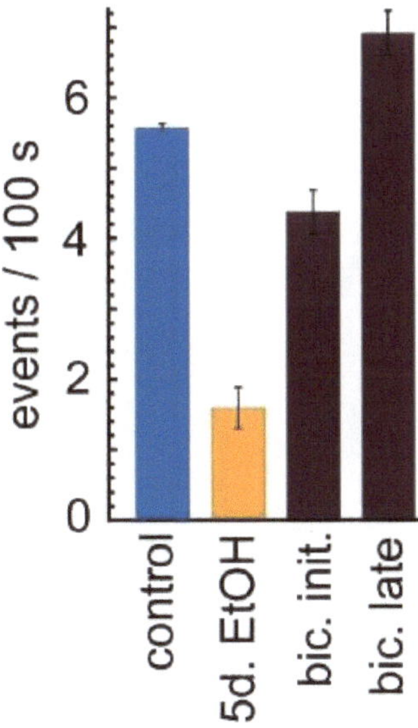

Fig. (21). Summary of effect of 10μM bicuculline (bic.) on cell activity, reduced by chronic exposure to 1% ethanol (EtOH).

Additional evidence for this assumption follows from an experiment analyzing the electrophysiological properties of cells following 5-day incubation with 1% ethanol (Fig. **22**). Still, the nature of enhanced activity due to 5, 12 and 24 hours of chronic exposure to ethanol remains unclear. We analyzed the effect of apamin on the enhanced activity, following alcohol withdrawal. As shown above, 12 hours-long incubation with 1% EtOH raised the activity (Fig. **22**).

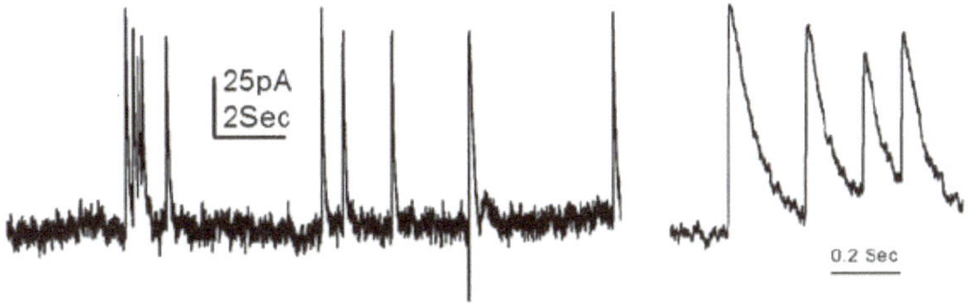

Fig. (22). Spontaneous inhibitory synaptic currents are not affected by 5 days of exposure to 1% ethanol. A sample illustration of spontaneous bursts of outward currents and an expanded trace on the right of the same cell. (Modified from [10]).

On Fig. (**23**), acute effect of EtOH is blocked by apamin (as in Fig. **11E**). However, after chronic application and wash which nearly doubles the activity, apamin was still able to recover the initial activity levels below the dotted line (right part of the Figure). Acute ethanol (1%) under this condition also reduces the activity. This data may suggest that chronic EtOH saturates the activity of SK channels in a long-term way, so that they steadily increase and could not be activated by EtOH any longer but are still blocked by apamin.

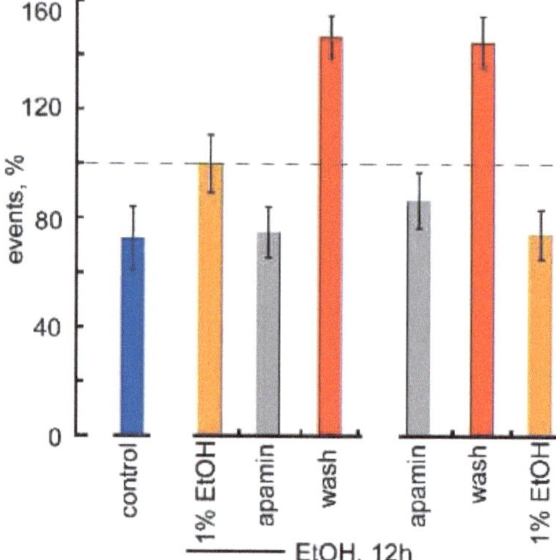

Fig. (23). Acute effect of 1% ethanol (EtOH) and apamin (40 nM) after chronic application of ethanol (EtOH).

The following experiment tested this suggestion (Fig. **24**). The activity enhanced by chronic EtOH was reduced by acute 1, 1.5 and 2% ethanol. We hypothesize that under the conditions of saturated SK-channel activity, acute alcohol can only enhance the GABAergic transmission in culture, as shown on Fig. (**7**).

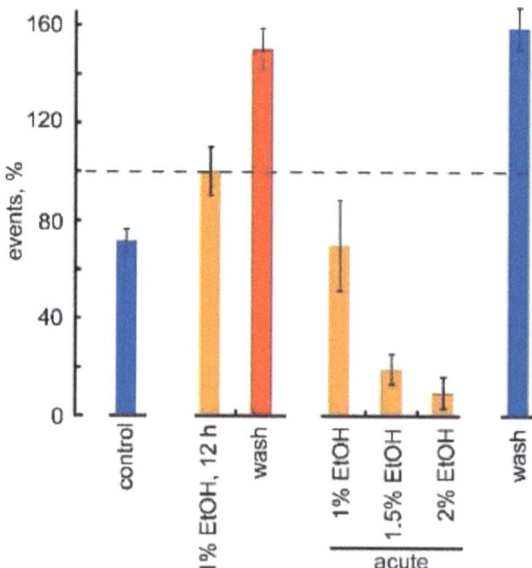

Fig. (24). Acute effect of 1, 1.5 and 2% ethanol (EtOH) on network activity following withdrawal from chronic EtOH.

An important issue is related to the target of both facilitative and suppressive actions of chronic alcohol and the acute effects of EtOH and apamin. We have treated the culture with 1% EtOH for 12 hours and then recorded its calcium transients after EtOH withdrawal and its extensive wash under four conditions: in control, 1% acute EtOH, 40 nM apamin, and finally, in apamin+EtOH. Recordings were done at two key sites of a neuron: at cell body and dendritic spines – the postsynaptic structures of synapses. Examples of synaptic activity and the summary of results are shown on Fig. (**25**).

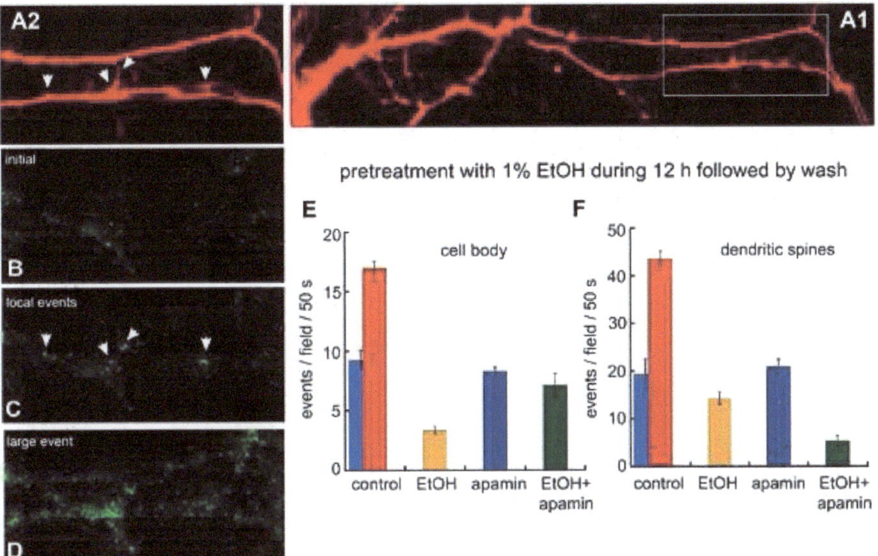

Fig. (25). A1 – dendritic arbor of a DsRed-transfected cell with several dendritic spines. An enlarged fragment of A1 in a white frame is shown in A2. B, C and D are single frames of calcium imaging from A2 fragment during initial state, local events in several spines marked with arrows and a large event. Scale bar i-3 microns. E, F – calcium events in cell bodies and in dendritic spines per 50 s for each experimental condition. (Also see [105, 106]).

The initial levels of activity increased proportionally in cell bodies (from about 9 events to almost 17 events per minute) and in dendritic spines (from 20 to 42 events) following 12 h incubation with 1% EtOH. Both acute EtOH (1%) and apamin (40 nM) reduce the levels of activity. Interestingly, combination of two treatments was much more efficient at synaptic areas than at cell bodies. Overall, these data support the suggestion that spontaneous activity arisen after withdrawal of chronic EtOH is sensitive to both acute ethanol and apamin as well as to their combination, especially at the postsynaptic area.

Regarding dendritic spines, we could not detect any significant changes in their density or morphology following 12 – 24 hours of chronic EtOH (data not shown). In contrast, 5 days of incubation, associated with a strong and permanent reduction in spontaneous activity led to predominance of thin and long spines, and to reduction in the number of mature mushroom spines (see [104 - 106]). These data are summarized in Fig. (**26**).

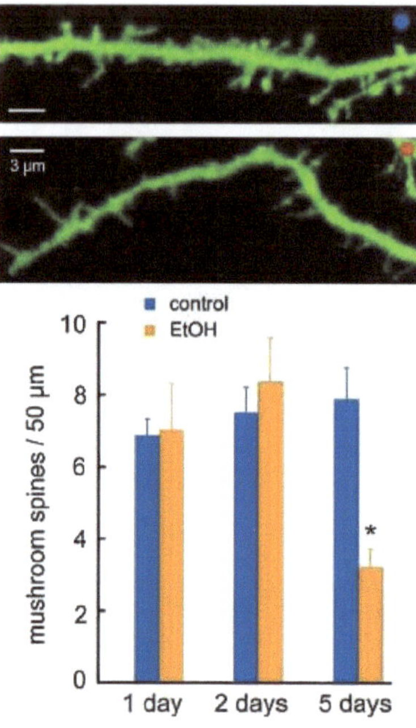

Fig. (26). Upper panel: examples of dendritic arbor with spines in control (upper image) and following 5 d of 1% EtOH (lower image). Lower panel: change in the number of mushroom dendritic spines after 5 days of chronic EtOH application. (Modified from [10]). (Also see [105, 106]).

In vivo Acute and Chronic Experiments

One of objective measures of the effect of alcohol under *in vivo* conditions, which provides clear quantitative results, is the rotarod, in which the time of animal retention on a rotating rod is measured. Holding on the rod is a matter of several brain functions, including the vestibular and cerebellar mechanisms. Still, an involvement of hippocampus and motor areas of cerebral cortex in the retention is also indicated.

We first established a correlation between the amount of 12% alcohol intraperitoneal injection (per animal weight) and its concentration in blood. Two concentrations were set according to pilot experiments: 0.05% and 0.1% in blood. Higher concentrations were found to be less instrumental because of very unstable position of animal on the rod and a quick fall. 1 month-old littermate male mice were used. Both concentrations of EtOH have been tested in acute and chronic exposure experiments. Results are shown on Figs. (**27A & B**).

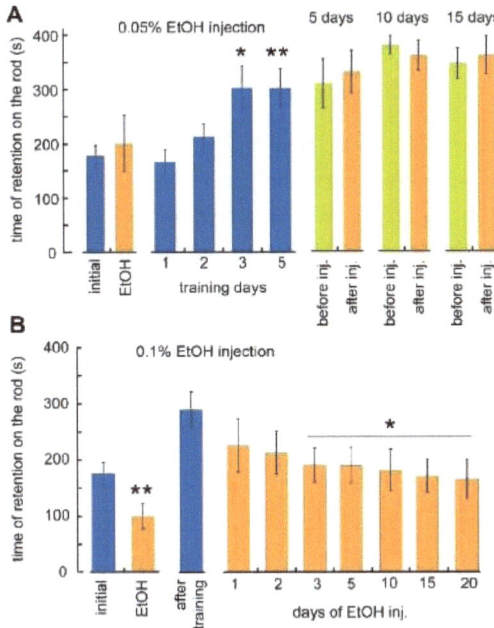

Fig. (27). Acute and chronic exposure to 0.05% and 0.1% ethanol (EtOH) in mice retaining on rotarod *In vivo*. Rod with a diameter of 6 cm, placed at the height of 60 cm from the floor is rotating at the speed of 10 turns/min.

Data show that initial 0.05% EtOH concentration in the blood of untrained mice did not change the suspension time (panel A, left). Training of mice on rotarod was done twice a day during five sequential days, in which animals were not injected. Following the training their ability to hold on the rod rose from 180 to about 300 s (A, middle part). During next 15 days, animals were tested on the rod, then injected with EtOH and tested again (A, the right part). Data do not reveal any significant differences neither between injected and non-injected state of the animals nor a reduction in performance during all the 15 days of the chronic treatment.

Substantially different results were obtained with 0.1% EtOH. Its acute effect reduced the untrained mice performance from about 180 to 100 s (panel B, left). Training process was similar to that, shown on the panel A, with only the "after training" column placed. Chronic exposure to 0.1% EtOH after the 5 days of training revealed clear yet insignificant time of retention during first two days of injection and a progressing reduction of the retention time during all 20 subsequent days of experiment (B, right part).

PLANT FLAVONOIDS AND ALCOHOL

Overview

In the scientific literature there is fragmented and insufficient information about the therapeutic effect of plant flavonoids (Fl's) (or extracts containing Fl's) on alcohol intoxication of the brain. The process, apparently, involves antioxidant properties, but their direct or indirect influence remains largely unknown. Occasionally, out of a wide range of these substances, catechins (monomers), as well as oligomers and polymers of procyanides are isolated. Their presence is documented in numerous foodstuffs such as red wine, fruit juices, tea, *etc*. They all include flavanols with a characteristic ketone group (flavan-3-ol). It is doubtful that flavonoids reach significant concentrations in the brain. The explanation of their action may include involvement in fine signaling pathways that respond to weaker influences.

Historically, the biological and pharmaceutical activities of Fls have been correlated with their antioxidant effect: either by direct influence or by changing the redox potential of the cell [109]. According to the modern view, the antioxidant ability of Fls with donation of a hydrogen atom in itself is not yet capable of explaining their bioactivity *In vivo*. Some hypotheses were proposed to explain the activity of Fls: 1) modulation of intracellular signaling cascades; 2) effects on gene expression and 3) interactions with mitochondria [110 - 112].

Flavonoids are polyphenolic compounds, usually of plant origin. They consist of two aromatic carbon rings and one benzene ring. The main groups of Fls are:

1. flavonols (kaempferol, quercetin);
2. flavones (apigenin, luteolin);
3. isoflavones (diazein, genistein);
4. flavanones (hesperetin, naringenin)
5. flavanols (catechin, epicatechin, EGGG);
6. anthocyanidins (pelargonidin, cyanidin, malvidin) [113].

Do Fls Penetrate the Blood-brain Barrier (BBB)?

Functions of BBB include control over the influx of foreign substances into the brain, as well as the maintenance of the internal microenvironment [114]. Complex studies have shown that many Fls freely penetrate the BBB. Moreover, it was found that their ability to do so depends on the degree of fat solubility. Thus, the capture of less polarized O-methylated metabolites is more likely than the capturing of their more polarized precursors. Nevertheless, water-soluble forms (for example, glucuronides) are able to overcome BBB by active transport [115]. Experiments in animals have shown that tea flavanol EGCG, administered orally, penetrates into brain tissue [116]. Indirectly, the complex effect of Fls on the whole brain was confirmed by cognitive tests. Nevertheless, it was found that under *in vivo* conditions they accumulate in comparatively small (micro- and nanomolar) concentrations, which is clearly insufficient for a direct antioxidant effects [117], for which it requires much larger, - millimolar doses of substances.

Effects of Fls on Memory and Cognitive Abilities

It has been shown that many Fls reduce neurotoxicity and improve cognitive abilities of animals in the experiment: in particular, they reduce the time of searching for a hidden platform in the Morris watermaze [118]. The mechanism of this effect is unknown: a number of hypotheses are considered. According to one of them, Fls improve the supply of oxygen to the brain [119], which is especially important for the functionally higher brain regions, or can contributes to neuregenesis [120] and to increase in the number of synapses [121]. The formation of long-term memory, which requires mRNA and protein synthesis, is controlled by cyclic AMP (cAMP) -dependent protein kinase (PKA), calcium-Calmodulin kinase, protein kinase C (PKC) and mitogen-activated protein kinase (MAPK). These factors lead to activation of the signaling protein cAMP-response element-binding (CREB), which is a transcription factor, and attaches itself to the promoter region of many important genes responsible for synaptic plasticity [122]. It is believed that the Fls directly interact with the signaling pathways of MAPK and thus activate CREB [123, 124].

Another target of Fls may be the brain derived neurotrophic factor (BDNF) which is required for the viability of central neurons [125, 126]. Alcohol also has similar effects to those of BDNF [127]. Conversely, an increase in the level of BDNF leads to an improvement in memory by enhancing the translation of proteins. Morphologically, BDNF rise is expressed in the increase in the size of dendritic spines, but whether Fls can cause such visible changes remains unexplored. Since the size of dendritic spines is correlated with cognitive abilities, Fls should be tested as potential “enhancers” of mental activity both in control and in a case of chronic influence of alcohol intoxication [see for review 128].

Another possible locus of action of Fls is on specific excitatory or inhibitory ion channels. For example, a direct effect of flavonoid quercetin on acetylcholine receptor-mediated ion currents has been reported [129]. Flavonoid baicalein extracted from skullcaps, was able to reduce glutamate release in rat hippocampus, protecting neurons from cytotoxicity [130]. Multiple effects are described for $GABA_A$ receptor channel pharmacology influenced by different Fls, for example, by apigenin [131]. Specifically some flavonoid glycosides, such as linarin, are sedative and anticonvulsant agents likely interacting with $GABA_A$ receptors [132]. Calcium-activated potassium channels, related to cell resting potential and stages of repolarization (as discussed above) can also serve a potential target for Fls. Thus, there is evidence that flavonoid quercetin may modulate vasodilatation by acting on Ca^{2+}-dependent SK channels [133]. Based on published sources, we do not yet have direct indications of the SK-channel modulation by Fls, but this effect requires experimental verification.

Suppression of Neural Inflammations and Alcohol Intoxication by Flavonoids

Neuroinflammatory and alcohol-intoxication processes in the brain can lead to massive damage and death of neurons, as in Alzheimer's disease [134, 135], or ischemic stroke. The main factor in this case is the production of nitric oxide on the background of increased expression of inducible NO synthase (iNOS). In particular, NO is capable of selectively inhibiting mitochondrial respiration through cytochrome C oxidase, which leads to the termination of ATP synthesis. Thus, the uncontrolled growth of iNOS production in glial cells is the main step towards inflammatory neurodegeneration. So the importance of controlling this path becomes obvious. In particular, an effective inhibitor of iNOS production is structured homologous to some of the Fls, indicating their possible anti-inflammatory effect. It has also been shown that flavanols, flavones and flavonols are capable of inhibiting NO production [see 5 for review].

Flavonoid-mediated Modulation of Neurons via Affecting Signaling Pathways

Phosphorylation or dephosphorylation of key molecules and modulation of the corresponding genes expression govern intracellular signaling pathways. Fls can interact with the zones of ATP docking on the key protein structure elements. In addition, it can reduce the effect of excitatory neurotoxicity through direct suppression of calcium intervention, possibly through enhanced synthesis of the GluR2 subtype of the AMPA receptor that does not conduct calcium. An alternative way is to suppress cellular kinases, usually activated by increased calcium [113].

The desensitization of the excitatory receptors by Fls is also proposed. Indeed, a number of receptors possessing specific binding zones of Fls. have been described in cortical neurons: in particular, these are adenosine and GABA receptors. In addition, monomeric and dimeric flavanols display nanomolar affinity to testosterone receptor which means that they can act *via* steroid type receptors to modulate the expression of genes mediated by CREB. Since a direct anomalous effect of alcohol on a number of neuronal brain receptors has been documented [136], we consider it necessary to pay special attention to this sector of Fls influencing particular receptors/channels.

The following is a brief summary of data regarding the interaction of flavonoids with nervous system.

Common Ways to Treat Alcoholism

Many patients with alcoholism undergo treatment reluctantly or do not wish to be treated at all, because they do not consider themselves unhealthy. However, even in case of their consent, there is a very limited number of effective anti-alcoholism medication.

Detoxification: Treatment of alcoholism, as a rule, begins with a detoxification program that lasts from four to seven days. In this case, sedatives are used to prevent shivering, agitation, mind confusion, hallucinations or other symptoms of withdrawal [137].

Oral preparations: Alcohol-sensitizing drug disulfiram (Antabuse) does not treat alcoholism, but only reduces addiction to alcohol, causing negative physiological reactions, such as hot flushes of nausea, vomiting and headache. Naltrexone (ReVia), a drug long known in the market, also blocks addiction to alcohol. Acamprosat (Campral) also removes alcoholic cravings, but unlike previous ones does not cause painful conditions [138].

Unfortunately, at present there are practically no drugs on the pharmaceutical market that improve nervous functions of patients suffering from alcohol abuse. One of the leading centers for the study and drug development - National Institute of Health - published a report titled "*In vivo* medication development for alcohol-related conditions" where unfavorable state in this field is reflected: "*There is a very significant need to develop treatments for the prevention and amelioration of the cognitive disturbances and structural brain damage associated with alcohol consumption. Among excessive drinkers, there is a wide spectrum of cognitive disturbances associated with chronic ethanol consumption, ranging from mild cognitive disturbances such as reduced attentional and visuospatial abilities to severe amnesia, dementia and psychosis. Thus, medications to improve cognitive function in alcoholics, particularly in alcoholic dementia and Korsakoff's psychosis, would lead to enrichment in quality of life of alcoholics as well as reduction in costs of long-term institutionalization. Recent studies have suggested that some medications can improve memory to a clinically meaningful degree in some patients with alcohol-induced amnesia. Unfortunately, very little research has been conducted on developing pharmacological cognitive enhancers or neuroprotective agents, a topic of major concern*" [139 - 142].

Effects of Plant Extracts and Specific Flavonoids on Neuronal Activity: A Screening Study

Screening new biologically active substances of natural origin that have been widely used during centuries in traditional medicine in order to find new drugs is a key objective of modern pharmaceutical research. Many current therapies for neurological disorders lack specificity and are associated with drug dependence and tolerance [143 - 145]. Of particular interest are drugs derived from little-known or traditional medicinal plants, containing a mixture of active substances, which demonstrate a large therapeutic range of properties. For instance, some herbal sedatives strengthen inhibitory processes and/or reduce excitation without causing muscle relaxation, ataxia, sleepiness and drug dependence [146, 147]. They also may enhance the effect of analgesics, anesthetics, and anti-epileptic and nootropic drugs and facilitate the normal onset of sleep [146 - 149]. They also may enhance the effect of analgesics, anesthetics, and anti-epileptic and nootropic drugs and facilitate the normal onset of sleep [146 - 149].

Several widespread species of the genus *Melampyrum Linnaeus: Melampyrum sylvaticum* and *Melampyrum pratense* (Mp) have sufficient resource base in Europe [150]. According to some studies Mp may affect the nervous system [151, 152]. Due to their unique properties, these plants are widely used in folk medicine as sedatives and anticonvulsants [151 - 153].

Above ground plant parts are used for the preparation of aqueous extracts (tinctures, decoctions), which are prescribed in small doses as an effective treatment in anti-inflammatory, cardio-vascular and neurological diseases, particularly as sedatives and anxiolytics [152 - 154].

The wide application in folk medicine contrasts with rather few studies on the chemical and pharmacological properties of *Melampyrum*. This plant contains a broad range of biologically active compounds, including flavonoids, iridoids and alkaloids [151, 152, 154 - 157].

Particularly, it has been found that Mp contains hyperoside, luteolin, cinaroside, apigenin, known to have multiple effects on the central nervous system. Neuroprotective [158 - 160], antidepressant [161] and anticonvulsive [162] properties of these compounds have been demonstrated. Luteolin could also attenuate diabetes-associated cognitive decline [163]. A function of flavonoids as monoaminergic modulators have been proposed: both luteolin and apigenin facilitate the function of monoamine transporter [164]. Apigenin alters serotonin and dopamine levels in distinct rat brain regions, and is effective in several models of depression [165]. Controversy remains in the literature regarding the effect of apigenin on GABAergic neurotransmission. This flavonoid was shown to be a ligand for the central benzodiazepine receptors exerting anxiolytic and slight sedative effects [166]. It also reduces glutamatergic activity and calcium transients in cultured hippocampal neurons [167]. But other studies argue that this compound reduces the GABA-induced chloride ion current and therefore acts as negative allosteric modulator of GABA [168]. When injected intraperitoneally, apigenin reduced locomotor activity in open field test, but did not demonstrate anxiolytic, myorelaxant or anticonvulsant activities in rats [169]. It is also possible that GABA responses can be enhanced by apigenin only in the presence of the main positive modulator such as diazepam [170].

In fact, the direct effects of *Melampyrum pratense* extract or of its main flavonoid substances on the effects of alcohol on neuronal activity have never been investigated. Moreover, the combination of several active compounds in plant extracts may produce complex effects different from those of single specific molecules [170]. We have now performed a screening study of extracts from Mp as well as its main flavonoids hyperoside, cinaroside, apigenin and luteolin on neuronal activity modified by alcohol and recorded from rat hippocampal cultures.

Extraction and Content of Flavonoids in Melampyrum Sylvaticum and Melampyrum Pratense

Vegetable raw material was milled to a particle size passing through a sieve with openings of 10 mm in diameter. The dust-free raw powder was mixed with distilled water at a ratio of 1:10, on a boiling water bath under reflux for 1 h. The final concentration of the extract in stock solution which we added to the recording medium in μl/ml was 0.1 mg of the dry extract per 0.3 μl of the stock solution (or 0.33 mg/1μl). The extracts contained a complex of biologically active substances the main groups of which were flavonoids, iridoids and amino acids. The overall content of flavonoids and iridoids in extracts of *Melampyrum sylvaticum* and *Melampyrum pratense* is about several percent of the dry matter. Amino acids were found in very small amounts of less than 1% in the extract. Additionally these values varied significantly depending on the way of extraction: water-based or alcohol-based. These data are summarized in Table **1**.

Table 1. Content of some biologically active substances in Melampyrum sylvaticum and Melampyrum pratense.

Extract		Flavonoids (%)	Iridoids (%)	Amino Acids (%)
Melampyrum sylvaticum	water	2.9	3.0	0.4
	alcohol	2	3.5	0.8
Melampyrum pratense	water	6.9	5.0	0.3
	alcohol	5.2	6.5	0.7

According to the liquid chromatography pattern (not shown here), three main flavonoids were found in all four extracts: quercetin (m.w. 302.2), hyperoside (m.w. 464.4) and cinaroside (m.w. 448.4). Two additional flavonoids were found in much smaller concentrations: apigenin (m.w. 270.2) and luteolin (m.w. 286.2). The last two components are poorly soluble in water, their concentration is reported to be higher in the ethanol extracts of Mp and Ms. The approximate quantitative content of several individual flavonoids is shown in Table **2** as percent. Table **3** shows concentration of the same flavonoid in μM in 1 μl of extract diluted in 1 ml of the recording solution.

Table 2. Percent of active flavonoids in dry extract of Melampyrum sylvaticum (Ms) and Melamphyrum pratense (Mp).

Flavonoids (%) in Dry Extract of **Ms and Mp**	*Method of Extraction*			
	Water Extraction		*Alcohol Extraction*	
	Ms	**Mp**	**Ms**	**Mp**
hyperoside	0.56	1.8	0.16	1.02
cinaroside	0.4	0.5	0.3	0.7
apigenin	0.01	0.01	0.15	0.2
luteolin	0.06	0.09	0.25	0.18

Table 3. Concentration of active flavonoids in 1 μl extract of Melamphyrum pratense, diluted in 1 ml of recording medium (1:1000).

Flavonoids (in μM) in 10 μl of Extract, Diluted in 1 ml of Recording Medium.	*Method of Extraction*			
	Water Extraction		*Alcohol Extraction*	
	Ms	**Mp**	**Ms**	**Mp**
hyperoside	4	12.2	1.1	6.8
cinaroside	3	3.7	2.2	5.1
apigenin	0.12	0.12	1.8	2.4
luteolin	0.7	1.1	2.9	2.1

It should be mentioned that following either method of extraction the outcome of flavonoids was relatively low compared to that revealed by chromatography. Additionally, some flavonoids, including very common quercetin and several others have not been included into the table. Many flavonoids are present in extracts in trace concentrations and cannot have any significant effect on the activity of biological systems. We tested a wide range of quercetin concentrations for the ability to affect the spontaneous activity of neurons in the control or in the presence of various doses of alcohol. No statistically significant effect was detected in any of the combinations.

Effects of Extracts from Melamphyrum Pratense and their main Active Flavonoids: Hyperoside, Cinaroside and Luteolin on Neuronal Activity

Effect of the range of concentrations of four listed flavonoids on neuronal spontaneous activity has been tested and summarized in Table **4** as percent of the basal level, taken as 100%. Taking into consideration the similar but overall higher proportion of main active flavonoids in both water and alcohol extract of *Melamphyrum pratense* we have conducted several experiments using the extracts of this plant.

Table 4. Screening of the concentration range of main flavonoids from Melamphyrum pratense for their effect on spontaneous activity of cultured neurons.

Hyperoside		Cinaroside		Apigenin		Luteolin	
Con.	**Activity (%)**	**Con.**	**Activity (%)**	**Con.**	**Activity (%)**	**Con.**	**Activity (%)**
1	101.5±5.1	1	96.6±13.9	1	100.7±10.6	0.5	151.7±8.6
2	91.8±14.2	2	84.2±14.8	2	106.6±9.3	1	213.8±15.5
4	83.5±7.5	3	25.9±6.5	4	104.6±11.9	1.5	242.2±20.7
6	61±8.3	4	33.3±3.7	6	117.9±9.2	2	115.5±11.2
8	47.5±4.2	6	44.5±10.2	8	125.8±14.3	4	58.7±6.4
10	36.7±3.3	8	81.5±3.6	10	160.3±15.2	6	27.3±4.03
15	26.7±4.5	10	107.4±6.5	15	168.2±16	8	8.1±3.01
30	22.5±6.2	15	127.8±12.1	30	186.5±19.8	10	0
50	4.5±2.2	25	168.5±14.8	-		15	0
70	0.4±1.7	30	77.8±5.5	-		30	0
-	-	50	17.6±1.8	-		50	0
-	-	70	4.6±3.7	-		70	0
wash	0	wash	40.7±9.25	wash	106.5±11.9	wash	69.8±6.9

Based on data in Table **4**, it can be predicted that very low levels of water-based MP extract, such as 0.4 µl/ml in recording medium, will produce relatively small inhibition of activity, induced by hyperoside (about 4µM) and cinaroside (about 1.5 µM), and no effect will be made by apigenin (0.12 µM) which has insufficient effect at less than 10 µM. On the other side, 0.5 µM of luteolin will have a pronounced facilitating effect, so that overall activity will go up. When the concentration of extract doubles (0.8 µl/ml), a significant inhibition will be obtained from hyperoside and cinaroside (about 9 and 3 µM, respectively), while the action of luteolin (at about 0.9 µl/ml) will partly compensate the "downshift". Higher doses of water extract from Mp (1.5-2.0 µl/ml) will effectively inhibit the activity mainly due to 25µM of hyperoside, while cinaroside at 8 µM of and luteolin at 2 µM of will have no significant effect (Fig. **28**, top panel). Alcohol extracts of Mp may reveal somewhat longer facilitation phase due to lower hyperoside, and higher cinaroside #x0026; luteolin in the tincture. Thus, even at the range of 1.5-2.5 µl/ml content of Mp extract in the recording medium, hyperoside seems to be less efficient as the activity suppressor, while luteolin will remain about neutral or slightly inhibitory. On the contrary, cinaroside (15-20 µM) has a tendency to significantly increase the level of spontaneous discharges (Fig. **28**, bottom panel). At the stages of higher concentrations, more than 2 µl/ml both extracts will turn to suppress the activity mainly due to hyperoside (Fig. **29A**). Luteolin reveals complex bi-phasic effect facilitating the cell activity at very low concentrations and becoming a strong inhibitor right after that beginning from 4-6 µM (Fig. **29C**). Cinaroside also produces a complex effect, at first slightly suppressing and then facilitating cell activity (Fig. **29B**). The second stage is more important for the alcohol Mp extract as it contains significantly higher doses of the flavonoid compared to the water extract. It may be the reason that the alcohol extract has a prolonged facilitating effect compared to water extract as shown on Fig. (**28**) (bottom panel). Initial doses of hyperoside slightly and gradually suppress the activity. Relatively high concentrations of hyperoside (higher than 20 µM) seem to be toxic to the cultured cells. As shown on Table **4**, no recovery of activity is observed following the washout of hyperoside. In contrast, complete recovery can be seen following 25-30 µM of cinaroside and 15 µM of luteolin. Nevertheless, partial recovery can be found even following the application of 70µM of both flavonoids. As mentioned above, apigenin plays a minor role in the formation of the pattern of neuronal activity shaped by the complex of flavonoids in a given extract. Apigenin is found at higher concentration in the alcohol extract of Mp due to its lower solubility in water. This flavonoid can be responsible for the later stages of enhanced activity and for its slower decay at very high concentrations of the extract such as 1.5-3 µl/ml when the water extract almost completely suppress the activity.

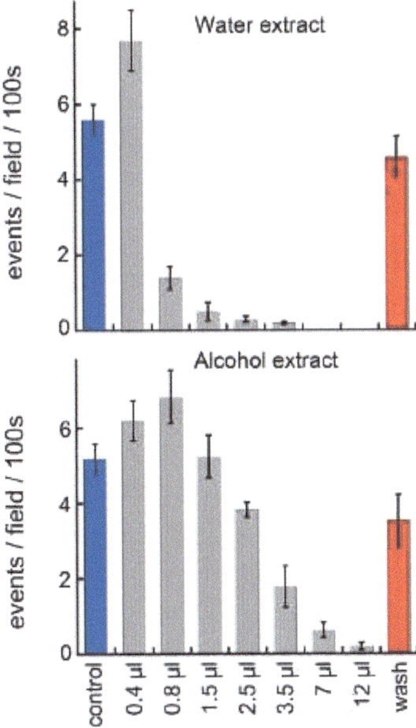

Fig. (28). Effects of different concentrations of water and alcohol extracts of Melamphyrum pratense on spontaneous activity of cultured hippocampal neurons.

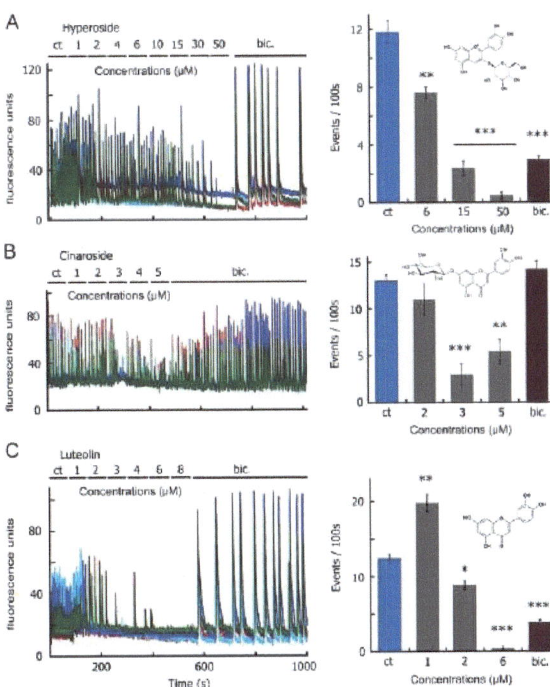

Fig. (29). Effects of the hyperoside, cinaroside and luteolin at the range of concentrations on cultured hippocampal cell activity in control and in the presence of bicuculline. (Modified from [171]).

An important issue in the context of antagonizing the pathological activation induced by low doses of EtOH is the sedative GABAergic effect of extract from Mp and their main active flavonoids. Fig. (**29**) illustrates the effect of individual flavonoids (hyperoside, cinaroside and luteolin) in the presence of bicuculline – a selective blocker of $GABA_A$ receptor.

Panel A of Fig. (**29**) (on left) shows the inhibitory effect of increased concentrations of hyperoside and the partial recovery in the presence of 50 μM flavonoid and 10 μM bicuculline (on right). This concentration of flavonoid corresponds to about 4 μl of water Mp extract diluted in 1 ml of recording medium. Panel B of the figure demonstrates a complete recovery of activity in bicuculline in the presence of 5 μM cinaroside related to 1.8 μl of extract. Its higher concentrations become potentiating rather than depressing the activity. As mentioned above, luteolin increases the rate of calcium events at low concentrations and becomes highly inhibitory at 6 μM which equals to about 3 μl/ml. Bicuculline only partly recovers the rate but as with hyperoside significantly amplifies the amplitude of calcium events (Fig. (**29C**), left and right).

We conclude that water extract of Mp is efficient in suppressing the cell activity at much lower concentrations than alcohol extract. Fig. (**30**) demonstrates the partial recovery of cell activity following 1.2 μl of water Mp extract in the presence of bicuculline.

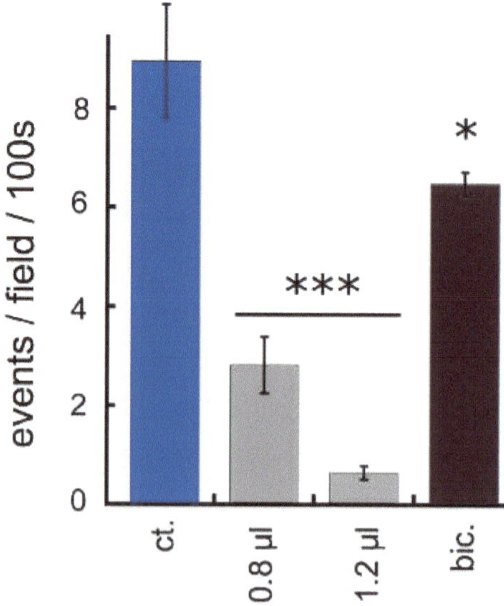

Fig. (30). Effect of water extract of Melamphyrum pratense in the presence of bicuculline (bic.). (Modified from [171]).

Water Extract from Melamphyrum pratense and Alcohol

It has been shown in chapter 2 that lower doses of EtOH ranging between 0.25 to 1.5% increase the rate of neuronal activity in the cultured hippocampal neurons as well as restrict the retention time of intact animals on the rod. Sedative effect *Melamphyrum pratense* may eliminate these pathological actions of EtOH as it is suggested by traditional medicine.

We therefore tested the cellular effects of EtOH in the presence of both Mp water and alcohol extracts. As shown in Fig. (**28**), low (0.4 μl) water extract and 0.4-0.8 μl alcohol extracts excite rather than inhibit neuronal activity. We made sure that mentioned potentiation does not share with EtOH the same pathway of excitation (data not shown) and skipped these doses, focusing on ones, which typically suppress the activity. The two doses: 0.8 and 1.5 μl/ml were tested with water extract of Mp and 1.5, 2.5, 3.5, 7 and 12 μl/ml – for the alcohol extract. Results are presented in Fig. (**31A** & **B**).

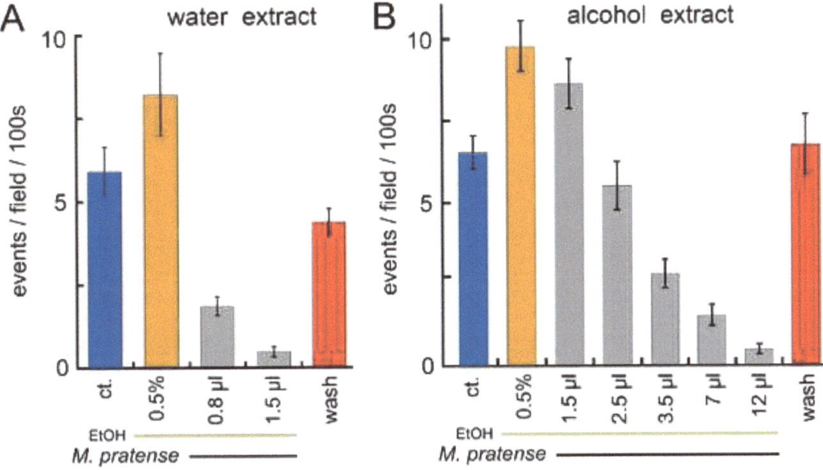

Fig. (31). Effects of water (A) and alcohol (B) extracts of Melamphyrum pratense on ethanol (EtOH) - enhanced neuronal activity.

Panels A&B of Fig. (**31**) indicate anti-ethanol activity of both extracts: water and alcohol-based ones. Already 0.8 μl/ml on panel A and 2.5 μl/ml on panel B reduce the excitation of low EtOH. Remarkably, washout of both extracts and the EtOH recover the initial levels of cellular activity. Yet, Fig. (**30**) shows that Mp extracts mainly work through enhancement of GABAergic transduction, so that bicuculline is able to reverse the extract-induced silencing of calcium bursts. Therefore, it may be hypothesized that the putative elimination of the excitatory effect of low EtOH may simply have an overall sedative nature unrelated to a specific anti-alcohol activity of both extracts. In order to test the last statement, we performed the opposite experiment in which EtOH is added not prior but after the application of Mp extracts. Results of such experiments are shown in Fig. (**32**).

Panels A and B of Fig. (**32**) suggest that both extracts at the concentrations of 0.8 μl/ml and 2.5 μl/ml, respectively, significantly reduce the level of spontaneous activity in the culture. Nevertheless, in both cases, a typical range of effects, produced by EtOH can be seen. More detailed analysis is performed on the panel A with water extract of Mp. Thus, 0.5-1.5% ethanol could gradually increase the level of activity even in the presence of the extract while the higher doses (2-3.5%) bit by bit suppressed the activity and finally 4% of EtOH completely blocked it. Again, this complex effect was washable. A similar yet less detailed analysis is shown in panel B with the alcohol extract for which some selected concentrations of EtOH: 0.5, 1, 2 and 3% have been tested with about the same outcome.

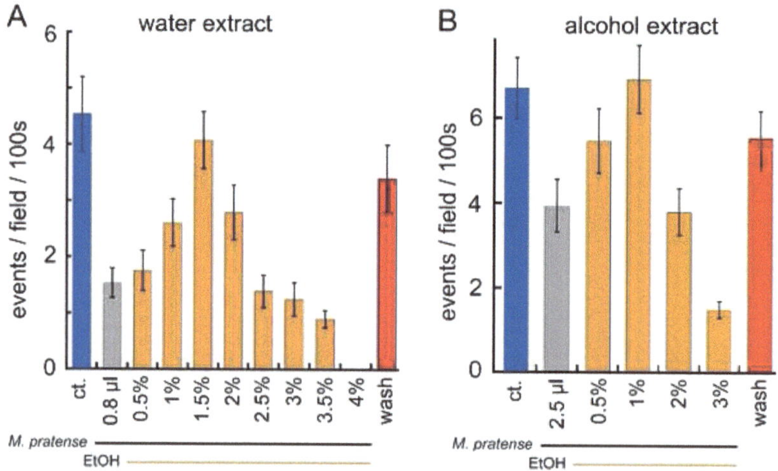

Fig. (32). Water Melamphyrum pratense extract (A) and its alcohol extract (B) (at 0.8 and 2.5 μl/ml, respectively) do not affect the overall pattern of neuronal activity shaped by the range of concentrations of ethanol (EtOH).

We therefore conclude that despite several indications from folk medicine, no specific ethanol-related activity of water and alcohol extracts of *Melamphyrum pratense* can be documented. Mp has a complex effect on the levels and patterns of spontaneous calcium events in cultured hippocampal culture, which can be partly explained by the specific and as well complex activities of its constituent active flavonoids: hyperoside, cinaroside, luteolin and apigenin. At the same time we do not exclude some additional effects of the minority rare flavonoids, iridoids and other biologically active substances that can be found the either of extracts and in the plant itself. Thus, hyperoside and apigenin have unidirectional effects on the neuronal activity; on decreasing and the other – increasing the spiking rate but having quite different threshold of activity. In contrast to this, cinaroside and luteolin have more complex pattern of activity. Depending on their particular concentrations, they can either facilitate or suppress the activity. Not all but some of depressive effects of listed flavonoids are realized through GABAergic system as the experiments with $GABA_A$ blocker bicuculline show. The nature of facilitative effects of the flavonoids remains unknown. Their study was out of the scope of our work. The only clear conclusion to which we could come up with after this screening part is that the extracts we studied do not have a specific anti-alcohol effect and, therefore, cannot be proposed as a prospective model of the drug for alcohol intoxication caused by its relatively low and the intermediate acute doses. Further studies will be required for a more exhaustive description of the effects *Melamphyrum pratense* on neuronal activity in hippocampal culture.

Alcohol-related Effects of Acetylpectolinarin from *Linaria*: *In Vivo* and *In Vitro* Studies

Overview of Linaria Mill

The genus *Linja* Mill. has been traditionally related to the figwort family (*Scrophulariaceae* Juss), although in recent studies it rather corresponds to a plantain family (*Plantaginaceae*) [172, 173]. Representatives of this family are distributed throughout the globe and includes about 200 genera and up to 3,000 species, mostly herbaceous plants, sometimes semi-parasitic, rarely parasitic; sometimes shrubs, very rarely - trees.

The genus *Linaria* includes 150 species and widely distributed in large territories in Eurasia and North Africa. Some types of *Linaria* found in North America, are considered extraneous [174]. In Europe, 70 species of *Linaria* are identified [175] and in the Caucasus, according to various estimates, there are 20 to 38 species.

The genus *Linaria* remains difficult systematically, despite numerous trials. Until now, there is no clear understanding of the division of the genus into sections as well as the boundaries of individual species. The first taxonomist of the genus was K. Linnaeus (1753). He included species of the genus *Linaria* in the genus *Antirrhinum* and divided them into 4 groups according to the leaf arrangement. Then P. Miller in 1768 returned the family name *Linaria* and proposed the way to combine the species [176].

Yellow toadflax or butter-and-eggs (*Linaria* Mill.) is widespread in most of Europe, northern Asia where it forms thickets, most abundant in the forest and forest-steppe zones. In addition, the plant is found in meadows, steppe slopes, in forests, on fringes, sandy and pebble banks of rivers, in garbage places, in fields, gardens, along the edges of roads and railroad embankments: singly, sparsely or in small groups. *Linaria* prefers loose soils, rarely it can be found in crops of cereal crops along the margins of fields, near the borders, on poorly treated sites where the proper agricultural technology is not applied. It is mainly a plant of ruderal habitats.

Yellow toadflax is a perennial herbaceous plant 30-90 cm high with a long, thin, woody rhizome. The main root penetrates into the soil at 80-100 cm. Stem is straight, glabrous, simple or branched, with a large number of leaves to the inflorescence. Leaves alternate, have linear-lanceolate shape with smooth edge, sharp, narrowed at the base and sessile. The axes of the inflorescence, pedicels, and sometimes the calyxes are glandular and pubescent. Flowers are light yellow, zygomorphic, collected in dense, long terminal brushes. Bracts are lanceolate, longer or equal to the pedicels. Calyx is 3 mm long, five-trimmed with lanceolate, thin-pointed fractions. Corolla is corolla is bilabergial, 20-30 mm long with a closed throat, pale yellow with an orange spot on the convex part of lower lip. Number of stamens is four; two of them are longer. Pestle has an upper bilocular ovary, long column and a small stigma. Fruit has a shape of oblong, smooth capsule, 9-10 mm long, 2-3 times longer than calyx. Seeds are 2.5 - 3 mm in diameter, elongated-kidney-shaped, black-gray or black, shining, with rather wide, uneven wings. The wing with small denticles along the edge completely covers the seed. The seed from the convex side is uniformly lumpy, and from the concave – is smooth or with few obtuse hemispherical tubercles [177].

Chemical constituents of genus *Linaria* are well studied [178] but still little is known about the biological activity of substances belonging to different classes of their active compounds. Biologically active substances of Yellow toadflax are mainly represented by flavonoids and iridoid glycosides. One of the most interesting and potentially useful groups belongs to phenolic compounds. Flavones are present in different species of *Linaria*. T. Klobb first identified one of them, known as pectolinarin, more than a hundred and ten years ago [179]. Thus, for a long time, information about the study of flavonoids in *Linaria* was limited to reports regarding the isolation of linarin and pectolinarin. During the 20th century, several different pectolinarine derivatives have been identified in L. vulgaris [180]. Particularly, Bankovskii and his colleagues first identified acetypectolinarine in early 1970th [181, 182]. Using chemical (acetylation, periodate oxidation) and physical methods (NMR spectroscopy), it was found that acetylpectolinarin belongs to a small group of acylated flavonoid glycosides [183,

184]. It is pectolinarine acylated with a single acetic acid residue over a carbohydrate substituent and has the structure of 7-0[6-0-(4-acet-l-α-L-rhamnopyranosyl)] - β-D-glucopyranosido-5-hydroxy-6,4 '-dimeto-Xi-fla vone.

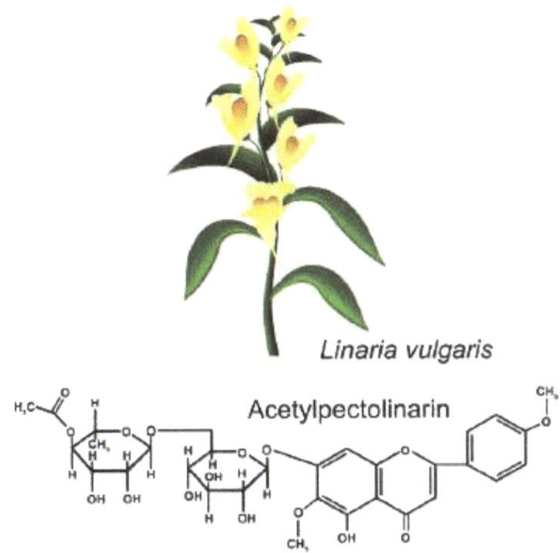

Fig. (33). The 7-0[6-0-(4-acetyl-α-L-rhamnopyranosyl)] - β-D-glucopyranosido-5-hydroxy-6,4 '-dimeto-Xi-flavone.

It has been established that species of the genus *Linaria*, including *L. vulgaris*, are the most promising sources of raw materials for the preparation of pectolinarine and acetylpectolinarin (ACP [185]). During studies of the flavonoid composition of various organs of *Linaria* vulgaris, it was established that the roots and stems of the plant do not contain flavonoids. Chromatographic analysis proved the presence of acacetin, pectolinarigenin, tylianin, linaroside, linarin, pectolinarin, acetylpectolinarin in leaves and flowers [136]. Some authors [185] studied the accumulation of acetylpectolinarin in different plant organs, depending on the phase of development. The maximum amount accumulates in leaves, buds and flowers: 5% in average. In roots and in stems the flavonoid is practically absent, while reaching about 3% in fruits. In leaves, the maximum content of acetylpectolinarin is reached in the vegetative phase (12%) and then its amount gradually decreases to the fruiting phase. In stems, the maximum content of acetylpectolinarin is noted during the growing season, somewhat less during flowering and fruiting. In flowers, however, the content of acetylpectolinarin is greater in the fruiting phase than in the flowering phase.

Yellow toadflax has an unpleasant odor, which is enhanced by drying. The taste of raw materials is sharp, brackish-bitter. According to toxicology studies, flavonoid acetylpectolinarin, isolated from the plant, refers to low-toxic compounds. Its LD50 with subcutaneous administration is calculated as 825 mg/kg. With long-term administration of for 30 days, there were no deviations in the condition of the experimental animals. Following autopsy, no pathological changes were noted in the internal organs.

L. vulgaris has a wide use in traditional medicine, including treatment of coughs and asthma, providing analgesic, sedative and sleep-enhancing effects in central nervous system [178, 186]. However, most promising were numerous indications that L. vulgaris extract and tincture affect drunken and hangover conditions [187, 188]. They are widely used in Russian traditional medicine to treat the spectrum of hangover symptoms such as vertigo, headache, drunken behaviors, and as a sedative. A brief screening of the plant extracts revealed that ACP was known but never investigated [178]. We shall demonstrate herein that ACP exerts an anti-alcoholic effect at a low dose that has no other noticeable effect on neuronal network activity. This action is likely to be mediated by an interaction with SK potassium channels.

Extraction of Acetylpectolinarin (ACP) and the Qualitative Analysis

Molecular formula of ACP is $C_{31}H_{36}O_{16}$, and the molecular mass is 664.6. For preparation, 50.0 g of herb, ground to the size of particles passing through a sieve with holes of 2 mm in diameter, three times extracted with 400 ml of ethyl alcohol 96%. The extracts were combined and evaporated, the residue was dissolved in a minimum amount of a dioxane-water mixture (1: 1) and mixed with 10 g of silica gel. It was dried in a vacuum oven at 40 °C, applied to a column 30 mm in diameter, prepared from 40 g of silica gel. The column was washed with one liter of carbon tetrachloride, after which the acetylpectolinarin was eluted with a chloroform-methanol mixture (96: 4). The eluate was collected in 200 ml portions and TLC in a solvent system of ethyl acetate-ethanol-water (100: 27: 13) examined its component composition. Portions, on the chromatograms of which, after treatment with a 5% alcohol solution of aluminum chloride, one spot of yellow appeared with a value of R_f 0.68 ± 0.01, combined, the eluent was distilled off, and the residue was dried in a vacuum oven at 40 °C. After recrystallization in ethanol, 96% of a white crystalline powder of light yellow color was isolated. The melting point of the obtained substance is 242-244 °C. For details of extraction and ACP verification, see [189].

The powder is soluble in ethanol 95% when heated in a water bath to 30 °C and easily soluble in chloroform. When dissolved, it forms turbid solutions. Very easily soluble in dimethylsulfoxide, forming a clear solution. Almost insoluble in the water.

A 0.1% solution in ethyl alcohol 95% forms a yellow stain with a 1% ethanolic solution of aluminum chloride and a 10% ethanolic sodium hydroxide solution and a dark green color with an ethanol 0.5% solution of trichloride iron. The Shinoda's test (cyanidin reaction) gives a red color of the solution and a red color in the aqueous layer is preserved following the addition of octanol, which proves the glycosidic structure of the substance.

Chromatographic analysis of the obtained substance by TLC was carried out according to the following procedure: 0.05 ml of a 0.1% solution in an ethyl alcohol 95% was applied using micropipette to the starting line of a plate prepared for chromatography, held in air for 10 minutes. Then it was chromatographed in a chamber in a solvent system of ethyl acetate-ethanol-water (100: 27: 13) until the solvent reaches the front line of 15 cm. The chromatogram was removed from the chamber, dried and treated with an alcohol solution of aluminum chloride, 5%. After drying, one yellow spot appeared with an R_f value of 0.68 ± 0.01.

To prove the structure of the substance, IR and NMR spectroscopy methods were used. The infrared spectrum (Fig. **34**) was taken using Specord M-80 in vaseline oil. The infrared spectrum of the substance has absorption bands of valence vibrations of hydroxyl groups at 3400 cm^{-1}, carbonyl ester group at 1724 cm^{-1}, ketone carbonyl at 1664 cm^{-1}, double bonds at 1612 cm^{-1}.

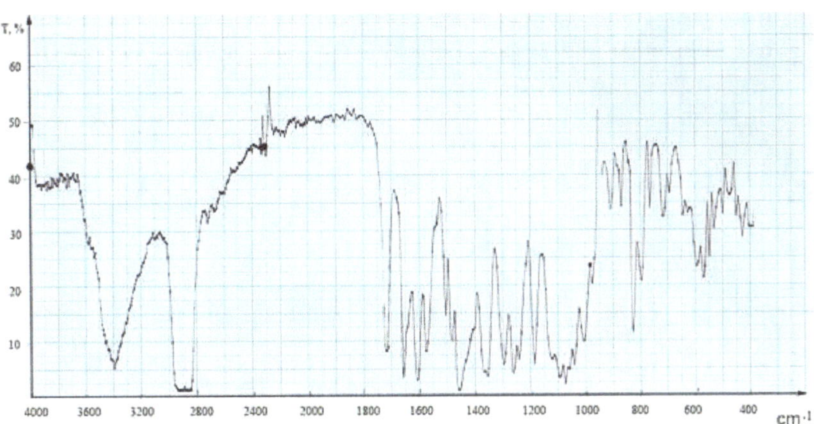

Fig. (34). Infrared (IR) spectrum of Acetylpectolinin.

The proton NMR spectra were recorded using Bruker-300 spectrophotometer with working frequency at 300 MHz. Tetramethylsilane (TMS) was used as an internal standard. In the proton NMR spectrum (Fig. **35**), the following signals are clearly seen: signals of protons -OCH3 groups (3.78, 3.86 ppm); signals of protons of a para-substituted aromatic ring (two doublets at δ = 7.15 ppm and δ = 8.05 ppm, J

= 8.9 Hz); proton signal -$COCH_3$ (singlet at δ = 1.97 ppm), proton signal of OH group of flavone (singlet at δ = 12.94 ppm); proton signals at the third and eighth carbon atoms (singlets at δ = 6.99 ppm and δ = 6.41 ppm, respectively); the signal of the -CH_3 group (doublet at δ = 0.86 with J = 6.3 Hz), the signals of ten methine protons; one methylene group (trivalent functional group =CH−, derived formally from methane); and five hydroxyl groups in the interval from 5.50 ppm up to 3.20 ppm.

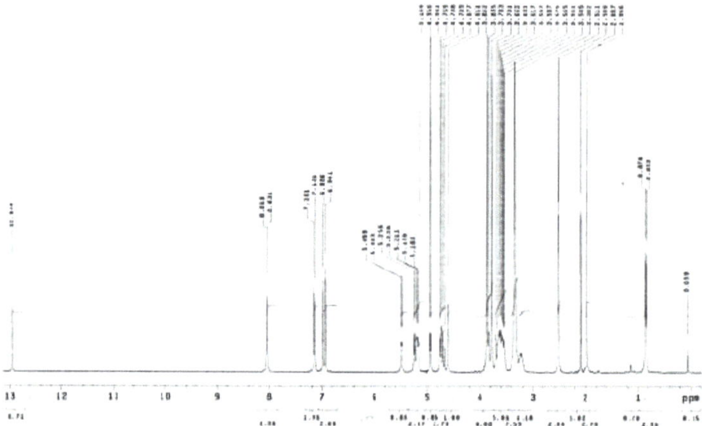

Fig. (35). Proton NMR spectrum of Acetylpectolinarin.

The UV spectrum of the acetylpectolinarin alcohol solution (1: 100) has two absorption maxima - shortwave (273 nm) and longwave (332 nm) (Fig. **36**).

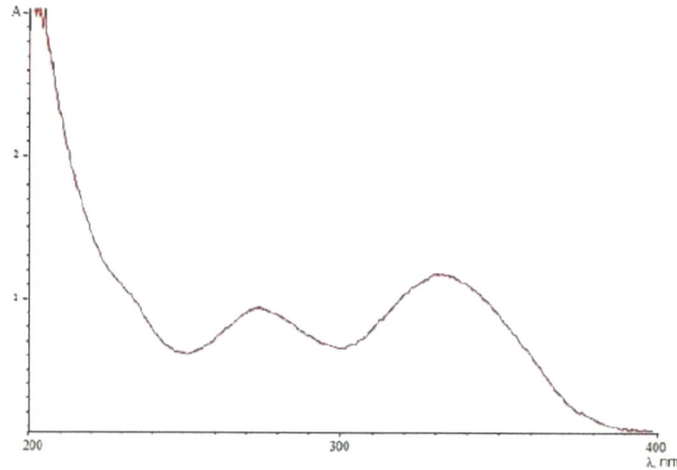

Fig. (36). Ultraviolet (UV) spectrum of Acetylpectolinarin.

Anti-alcohol Effect of Acetylpectolinarin In Vivo

As it has been shown in paragraph 2.5, two different concentrations of EtOH: 0.05% and 0.1% measured in the blood of animals tested after intraperitoneal injection, had very different acute and chronic effects. Thus, lower 0.05% concentration did not decrease and in some experiments even significantly increased the retention time on the rotarod. Chronic injection of this concentration of alcohol during 15 sequential days also did not have any restricting effect of the time spent on the rod. In contrast, the double dose of 0.1% of alcohol measured in the blood had a clear and significant effect, shortening the time of retention under both acute and chronic conditions (Fig. **27**).

Therefore, in the following set of experiments we used the higher 0.1% EtOH and in some control experiment also 0.3%. In order to investigate the possible anti-alcoholic potential of ACP flavonoid, we injected animals intraperitoneally with ACP solution according to 10mg/kg of the mice weight, 10 minutes prior to the alcohol injection. Experiment on rotarod was performed after next 30 minutes. In the case of chronic *In vivo* experiment, mice were first trained to retain on the rotarod during 5 sequential days (Fig. **28A**) and then the same procedure of injection was routinely performed every day during next 20 days using two groups of animals: one receiving only alcohol and the other – ACP #x0026; alcohol. Results of these results are presented in Fig. (**37A-C**).

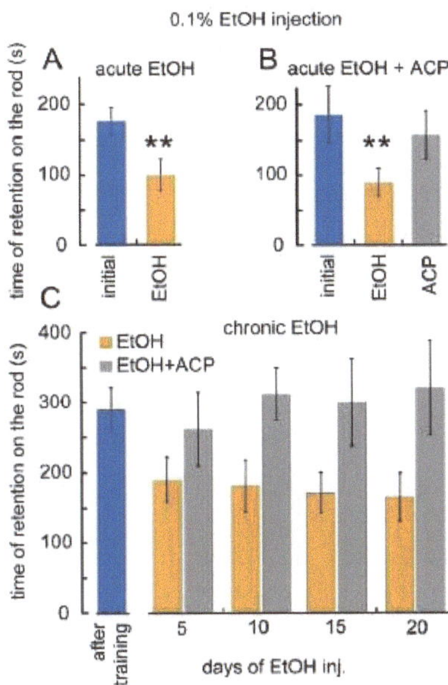

Fig. (37). Acute and chronic effects of 0.1% ethanol (EtOH) and EtOH + Acetylpectolinarin (ACP) on the retention time on rod.

Panel A shows the significant reduction of the time of retention on rotarod for naïve (untrained) mice in acute experiment in control (blue) and after EtOH injection. Panel B demonstrates another set on animals which are able to stay on the rod for about 180s, while after EtOH this time is reduced to about 85s. Prior injection of animals with ACP could elongate and almost completely recover the time until 160s.

After 5-day training twice a day the retention time of mice in control increased to about 290s and daily alcohol injection could reduce this time to about 190s after 5 days and to 255s after 20 days of treatment. Nevertheless, injection of ACP 10 minutes prior to EtOH could completely recover the initial retention time until 265s on the 5th day of the treatment and until 315s on the 20th day (Fig. **37**).

Another important issue is the age-dependent effect of different concentrations of EtOH and the ability of ACP to treat alcohol-induced toxicity at different stages of mice development. To clarify these questions we used four groups of mice at the age of 20, 25, 30 and 35 days. Each group was used only once. Mice in all the groups were not trained on rotarod before. Each group was additionally divided into 5 subgroups of 6. The first group served as control, injected with vehicle. Two other groups were injected with low and high EtOH, (0.1 and 0.3% in the blood). In two additional groups 10mg/kg ACP was injected 10 minutes prior the introduction of corresponding doses of alcohol. Animals were retested on rotarod half an hour after the injections and the results are presented on Fig. (**38**).

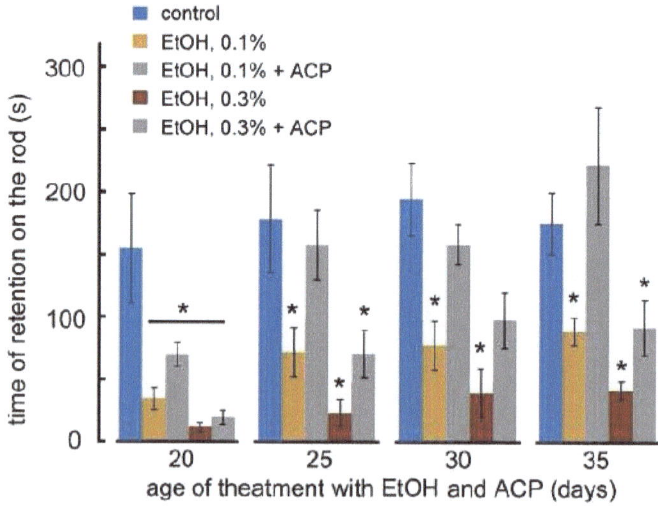

Fig. (38). Dependence of the retention time on the rotarod on the age of mice and concentration of ethanol (EtOH) as well as ability of Acetylpectolinarin (ACP) to block the toxicity of alcohol depending on both the age and the dose of EtOH.

Apparently, alcohol has stronger effect on the younger mice (20 days-old), compared to the older group of 30-35 day-old mice. This effect was more obvious with the lower, than with 0.3%,EtOH. Thus, retention time in the younger group with 0.1/0.3 EtOH was 30 and 10s, correspondingly, while for the oldest group is was about 85 and 45s. The same tendency was seen for ACP pretreated animals. Flavonoid had relatively little anti-toxic effect in the young 0.1% group and no significant change could be observed for 0.3%-treated mice. ACP was able to completely recover the initial time spent on the rod for 25-35-days-old mice but had relatively smaller effect on the 0.3% treated group.

Acute and Chronic Effects of Acetylpectolinarin on the Activity of Cultured Hippocampal Neurons

In the next few paragraphs, we describe the effects of ACP with its ability to prevent alcohol-induced intoxication in cultured neuronal networks as well as analyze some preliminary hypothesis related to the molecular mechanisms of the activity of this flavonoid, extracted from *Linaria*.

Acute Effects of LVE on Spontaneous and Induced Activity of Hippocampal Neurons

We first tested the extract of *Linaria* (LVE) in control condition. We applied 0.5, 1, 2, 5, 10 and 20 µl of the stock solution of LVE diluted 1:1000 in the recording medium. Results of this examination are presented in Table **5**.

Table 5. Effect of different concentrations of *Linaria* extract (LVE) diluted 1:1000 in recording medium, on neuronal activity in control conditions.

Rate of calcium events/100s	control	Concentrations of LVE (µl) in recording medium (1:1000)					
		0.5	1	2	5	10	20
	14.2±0.3	13.8±0.3	14.0±0.4	13.2±0.4	11.7±0.15	7.9±0.45	4.1±0.2

All the doses of LVE could be successfully washed out with the complete recovery of the initial level of activity without any visible neurotoxicity such as the rise of basal calcium levels or cell death. The first four concentrations did not change the network activity while 5 and 10 µl of LVE reduced it significantly and we therefore excluded them from farther investigations.

We next examined the effects of LVE on the sequential phases of the hippocampal network activity in presence of increasing concentrations of EtOH. As shown in the previous paragraphs, low doses of EtOH typically increase the level of spontaneous discharges and its higher dosed have an opposite effect.

Thus, here ethanol at the dose of 0.5% increased the cell basal activity up to 19.7±0.67, while 3% decreased it to 2.4±0.07. Addition of LVE could affect the increased but not the decreased levels of activity. These results are summarized in Table **6**.

Table 6. Effect of *Linaria* extracts (LVE) on neuronal activity in presence of low and high ethanol (EtOH).

Treatments	EtOH (%)	LVE (µl) in recording medium (1:1000)				
		0	0.5	1	2	5
Rate of calcium events/100s	0.5	19.5±0.67	17.6±0.6	13.8±0.44	13.0±0.51	11.2±0.18
	3	2.4±0.07	2.5±0.16	2.2±0.21	1.8±0.12	1.1±0.09

Content and Acute Effects of ACP Under Control Conditions

We next hypothesized that the anti-alcohol effect of the three weaker solutions of LVE (0.5, 1 and 2 µl/ml of recording medium) can be explained by the presence of its main flavonoid ACP. In order to test this assumption we first estimated the content of ACP in LVE. Results are summarized in Table **7**.

Table 7. Estimated concentration (µM) of Acetylpectolinarin (ACP) in *Linaria* extract (LVE), diluted in recording medium (µl/ml)

LVE (µl/ml)	0.5	1	2	5	10	20
ACP (µM)	3.5	7	14	35	70	140

ACP is purely diluted in water and easily dissolved in organic solvents such as dimethylsulfoxid (DMSO). We have used 5mM stock solution of ACP in DMSO in order to investigate the effects of various concentrations of ACP on spontaneous network activity (Fig. **39**). The same cultures were exposed to increasing concentrations of the drug.

Apparently, there was no effect of ACP at 1-30µM concentrations, while 60-120 µM could gradually reduce the level of activity. In fact, only in the presence of 100 and 120 µM of ACP the reduction was statistically significant. Washout of flavonoid could shortly and slightly enhance the activity (first wash panel on Fig. **39**) but a few tens of seconds later, it returned to the initial level.

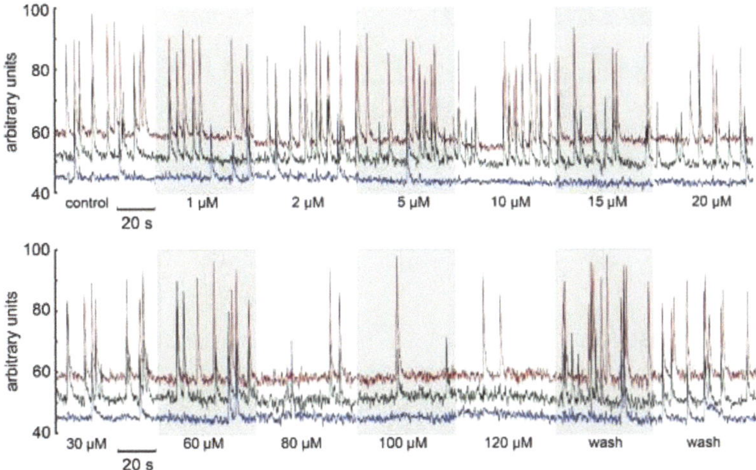

Fig. (39). Dose-dependent effects of acetylpectolinarin (ACP) on spontaneous activity in the cultured networks. (Modified from [107]).

These results are summarized in Fig. (**40A**). Thus, lower doses of ACP did not change either rate or the amplitude of the network activity except for first 3 min of application (Fig. **40B**). This observation is similar to the effect of apamin, described in the paragraph 2.3.3 (Fig. **8**) which also briefly elevates the level of cell activity followed by a complete recovery in 10 minutes of exposure. Additionally there was no significant effect of ACP on the burst decay time (not shown).

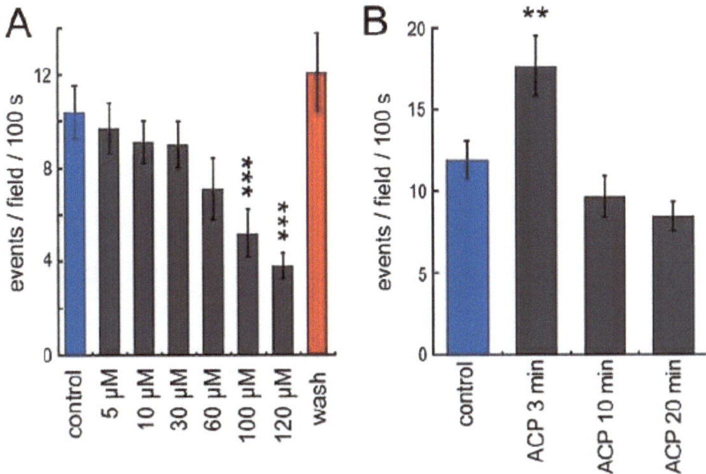

Fig. (40). The rates of bursts at the range of Acetylpectolinarin (ACP) concentrations: 5, 10, 30, 60, 100 and 120 µM (A). Change of the rates of bursts in the presence of 10 µM ACP at 3, 10 and 20 min following application (B). (Modified from [107]).

Alcohol-related Acute Effects of ACP

It was shown above that the extract of *Linaria* could antagonize the disinhibiting effect of alcohol. We therefore studied the effects of several concentrations of ACP on the action of low EtOH on network activity.

As seen before, moderate (0.25 and 0.5%) ethanol caused an increase in the number of network bursts. This increase was completely blocked by ACP, at both EtOH concentrations.

Fig. (**41A**) demonstrates the traces of three neurons marked on panel B (left). Application of low, 0.25% EtOH increased the frequency of spikes, a representative example of which is shown in panel B middle and right (as net change of fluorescence). Sequential addition of 10 μM ACP brings the activity back to baseline, which remains almost unchanged following washout of both compounds. During the next part of the same experimental set, two sequential EtOH doses of 0.25 and 0.5% are added creating a new increase of activity. And again, ACP effectively blocks this increase. Results of this trial are displayed in the figure panel C.

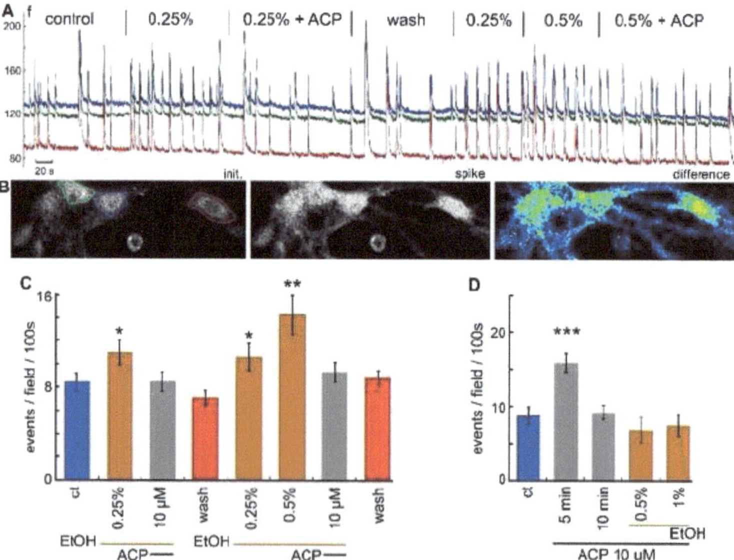

Fig. (41). Acetylpectolinarin (ACP) blocks enhancing effect of ethanol (EtOH) on spontaneous activity. A&B – examples of neuronal activity. C – ACP blocks the effect of EtOH. D – ACP prevents the enhancing effect of EtOH. (Modified from [107]).

An opposite experimental sequence is presented on panel D, where a dose of 10 μM ACP was added prior to ethanol. Interestingly, the initial effect of ACP, seen here and in Fig. (**40B**), is to cause an increase in rate of network bursts within 3-5 minutes after onset of exposure to the drug, but this effect subsided after 10 minutes of exposure, at which time, the blockade of ethanol effect was highly significant. After complete recovery, in the presence of flavonoid in recording medium, 0.5 and 1% of alcohol were consistently added to the same set of neurons, but this time – without any additional modification of the basal activity. It should be noted that 10 μM of flavonoid corresponds to about 1.5 μl of LVE, as follows from Table **7**.

As seen above, high ACP suppressed network bursts, additionally decreasing the amplitudes of events (see Fig. **39**, and also Fig. **42A**).

If high, 100 μM ACP is used after the lower 10 μM concentration has abolished the alcohol-induced facilitation, it will act as it would be alone, by decreasing both the rate and the amplitudes of recorded calcium events. This result indicates that additional suppressive effect of ACP is not alternated by the presence of alcohol and may act through the same biochemical pathway as the lower dose. Still, this elevated portion of ACP does not seem to be toxic and can be successfully washed out as shown on the Fig. (**42B** & **C**).

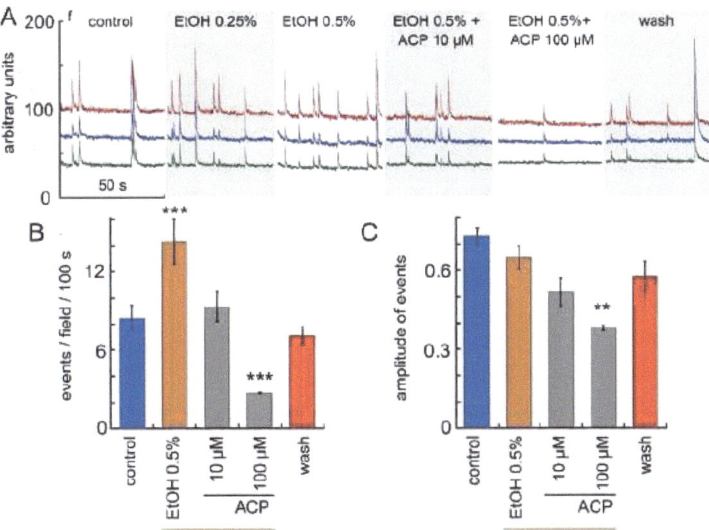

Fig. (42). Presence of ethanol (EtOH) does not affect the ability of high Acetylpectolinarin (ACP) to suppress the rate of neuronal activity and decreases the amplitude of events. (Modified from [107]).

Facilitative responses of particular neuronal networks to alcohol may differentiate significantly, being low or moderate in some cases and very strong in some others. Figs. **43A** & **C** brings an example of a very strong response of a network to the range of EtOH concentrations.

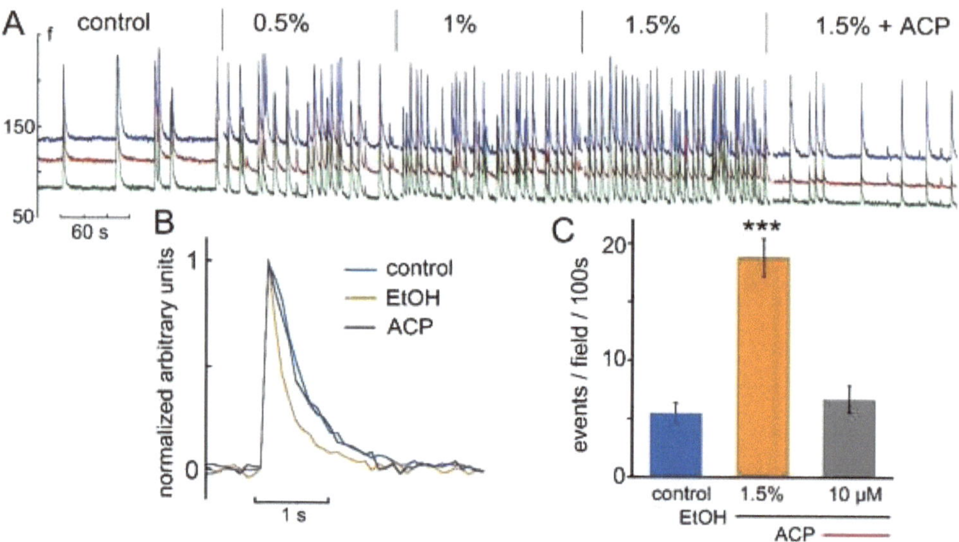

Fig. (43). Acetylpectolinarin (ACP) counteracts the effect of EtOH to speed up the recovery of calcium spikes associated with the network bursts.

Recorded traces of three neighboring neurons shown on panel A show about 3-fold increase of the rate with 0.5% EtOH and about 4-fold – following 1.5%. Once again, addition of flavonoid was able to block this increase. In addition, ACP counteracted the effect of ethanol to speed up the recovery of the elevated calcium spikes associated with the network bursts, as seen above with alcohol alone (paragraph 2.3.1, Figs. **2C** and **3**) as well as for alcohol + apamin (paragraph 2.3.3, Fig. **9** and 11C). These data suggest that apamin and ACP share same molecular and cellular pathway, antagonizing the alcohol-induced disinhibition.

Finally, we examined the effect of ACP on the suppression of activity produced by high concentration (3%) of ethanol (Fig. **44**). Using a range of ACP concentrations, we were unable to affect the suppression of activity produced by high ethanol, whether it was applied before or after the exposure to the drug. In fact, the high ACP concentration, applied together with ethanol, completely suppressed the spontaneous activity, to show a complete recovery after washout of both agents. None of doses of ACP, beginning from 5μM and up to 100μM could facilitate the suppressed activity. This effect corresponds to the LVE data summarized in Tables **5**, **6** & **7** and covering the range of ACP concentration in the extract from about 3.5 to 140 μM.

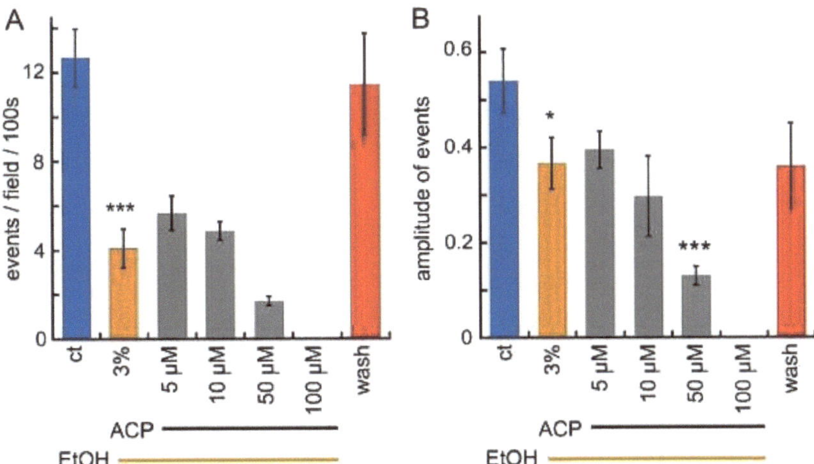

Fig. (44). Acetylpectolinarin (ACP) does not block the effect of high 3% ethanol (EtOH), which decreases network activity. Left is the number of events, right is the amplitude of events. (Modified from [107]).

Alcohol-related Chronic and Morphological Effects of ACP

One of major effects of chronic alcohol abuse, which the chronic EtOH *in vitro* mimics, is the withdrawal syndrome or so called chronic intermittent ethanol as it has been described elsewhere [94]. At the level of primary culture, this syndrome is reflected in two ways: 1) as an essential and long-term increase of spontaneous activity after alcohol withdrawal and 2) as a deep depression of activity, reduced to very low, abnormal levels. Both effects are seen with ethanol, completely absent from the recording medium and may last at least several hours. The origin of these two polar states lies in the duration of chronic alcohol pretreatment as well as in the concentration of the agent. Thus, lower (from 0.25 up to 1% EtOH) doses and shorter (from few hours and up to 1-2 days) treatments lead to enormous activation upon withdrawal, while higher concentrations, such as 2-3% and extended, 2-5 day-long application bring the neuronal network to the highly reduced levels of activity. These data were described in paragraph 2.4, Figs. (**14-19**). We have also shown that the depressive phase of chronic alcohol influence is related to inhibitory cells and sensitive to $GABA_A$ blocker bicuculline (Figs. **20-22**). Finally, we have shown, that the state of abnormal activation following alcohol withdrawal after shorter treatment is sensitive to SK-channel blocker apamin, indicating that even after removal of EtOH, SK channels remain excessively activated or, alternatively, the number/density of these channels were upregulated at least in some cells.

In this context, ACP was found to reduce the cellular EtOH withdrawal syndrome when introduced after the removal and washout of 0.5% ethanol, which was incubated with the cultures during 24 hours (data not shown). Interestingly, ACP could reduce the elevated neuronal activity only during its perfusion with the recording medium. After removal of ACP, the activity recovers.

More interesting are the results showing that ACP can prevent neurotoxic effects of chronic alcohol following the joint long-term incubation of both compounds. It was found that 10μM ACP does not induce neurotoxicity or cell death. Results of this preliminary experiment are shown in Figs. (**45A** & **B**).

It can be seen that the flavonoid was able to prevent the chronic alcohol-induced potentiation of neuronal activity induced by its withdrawal. More experiments should be carried out to clarify the ability of ACP to prevent depressive effect of long-lasting incubation with EtOH, such as shown in Fig. (**19**), right part of each panel. Particularly, our preliminary results suggest that incubation with 1% EtOH during 5 days in the presence of ACP may be instrumental in preserving the initial level of mushroom dendritic spines (see [104 - 106]), typically reduced during this treatment in the absence of flavonoid, as shown in Fig. (**26**), right column.

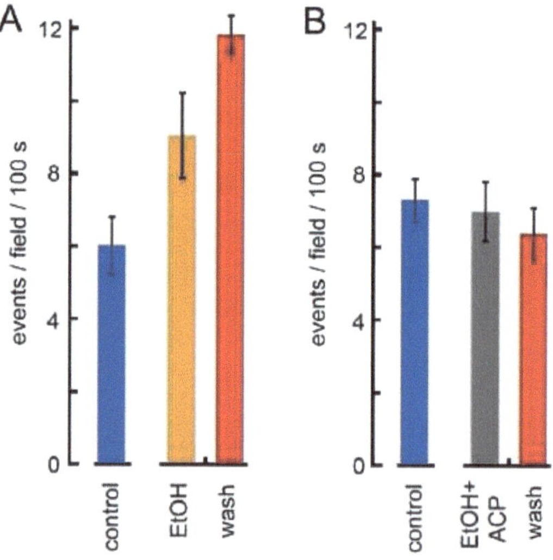

Fig. (45). Chronic effect of 0.5% ethanol (EtOH) applied for 24 hours and washed out (A) versus the same experimental set performed in the presence of 10 μM Acetylpectolinarin (ACP).

The Ways Flavonoids Eliminate the Effects of Alcohol

ACP Probably Acts via SK Channels

In an attempt to examine the mechanisms through which ACP exerts its effect on low ethanol concentrations, we return to previous studies (paragraph 3.2.3) which implied that ethanol acts *via* an effect on SK potassium channels. We performed these experiments, to find that apamin (20 or 40 nM) an SK channel blocker, at low concentrations suppressed the increase in network activity produced by low EtOH (Figs. **11** and **12**).

It was shown that apamin also increased the decay time of the network spikes, as expected from its action to block SK channels.

We examined the interaction between ACP and 1-EBIO, an SK channel opener. It was shown that 1-EBIO at low concentrations of 200-1000nM by itself caused a large increase in spontaneous network activity (Fig. **13A** and Fig. **46C**). At higher concentrations 1-EBIO gradually decreased the number of events as well as their amplitude (Figs. **13A** & **B**). Both of these effects: potentiation and depression could be blocked by 40nM apamin. Moreover, 1-EBIO and ethanol had similar impact on the duration of spontaneous events, speeding up the decay time, an effect that blocked by apamin (panels C&D).

Fig. (**46**) provides a direct comparison of the recovery of initial level of spontaneous neuronal activity, assisted by 40 nM apamin (panel C) and by 10μM flavonoid ACP (panel D).

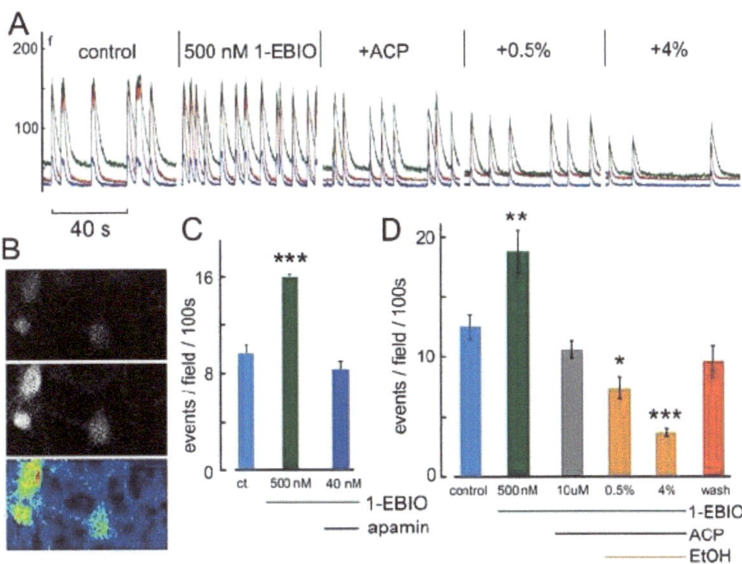

Fig. (46). 1-EBIO, an agonist of SK-channels acts similarly to low doses ethanol (EtOH) and is antagonized by Acetylpectolinarin (ACP). (Modified from [107]).

Background impulse activity of three neurons, shown on panel B was traced on panel A, left, as green, red and blue lines. 500nM 1-EBIO increased the activity in a manner similar to the influence of alcohol and ACP was able to block this potentiation. Interestingly, further application of 0.5% EtOH in the presence of 1-EBIO and ACP decreased rather than increased the activity and this phenomenon manifested itself even more in the presence of 4% EtOH. Summarizing, the effect of 1-EBIO was abolished by apamin and ACP as expected from a SK channel blockers. Low concentrations of ethanol, in presence of ACP, were unable to elevate network frequency (Fig. **46D**), indicating that 1-EBIO and ethanol share the same channel, which is blocked by ACP.

Active Flavonoids of Mp Probably Act via $GABA_A$ Channels

Our experiments indicate that *M. pratense* may act by facilitating responses to GABA, perhaps not at the synaptic site, as the size and kinetics of the sIPSCs were not changed significantly by presence of the drug, but perhaps on the extra synaptic sites (Fig. **47**).

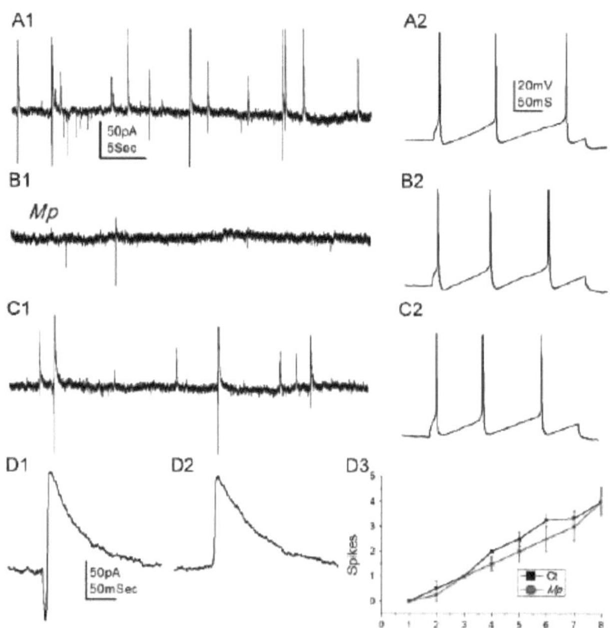

Fig. (47). Effects of Melampyrum pratense (Mp) (2µl/ml) on spontaneous activity and action potentials evoked by depolarizing current pulses in current clamped hippocampal neurons. (A1) Voltage clamped neuron, held at -50 mV, to show inward deflections of sEPSCs, and outward deflections of sIPSCs before, during (B1) and after washout of Mp (C1). A2, B2, and C2 are of the same neuron, corresponding to A1, B1 and C1, which was current clamped around its resting potential (-60 mV), responding to depolarizing current pulses that evoked action potentials. (D1 and D2) Spontaneous IPSCs, shown in an expanded scale, to demonstrate the similarity of their size and decay time constant, before and during exposure to Mp. (D3) Number of spikes (on ordinate), evoked by single or several depolarizing current pulses (on abscissa) (from [171]).

These sites may not result in a massive action on intrinsic and synaptic properties of the recorded neurons, but are sufficient to reduce network activity. Alternatively, the drug may act primarily at the benzodiazepine-modulating site, which may not be expressed under standard recording conditions. Further experiments are needed to explore further the possible GABA site where these drugs may interact.

The present results confirm and provide a tentative basis for the medicinal action of Mp long used in folk medicine in regions of the world, which are enriched with this plant, and suggest that further explorations may provide a more directed indications for this plant extract. An aqueous extract of the herbal plant Mp has distinct, biphasic, concentration dependent action on spontaneous network activity of cultured hippocampal neurons. Flavonoid compounds extracted from Mp mimic the facilitator as well as the depressive action of Mp.

Nevertheless, despite the fact that Mp extract as well as its active flavonoid components are able to produce sedative action on the background of alcohol intoxication, still this effect is not specific to particular ethanol activity and therefore is able to activate the neurons to a certain degree also at the presence of Mp or its flavonoids as shown in Fig. (**32**).

CONCLUSION

The present results describe for the first time a selective effect of the flavonoid extract acetylpectolinarin (ACP) on reactivity of cultured hippocampal neuronal networks to low concentrations of ethanol. Cultured neurons express spontaneous network bursts expressed as fast and simultaneous rise of intracellular calcium concentrations, associated with action potential discharges. When several neurons in the field of view exhibit simultaneously this rise in calcium, it indicates the presence of a network burst [190]. Imaging spontaneous fluctuations of calcium ions can thus provide a sensitive assay of drug effects on activity in a stable in-vitro system. We have used this system before to describe an effect of ethanol on network activity. Apparently, ethanol at low concentration facilitates network burst activity, while high concentration (above 2%) suppresses it. The facilitation is assumed to involve an interaction with SK channels, whereas the suppression involves activation of GABAergic inhibition. These observations corroborate and extend earlier observations on the effects of ethanol on brain activity and behavior. In the present study, we investigated a flavonoid extracted from *Linaria* vulgais, called acetylpectolinarin (ACP [191],) as well as the extract itself. Used in traditional medicine, this extract is suggested to exert a variety of biological activities [178], including a variety of symptoms of hangover, however the specific activities of ACP have not been studied as yet. In the present study we found that low concentrations of ACP have no effects on their own in the culture system, but they antagonize the facilitatory action of low, physiological concentrations of ethanol on network activity. This action of ethanol is similar to that produced by activation of SK channels with 1-EBIO, and both are antagonized by ACP, as well as by apamin, an SK channel blocker. Our test system does not have the cellular resolution to identify the exact molecular mechanism affected by ACP, but this work provides a solid biological basis for the antidote effect of ACP on excessive consumption of alcohol. Further studies are needed to extend these observations to animal brain and behavior.

CONSENT FOR PUBLICATION

Not applicable.

CONFLICT OF INTEREST

The authors declare no conflict of interest, financial or otherwise.

ACKNOWLEDGEMENTS

Declared none.

REFERENCES

[1] Global status report on alcohol and health 2014. http://www.who.int/substance_abuse/publications/global_alcohol_report/en/

[2] 2000.

[3] Moser MB, Rowland DC, Moser EI. Place cells, grid cells, and memory. Cold Spring Harb Perspect Biol 2015; 7(2)a021808
[http://dx.doi.org/10.1101/cshperspect.a021808] [PMID: 25646382]

[4] Hashemi Nosrat Abadi T, Vaghef L, Babri S, Mahmood-Alilo M, Beirami M. Effects of different exercise protocols on ethanol-induced spatial memory impairment in adult male rats. Alcohol 2013; 47(4): 309-16.
[http://dx.doi.org/10.1016/j.alcohol.2013.01.008] [PMID: 23683528]

[5] A hybridizing of effects as described at Alcohol's Effects from Virginia Tech and Federal Aviation Regulation (CFR) 9117: Alcohol and Flying 2007.

[6] Schuckit M. Four decades of research on the level of response to alcohol as a risk factor for alcoholism: from idea to prevention. Alcohol Alcohol 2013; 48(1): 2-2.
[http://dx.doi.org/10.1093/alcalc/agt072]

[7] Schuckit M. Risk factors for alcohol dependence. Alcohol Alcohol 2013; 48(1): 33-3.
[http://dx.doi.org/10.1093/alcalc/agt100]

[8] Nurmi M, Kiianmaa K, Sinclair JD. Brain ethanol levels after voluntary ethanol drinking in AA and Wistar rats. Alcohol 1999; 19(2): 113-8.
[http://dx.doi.org/10.1016/S0741-8329(99)00022-1] [PMID: 10548154]

[9] Korkotian E, Bombela T, Odegova T, Zubov P, Segal M. Ethanol affects network activity in cultured rat hippocampus: mediation by potassium channels. PLoS One 2013; 8(11)e75988
[http://dx.doi.org/10.1371/journal.pone.0075988] [PMID: 24260098]

[10] Korkotian E, Botalova A, Odegova T, Segal M. Chronic exposure to alcohol alters network activity and morphology of cultured hippocampal neurons. Neurotoxicology 2015; 47: 62-71. [http://dx.doi.org/10.1016/j.neuro.2015.01.005] [PMID: 25655208]

[11] Chin JH, Goldstein DB. Effects of low concentrations of ethanol on the fluidity of spin-labeled erythrocyte and brain membranes. Mol Pharmacol 1977; 13(3): 435-41. [PMID: 876032]

[12] Kalivas PW, Volkow ND. The neural basis of addiction: a pathology of motivation and choice. Am J Psychiatry 2005; 162(8): 1403-13. [http://dx.doi.org/10.1176/appi.ajp.162.8.1403] [PMID: 16055761]

[13] Lau CG, Zukin RS. NMDA receptor trafficking in synaptic plasticity and neuropsychiatric disorders. Nat Rev Neurosci 2007; 8(6): 413-26. [http://dx.doi.org/10.1038/nrn2153] [PMID: 17514195]

[14] Kelley AE. Memory and addiction: shared neural circuitry and molecular mechanisms. Neuron 2004; 44(1): 161-79. [http://dx.doi.org/10.1016/j.neuron.2004.09.016] [PMID: 15450168]

[15] Vengeliene V, Bilbao A, Molander A, Spanagel R. Neuropharmacology of alcohol addiction. Br J Pharmacol 2008; 154(2): 299-315. [http://dx.doi.org/10.1038/bjp.2008.30] [PMID: 18311194]

[16] Li Q, Fleming RL, Acheson SK, *et al.* Long-term modulation of A-type K(+) conductances in hippocampal CA1 interneurons in rats after chronic intermittent ethanol exposure during adolescence or adulthood. Alcohol Clin Exp Res 2013; 37(12): 2074-85. [http://dx.doi.org/10.1111/acer.12204] [PMID: 23889304]

[17] Bukiya AN, Kuntamallappanavar G, Edwards J, Singh AK, Shivakumar B, Dopico AM. An alcohol-sensing site in the calcium- and voltage-gated, large conductance potassium (BK) channel. Proc Natl Acad Sci USA 2014; 111(25): 9313-8. [http://dx.doi.org/10.1073/pnas.1317363111] [PMID: 24927535]

[18] Zorumski CF, Mennerick S, Izumi Y. Acute and chronic effects of ethanol on learning-related synaptic plasticity. Alcohol 2014; 48(1): 1-17. [http://dx.doi.org/10.1016/j.alcohol.2013.09.045] [PMID: 24447472]

[19] Richardson BD, Rossi DJ. Recreational concentrations of alcohol enhance synaptic inhibition of cerebellar unipolar brush cells *via* pre- and postsynaptic mechanisms. J Neurophysiol 2017; 118(1): 267-79. [http://dx.doi.org/10.1152/jn.00963.2016] [PMID: 28381493]

[20] Romero AM, Renau-Piqueras J, Pilar Marin M, *et al.* Chronic alcohol alters dendritic spine development in neurons in primary culture. Neurotox Res 2013; 24(4): 532-48. [http://dx.doi.org/10.1007/s12640-013-9409-0] [PMID: 23820986]

[21] Golub HM, Zhou QG, Zucker H, *et al.* Chronic alcohol exposure is associated with decreased neurogenesis, aberrant integration of newborn neurons, and cognitive dysfunction in female mice. Alcohol Clin Exp Res 2015; 39(10): 1967-77. [http://dx.doi.org/10.1111/acer.12843] [PMID: 26365148]

[22] Ariwodola OJ, Weiner JL. Ethanol potentiation of GABAergic synaptic transmission may be self-limiting: role of presynaptic GABA(B) receptors. J Neurosci 2004; 24(47): 10679-86. [http://dx.doi.org/10.1523/JNEUROSCI.1768-04.2004] [PMID: 15564584]

[23] Fleming RL, Manis PB, Morrow AL. The effects of acute and chronic ethanol exposure on presynaptic and postsynaptic gamma-aminobutyric acid (GABA) neurotransmission in cultured cortical and hippocampal neurons. Alcohol 2009; 43(8): 603-18. [http://dx.doi.org/10.1016/j.alcohol.2009.10.006] [PMID: 20004338]

[24] Sanna E, Talani G, Busonero F, *et al.* Brain steroidogenesis mediates ethanol modulation of GABAA

receptor activity in rat hippocampus. J Neurosci 2004; 24(29): 6521-30.
[http://dx.doi.org/10.1523/JNEUROSCI.0075-04.2004] [PMID: 15269263]

[25] Wakita M, Shin MC, Iwata S, Nonaka K, Akaike N. Effects of ethanol on GABA(A) receptors in GABAergic and glutamatergic presynaptic nerve terminals. J Pharmacol Exp Ther 2012; 341(3): 809-19.
[http://dx.doi.org/10.1124/jpet.111.189126] [PMID: 22434676]

[26] Valenzuela CF, Jotty K. Mini-Review: effects of ethanol on GABAA receptor-mediated neurotransmission in the cerebellar cortex - recent advances. Cerebellum 2015; 14(4): 438-46.
[http://dx.doi.org/10.1007/s12311-014-0639-3] [PMID: 25575727]

[27] Sun Y, Jiang SY, Ni J, *et al.* Ethanol inhibits histaminergic neurons in mouse tuberomammillary nucleus slices *via* potentiating GABAergic transmission onto the neurons at both pre- and postsynaptic sites. Acta Pharmacol Sin 2016; 37(10): 1325-36.
[http://dx.doi.org/10.1038/aps.2016.66] [PMID: 27498778]

[28] Lindemeyer AK, Shen Y, Yazdani F, *et al.* α2 subunit-containing GABA(A) receptor subtypes are upregulated and contribute to alcohol-induced functional plasticity in the rat hippocampus. Mol Pharmacol 2017; 92(2): 101-12.
[http://dx.doi.org/10.1124/mol.116.107797] [PMID: 28536106]

[29] Jensen JP, Nipper MA, Helms ML, *et al.* Ethanol withdrawal-induced dysregulation of neurosteroid levels in plasma, cortex, and hippocampus in genetic animal models of high and low withdrawal. Psychopharmacology (Berl) 2017; 234(18): 2793-811.
[http://dx.doi.org/10.1007/s00213-017-4671-0] [PMID: 28664280]

[30] Rose AK, Grunsell L. The subjective, rather than the disinhibiting, effects of alcohol are related to binge drinking. Alcohol Clin Exp Res 2008; 32(6): 1096-104.
[http://dx.doi.org/10.1111/j.1530-0277.2008.00672.x] [PMID: 18445111]

[31] Quinn PD, Fromme K. Individual differences in subjective alcohol responses and alcohol-related disinhibition. Exp Clin Psychopharmacol 2016; 24(2): 90-9.
[http://dx.doi.org/10.1037/pha0000065] [PMID: 26867000]

[32] Pickering C, Wicher G, Rosendahl S, Schiöth HB, Fex-Svenningsen A. A low ethanol dose affects all types of cells in mixed long-term embryonic cultures of the cerebellum. Basic Clin Pharmacol Toxicol 2010; 106(6): 472-8.
[http://dx.doi.org/10.1111/j.1742-7843.2009.00528.x] [PMID: 20074269]

[33] Carpenter-Hyland EP, Chandler LJ. Homeostatic plasticity during alcohol exposure promotes enlargement of dendritic spines. Eur J Neurosci 2006; 24(12): 3496-506.
[http://dx.doi.org/10.1111/j.1460-9568.2006.05247.x] [PMID: 17229098]

[34] Yool AJ, Gruol DL. Development of spontaneous and glutamate-evoked activity is altered by chronic ethanol in cultured cerebellar Purkinje neurons. Brain Res 1987; 420(2): 205-19.
[http://dx.doi.org/10.1016/0006-8993(87)91240-6] [PMID: 2890413]

[35] Tu Y, Kroener S, Abernathy K, *et al.* Ethanol inhibits persistent activity in prefrontal cortical neurons. J Neurosci 2007; 27(17): 4765-75.
[http://dx.doi.org/10.1523/JNEUROSCI.5378-06.2007] [PMID: 17460089]

[36] Brodie MS, Scholz A, Weiger TM, Dopico AM. Ethanol interactions with calcium-dependent potassium channels. Alcohol Clin Exp Res 2007; 31(10): 1625-32.
[http://dx.doi.org/10.1111/j.1530-0277.2007.00469.x] [PMID: 17850640]

[37] Basavarajappa BS, Ninan I, Arancio O. Acute ethanol suppresses glutamatergic neurotransmission through endocannabinoids in hippocampal neurons. J Neurochem 2008; 107(4): 1001-13.
[http://dx.doi.org/10.1111/j.1471-4159.2008.05685.x] [PMID: 18796007]

[38] Acevedo MB, Pautassi RM, Spear NE, Spear LP. Age-dependent effects of stress on ethanol-induced motor activity in rats. Psychopharmacology (Berl) 2013; 230(3): 389-98.

[http://dx.doi.org/10.1007/s00213-013-3163-0] [PMID: 23775530]

[39] Elibol-Can B, Dursun I, Telkes I, Kilic E, Canan S, Jakubowska-Dogru E. Examination of age-dependent effects of fetal ethanol exposure on behavior, hippocampal cell counts, and doublecortin immunoreactivity in rats. Dev Neurobiol 2014; 74(5): 498-513. [http://dx.doi.org/10.1002/dneu.22143] [PMID: 24302592]

[40] Van Skike CE, Botta P, Chin VS, *et al.* Behavioral effects of ethanol in cerebellum are age dependent: potential system and molecular mechanisms. Alcohol Clin Exp Res 2010; 34(12): 2070-80. [http://dx.doi.org/10.1111/j.1530-0277.2010.01303.x] [PMID: 20860615]

[41] McArdle P. Substance abuse by children and young people. Arch Dis Child 2004; 89(8): 701-4. [http://dx.doi.org/10.1136/adc.2003.040584] [PMID: 15269062]

[42] Liang J, Olsen RW. Alcohol use disorders and current pharmacological therapies: the role of GABA(A) receptors. Acta Pharmacol Sin 2014; 35(8): 981-93. [http://dx.doi.org/10.1038/aps.2014.50] [PMID: 25066321]

[43] Zheng M, Liu C, Pan F, Shi D, Zhang Y, Zhang Y. Antidepressant-like effect of hyperoside isolated from Apocynum venetum leaves: possible cellular mechanisms. Phytomedicine 2012; 19(2): 145-9. [http://dx.doi.org/10.1016/j.phymed.2011.06.029] [PMID: 21802268]

[44] Zeng KW, Wang XM, Ko H, Kwon HC, Cha JW, Yang HO. Hyperoside protects primary rat cortical neurons from neurotoxicity induced by amyloid β-protein via the PI3K/Akt/Bad/Bcl(XL)-regulated mitochondrial apoptotic pathway. Eur J Pharmacol 2011; 672(1-3): 45-55. [http://dx.doi.org/10.1016/j.ejphar.2011.09.177] [PMID: 21978835]

[45] Xu B, Li XX, He GR, *et al.* Luteolin promotes long-term potentiation and improves cognitive functions in chronic cerebral hypoperfused rats. Eur J Pharmacol 2010; 627(1-3): 99-105. [http://dx.doi.org/10.1016/j.ejphar.2009.10.038] [PMID: 19857483]

[46] Shen Y, Lindemeyer AK, Gonzalez C, *et al.* Dihydromyricetin as a novel anti-alcohol intoxication medication. J Neurosci 2012; 32(1): 390-401. [http://dx.doi.org/10.1523/JNEUROSCI.4639-11.2012] [PMID: 22219299]

[47] Ali Shah S, Ullah I, Lee HY, Kim MO. Anthocyanins protect against ethanol-induced neuronal apoptosis *via* GABAB1 receptors intracellular signaling in prenatal rat hippocampal neurons. Mol Neurobiol 2013; 48(1): 257-69. [http://dx.doi.org/10.1007/s12035-013-8458-y] [PMID: 23645118]

[48] Chen G, Bower KA, Xu M, *et al.* Cyanidin-3-glucoside reverses ethanol-induced inhibition of neurite outgrowth: role of glycogen synthase kinase 3 Beta. Neurotox Res 2009; 15(4): 321-31. [http://dx.doi.org/10.1007/s12640-009-9036-y] [PMID: 19384566]

[49] Penetar DM, Maclean RR, McNeil JF, Lukas SE. Kudzu extract treatment does not increase the intoxicating effects of acute alcohol in human volunteers. Alcohol Clin Exp Res 2011; 35(4): 726-34. [http://dx.doi.org/10.1111/j.1530-0277.2010.01390.x] [PMID: 21244439]

[50] Shannon EE, Staniforth ER, McNamara J, Bernosky-Smith KA, Liguori A. Response inhibition impairments predict alcohol-induced sedation. Alcohol Alcohol 2011; 46(1): 33-8. [http://dx.doi.org/10.1093/alcalc/agq080] [PMID: 21127353]

[51] Holdstock L, King AC, de Wit H. Subjective and objective responses to ethanol in moderate/heavy and light social drinkers. Alcohol Clin Exp Res 2000; 24(6): 789-94. [http://dx.doi.org/10.1111/j.1530-0277.2000.tb02057.x] [PMID: 10888066]

[52] Lovinger DM. Alcohols and neurotransmitter gated ion channels: past, present and future. Naunyn Schmiedebergs Arch Pharmacol 1997; 356(3): 267-82. [http://dx.doi.org/10.1007/PL00005051] [PMID: 9303562]

[53] Harris RA. Ethanol actions on multiple ion channels: which are important? Alcohol Clin Exp Res 1999; 23(10): 1563-70. [http://dx.doi.org/10.1097/00000374-199910000-00001] [PMID: 10549986]

[54] Aguayo LG, Peoples RW, Yeh HH, Yevenes GE. GABA(A) receptors as molecular sites of ethanol action. Direct or indirect actions? Curr Top Med Chem 2002; 2(8): 869-85. [http://dx.doi.org/10.2174/1568026023393426] [PMID: 12171577]

[55] Cardoso RA, Brozowski SJ, Chavez-Noriega LE, Harpold M, Valenzuela CF, Harris RA. Effects of ethanol on recombinant human neuronal nicotinic acetylcholine receptors expressed in Xenopus oocytes. J Pharmacol Exp Ther 1999; 289(2): 774-80. [PMID: 10215652]

[56] Roberto M, Nelson TE, Ur CL, Brunelli M, Sanna PP, Gruol DL. The transient depression of hippocampal CA1 LTP induced by chronic intermittent ethanol exposure is associated with an inhibition of the MAP kinase pathway. Eur J Neurosci 2003; 17(8): 1646-54. [http://dx.doi.org/10.1046/j.1460-9568.2003.02614.x] [PMID: 12752382]

[57] Davis TJ, de Fiebre CM. Alcohol's actions on neuronal nicotinic acetylcholine receptors. Alcohol Res Health 2006; 29(3): 179-85. [PMID: 17373406]

[58] Zhou Q, Verdoorn TA, Lovinger DM. Alcohols potentiate the function of 5-HT3 receptor-channels on NCB-20 neuroblastoma cells by favouring and stabilizing the open channel state. J Physiol 1998; 507(Pt 2): 335-52. [http://dx.doi.org/10.1111/j.1469-7793.1998.335bt.x] [PMID: 9518697]

[59] Tonner PH, Miller KW. Molecular sites of general anaesthetic action on acetylcholine receptors. Eur J Anaesthesiol 1995; 12(1): 21-30. [PMID: 7535690]

[60] Welsh BT, Goldstein BE, Mihic SJ. Single-channel analysis of ethanol enhancement of glycine receptor function. J Pharmacol Exp Ther 2009; 330(1): 198-205. [http://dx.doi.org/10.1124/jpet.109.154344] [PMID: 19380602]

[61] Sebe JY, Eggers ED, Berger AJ. Differential effects of ethanol on GABA(A) and glycine receptor-mediated synaptic currents in brain stem motoneurons. J Neurophysiol 2003; 90(2): 870-5. [http://dx.doi.org/10.1152/jn.00119.2003] [PMID: 12702707]

[62] Ye JH, Tao L, Ren J, *et al.* Ethanol potentiation of glycine-induced responses in dissociated neurons of rat ventral tegmental area. J Pharmacol Exp Ther 2001; 296(1): 77-83. [PMID: 11123365]

[63] Ziskind-Conhaim L, Gao BX, Hinckley C. Ethanol dual modulatory actions on spontaneous postsynaptic currents in spinal motoneurons. J Neurophysiol 2003; 89(2): 806-13. [http://dx.doi.org/10.1152/jn.00614.2002] [PMID: 12574458]

[64] Eggers ED, Berger AJ. Mechanisms for the modulation of native glycine receptor channels by ethanol. J Neurophysiol 2004; 91(6): 2685-95. [http://dx.doi.org/10.1152/jn.00907.2003] [PMID: 14762156]

[65] Siggins GR, Roberto M, Nie Z. The tipsy terminal: presynaptic effects of ethanol. Pharmacol Ther 2005; 107(1): 80-98. [http://dx.doi.org/10.1016/j.pharmthera.2005.01.006] [PMID: 15963352]

[66] Zhu PJ, Lovinger DM. Ethanol potentiates GABAergic synaptic transmission in a postsynaptic neuron/synaptic bouton preparation from basolateral amygdala. J Neurophysiol 2006; 96(1): 433-41. [http://dx.doi.org/10.1152/jn.01380.2005] [PMID: 16624993]

[67] Lu SM, Yeh HH. Ethanol modulates AMPA-induced current responses of primary somatosensory cortical neurons. Neurochem Int 1999; 35(2): 175-83. [http://dx.doi.org/10.1016/S0197-0186(99)00059-5] [PMID: 10406001]

[68] Roberto M, Schweitzer P, Madamba SG, Stouffer DG, Parsons LH, Siggins GR. Acute and chronic ethanol alter glutamatergic transmission in rat central amygdala: an *in vitro* and *in vivo* analysis. J Neurosci 2004; 24(7): 1594-603. [http://dx.doi.org/10.1523/JNEUROSCI.5077-03.2004] [PMID: 14973247]

[69] Wang J, Carnicella S, Phamluong K, *et al.* Ethanol induces long-term facilitation of NR2B-NMDA receptor activity in the dorsal striatum: implications for alcohol drinking behavior. J Neurosci 2007; 27(13): 3593-602. [http://dx.doi.org/10.1523/JNEUROSCI.4749-06.2007] [PMID: 17392475]

[70] Moriguchi S, Zhao X, Marszalec W, Yeh JZ, Narahashi T. Effects of ethanol on excitatory and inhibitory synaptic transmission in rat cortical neurons. Alcohol Clin Exp Res 2007; 31(1): 89-99. [http://dx.doi.org/10.1111/j.1530-0277.2006.00266.x] [PMID: 17207106]

[71] Mameli M, Zamudio PA, Carta M, Valenzuela CF. Developmentally regulated actions of alcohol on hippocampal glutamatergic transmission. J Neurosci 2005; 25(35): 8027-36. [http://dx.doi.org/10.1523/JNEUROSCI.2434-05.2005] [PMID: 16135760]

[72] Dopico AM, Lemos JR, Treistman SN. Ethanol increases the activity of large conductance, Ca(2+)-activated K+ channels in isolated neurohypophysial terminals. Mol Pharmacol 1996; 49(1): 40-8. [PMID: 8569710]

[73] Dopico AM, Chu B, Lemos JR, Treistman SN. Alcohol modulation of calcium-activated potassium channels. Neurochem Int 1999; 35(2): 103-6. [http://dx.doi.org/10.1016/S0197-0186(99)00051-0] [PMID: 10405993]

[74] Knott TK, Dopico AM, Dayanithi G, Lemos J, Treistman SN. Integrated channel plasticity contributes to alcohol tolerance in neurohypophysial terminals. Mol Pharmacol 2002; 62(1): 135-42. [http://dx.doi.org/10.1124/mol.62.1.135] [PMID: 12065764]

[75] Martin G, Puig S, Pietrzykowski A, Zadek P, Emery P, Treistman S. Somatic localization of a specific large-conductance calcium-activated potassium channel subtype controls compartmentalized ethanol sensitivity in the nucleus accumbens. J Neurosci 2004; 24(29): 6563-72. [http://dx.doi.org/10.1523/JNEUROSCI.0684-04.2004] [PMID: 15269268]

[76] Wynne PM, Puig SI, Martin GE, Treistman SN. Compartmentalized beta subunit distribution determines characteristics and ethanol sensitivity of somatic, dendritic, and terminal large-conductance calcium-activated potassium channels in the rat central nervous system. J Pharmacol Exp Ther 2009; 329(3): 978-86. [http://dx.doi.org/10.1124/jpet.108.146175] [PMID: 19321803]

[77] Dopico AM, Bukiya AN, Kuntamallappanavar G, Liu J. Modulation of BK channels by ethanol. Int Rev Neurobiol 2016; 128: 239-79. [http://dx.doi.org/10.1016/bs.irn.2016.03.019] [PMID: 27238266]

[78] Dopico AM, Bukiya AN, Martin GE. Ethanol modulation of mammalian BK channels in excitable tissues: molecular targets and their possible contribution to alcohol-induced altered behavior. Front Physiol 2014; 5: 466. [http://dx.doi.org/10.3389/fphys.2014.00466] [PMID: 25538625]

[79] Tonini R, Ferraro T, Sampedro-Castañeda M, *et al.* Small-conductance Ca2+-activated K+ channels modulate action potential-induced Ca2+ transients in hippocampal neurons. J Neurophysiol 2013; 109(6): 1514-24. [http://dx.doi.org/10.1152/jn.00346.2012] [PMID: 23255726]

[80] Chen S, Benninger F, Yaari Y. Role of small conductance Ca^{2+}-activated K^{+} channels in controlling CA1 pyramidal cell excitability. J Neurosci 2014; 34(24): 8219-30. [http://dx.doi.org/10.1523/JNEUROSCI.0936-14.2014] [PMID: 24920626]

[81] Brodie MS, Pesold C, Appel SB. Ethanol directly excites dopaminergic ventral tegmental area reward neurons. Alcohol Clin Exp Res 1999; 23(11): 1848-52. [http://dx.doi.org/10.1111/j.1530-0277.1999.tb04082.x] [PMID: 10591603]

[82] Brodie MS, Shefner SA, Dunwiddie TV. Ethanol increases the firing rate of dopamine neurons of the rat ventral tegmental area *in vitro*. Brain Res 1990; 508(1): 65-9. [http://dx.doi.org/10.1016/0006-8993(90)91118-Z] [PMID: 2337793]

[83] Hopf FW, Bowers MS, Chang SJ, *et al.* Reduced nucleus accumbens SK channel activity enhances alcohol seeking during abstinence. Neuron 2010; 65(5): 682-94. [http://dx.doi.org/10.1016/j.neuron.2010.02.015] [PMID: 20223203]

[84] Mulholland PJ, Becker HC, Woodward JJ, Chandler LJ. Small conductance calcium-activated potassium type 2 channels regulate alcohol-associated plasticity of glutamatergic synapses. Biol Psychiatry 2011; 69(7): 625-32. [http://dx.doi.org/10.1016/j.biopsych.2010.09.025] [PMID: 21056409]

[85] Chandler LJ, Harris RA, Crews FT. Ethanol tolerance and synaptic plasticity. Trends Pharmacol Sci 1998; 19(12): 491-5. [http://dx.doi.org/10.1016/S0165-6147(98)01268-1] [PMID: 9871410]

[86] Littleton J. Neurochemical mechanisms underlying alcohol withdrawal. Alcohol Health Res World 1998; 22(1): 13-24. [PMID: 15706728]

[87] Kliethermes CL. Anxiety-like behaviors following chronic ethanol exposure. Neurosci Biobehav Rev 2005; 28(8): 837-50. [http://dx.doi.org/10.1016/j.neubiorev.2004.11.001] [PMID: 15642625]

[88] Kumar S, Fleming RL, Morrow AL. Ethanol regulation of gamma-aminobutyric acid A receptors: genomic and nongenomic mechanisms. Pharmacol Ther 2004; 101(3): 211-26. [http://dx.doi.org/10.1016/j.pharmthera.2003.12.001] [PMID: 15031000]

[89] Kumar S, Porcu P, Werner DF, *et al.* The role of GABA(A) receptors in the acute and chronic effects of ethanol: a decade of progress. Psychopharmacology (Berl) 2009; 205(4): 529-64. [http://dx.doi.org/10.1007/s00213-009-1562-z] [PMID: 19455309]

[90] Marutha Ravindran CR, Mehta AK, Ticku MK. Effect of chronic administration of ethanol on the regulation of the delta-subunit of GABA(A) receptors in the rat brain. Brain Res 2007; 1174: 47-52. [http://dx.doi.org/10.1016/j.brainres.2007.07.077] [PMID: 17854781]

[91] Matthews DB, Devaud LL, Fritschy JM, Sieghart W, Morrow AL. Differential regulation of GABA(A) receptor gene expression by ethanol in the rat hippocampus versus cerebral cortex. J Neurochem 1998; 70(3): 1160-6. [http://dx.doi.org/10.1046/j.1471-4159.1998.70031160.x] [PMID: 9489737]

[92] Grobin AC, Matthews DB, Devaud LL, Morrow AL. The role of GABA(A) receptors in the acute and chronic effects of ethanol. Psychopharmacology (Berl) 1998; 139(1-2): 2-19. [http://dx.doi.org/10.1007/s002130050685] [PMID: 9768538]

[93] Kokka N, Sapp DW, Taylor AM, Olsen RW. The kindling model of alcohol dependence: similar persistent reduction in seizure threshold to pentylenetetrazol in animals receiving chronic ethanol or chronic pentylenetetrazol. Alcohol Clin Exp Res 1993; 17(3): 525-31. [http://dx.doi.org/10.1111/j.1530-0277.1993.tb00793.x] [PMID: 8392817]

[94] Cagetti E, Liang J, Spigelman I, Olsen RW. Withdrawal from chronic intermittent ethanol treatment changes subunit composition, reduces synaptic function, and decreases behavioral responses to positive allosteric modulators of GABAA receptors. Mol Pharmacol 2003; 63(1): 53-64. [http://dx.doi.org/10.1124/mol.63.1.53] [PMID: 12488536]

[95] Grobin AC, Papadeas ST, Morrow AL. Regional variations in the effects of chronic ethanol administration on GABA(A) receptor expression: potential mechanisms. Neurochem Int 2000; 37(5-

6): 453-61.
[http://dx.doi.org/10.1016/S0197-0186(00)00058-9] [PMID: 10871697]

[96] Weiner JL, Ariwodola OJ, Bates WH, *et al.* Presynaptic mechanisms underlying ethanol actions at GABAergic synapses in rat and monkey hippocampus. Alcohol Clin Exp Res 2005; 29: 187A.

[97] Peris J, Eppler B, Hu M, *et al.* Effects of chronic ethanol exposure on GABA receptors and GABAB receptor modulation of 3H-GABA release in the hippocampus. Alcohol Clin Exp Res 1997; 21(6): 1047-52.
[http://dx.doi.org/10.1111/j.1530-0277.1997.tb04252.x] [PMID: 9309316]

[98] Diaz MR, Christian DT, Anderson NJ, McCool BA. Chronic ethanol and withdrawal differentially modulate lateral/basolateral amygdala paracapsular and local GABAergic synapses. J Pharmacol Exp Ther 2011; 337(1): 162-70.
[http://dx.doi.org/10.1124/jpet.110.177121] [PMID: 21209156]

[99] Roberto M, Nelson TE, Ur CL, Gruol DL. Long-term potentiation in the rat hippocampus is reversibly depressed by chronic intermittent ethanol exposure. J Neurophysiol 2002; 87(5): 2385-97.
[http://dx.doi.org/10.1152/jn.2002.87.5.2385] [PMID: 11976376]

[100] Durand D, Carlen PL. Impairment of long-term potentiation in rat hippocampus following chronic ethanol treatment. Brain Res 1984; 308(2): 325-32.
[http://dx.doi.org/10.1016/0006-8993(84)91072-2] [PMID: 6541071]

[101] Fujii S, Yamazaki Y, Sugihara T, Wakabayashi I. Acute and chronic ethanol exposure differentially affect induction of hippocampal LTP. Brain Res 2008; 1211: 13-21.
[http://dx.doi.org/10.1016/j.brainres.2008.02.052] [PMID: 18423576]

[102] Stephens DN, Ripley TL, Borlikova G, *et al.* Repeated ethanol exposure and withdrawal impairs human fear conditioning and depresses long-term potentiation in rat amygdala and hippocampus. Biol Psychiatry 2005; 58(5): 392-400.
[http://dx.doi.org/10.1016/j.biopsych.2005.04.025] [PMID: 16018978]

[103] Korkotian E, Segal M. Lasting effects of glutamate on nuclear calcium concentration in cultured rat hippocampal neurons: regulation by calcium stores. J Physiol 1996; 496(Pt 1): 39-48.
[http://dx.doi.org/10.1113/jphysiol.1996.sp021663] [PMID: 8910194]

[104] Korkotian E, Segal M. Structure-function relations in dendritic spines: is size important? Hippocampus 2000; 10(5): 587-95.
[http://dx.doi.org/10.1002/1098-1063(2000)10:5<587::AID-HIPO9>3.0.CO;2-C] [PMID: 11075829]

[105] Korkotian E, Segal M. Spatially confined diffusion of calcium in dendrites of hippocampal neurons revealed by flash photolysis of caged calcium. Cell Calcium 2006; 40(5-6): 441-9.
[http://dx.doi.org/10.1016/j.ceca.2006.08.008] [PMID: 17064764]

[106] Korkotian E, Segal M. Synaptopodin regulates release of calcium from stores in dendritic spines of cultured hippocampal neurons. J Physiol 2011; 589(Pt 24): 5987-95.
[http://dx.doi.org/10.1113/jphysiol.2011.217315] [PMID: 22025667]

[107] Botalova A, Bombela T, Zubov P, Segal M, Korkotian E. The flavonoid acetylpectolinarin counteracts the effects of low ethanol on spontaneous network activity in hippocampal cultures. J Ethnopharmacol 2019; 30(229): 22-8.
[http://dx.doi.org/10.1016/j.jep.2018.09.040]

[108] Mulholland PJ, Hopf FW, Bukiya AN, *et al.* Sizing up ethanol-induced plasticity: the role of small and large conductance calcium-activated potassium channels. Alcohol Clin Exp Res 2009; 33(7): 1125-35.
[http://dx.doi.org/10.1111/j.1530-0277.2009.00936.x] [PMID: 19389201]

[109] Rice-Evans CA, Miller NJ, Paganga G. Structure-antioxidant activity relationships of flavonoids and phenolic acids. Free Radic Biol Med 1996; 20(7): 933-56.
[http://dx.doi.org/10.1016/0891-5849(95)02227-9] [PMID: 8743980]

[110] Williams RJ, Spencer JP, Rice-Evans C. Flavonoids: antioxidants or signalling molecules? Free Radic

Biol Med 2004; 36(7): 838-49.
[http://dx.doi.org/10.1016/j.freeradbiomed.2004.01.001] [PMID: 15019969]

[111] Spencer JP, Rice-Evans C, Williams RJ. Modulation of pro-survival Akt/protein kinase B and ERK1/2 signaling cascades by quercetin and its *In vivo* metabolites underlie their action on neuronal viability. J Biol Chem 2003; 278(37): 34783-93.
[http://dx.doi.org/10.1074/jbc.M305063200] [PMID: 12826665]

[112] Schroeter H, Boyd C, Spencer JP, Williams RJ, Cadenas E, Rice-Evans C. MAPK signaling in neurodegeneration: influences of flavonoids and of nitric oxide. Neurobiol Aging 2002; 23(5): 861-80.
[http://dx.doi.org/10.1016/S0197-4580(02)00075-1] [PMID: 12392791]

[113] Spencer JP. Flavonoids: modulators of brain function? Br J Nutr 2008; 99 E (Suppl. 1): ES60-77.
[http://dx.doi.org/10.1017/S0007114508965776] [PMID: 18503736]

[114] Abbott NJ. Astrocyte-endothelial interactions and blood-brain barrier permeability. J Anat 2002; 200(6): 629-38.
[http://dx.doi.org/10.1046/j.1469-7580.2002.00064.x] [PMID: 12162730]

[115] Aasmundstad TA, Mørland J, Paulsen RE. Distribution of morphine 6-glucuronide and morphine across the blood-brain barrier in awake, freely moving rats investigated by *in vivo* microdialysis sampling. J Pharmacol Exp Ther 1995; 275(1): 435-41.
[PMID: 7562582]

[116] Suganuma M, Okabe S, Oniyama M, Tada Y, Ito H, Fujiki H. Wide distribution of [3H](---epigallocatechin gallate, a cancer preventive tea polyphenol, in mouse tissue. Carcinogenesis 1998; 19(10): 1771-6.
[http://dx.doi.org/10.1093/carcin/19.10.1771] [PMID: 9806157]

[117] Halliwell B, Zhao K, Whiteman M. The gastrointestinal tract: a major site of antioxidant action? Free Radic Res 2000; 33(6): 819-30.
[http://dx.doi.org/10.1080/10715760000301341] [PMID: 11237104]

[118] Joseph JA, Shukitt-Hale B, Denisova NA, *et al.* Long-term dietary strawberry, spinach, or vitamin E supplementation retards the onset of age-related neuronal signal-transduction and cognitive behavioral deficits. J Neurosci 1998; 18(19): 8047-55.
[http://dx.doi.org/10.1523/JNEUROSCI.18-19-08047.1998] [PMID: 9742171]

[119] Francis ST, Head K, Morris PG, Macdonald IA. The effect of flavanol-rich cocoa on the fMRI response to a cognitive task in healthy young people. J Cardiovasc Pharmacol 2006; 47 (Suppl. 2): S215-20.
[http://dx.doi.org/10.1097/00005344-200606001-00018] [PMID: 16794461]

[120] Gage FH. Mammalian neural stem cells. Science 2000; 287(5457): 1433-8.
[http://dx.doi.org/10.1126/science.287.5457.1433] [PMID: 10688783]

[121] Harris KM, Kater SB. Dendritic spines: cellular specializations imparting both stability and flexibility to synaptic function. Annu Rev Neurosci 1994; 17: 341-71.
[http://dx.doi.org/10.1146/annurev.ne.17.030194.002013] [PMID: 8210179]

[122] Bourtchuladze R, Frenguelli B, Blendy J, Cioffi D, Schutz G, Silva AJ. Deficient long-term memory in mice with a targeted mutation of the cAMP-responsive element-binding protein. Cell 1994; 79(1): 59-68.
[http://dx.doi.org/10.1016/0092-8674(94)90400-6] [PMID: 7923378]

[123] Jung JS, Choi MJ, Lee YY, Moon BI, Park JS, Kim HS. Suppression of Lipopolysaccharide-Induced Neuroinflammation by Morin *via* MAPK, PI3K/Akt, and PKA/HO-1 Signaling Pathway Modulation. J Agric Food Chem 2017; 65(2): 373-82.
[http://dx.doi.org/10.1021/acs.jafc.6b05147] [PMID: 28032996]

[124] Abarikwu SO. Kolaviron, a natural flavonoid from the seeds of Garcinia kola, reduces LPS-induced inflammation in macrophages by combined inhibition of IL-6 secretion, and inflammatory

transcription factors, ERK1/2, NF-κB, p38, Akt, p-c-JUN and JNK. Biochim Biophys Acta 2014; 1840(7): 2373-81.
[http://dx.doi.org/10.1016/j.bbagen.2014.03.006] [PMID: 24650887]

[125] Murer MG, Yan Q, Raisman-Vozari R. Brain-derived neurotrophic factor in the control human brain, and in Alzheimer's disease and Parkinson's disease. Prog Neurobiol 2001; 63(1): 71-124.
[http://dx.doi.org/10.1016/S0301-0082(00)00014-9] [PMID: 11040419]

[126] Lu B, Nagappan G, Guan X, Nathan PJ, Wren P. BDNF-based synaptic repair as a disease-modifying strategy for neurodegenerative diseases. Nat Rev Neurosci 2013; 14(6): 401-16.
[http://dx.doi.org/10.1038/nrn3505] [PMID: 23674053]

[127] You C, Zhang H, Sakharkar AJ, Teppen T, Pandey SC. Reversal of deficits in dendritic spines, BDNF and Arc expression in the amygdala during alcohol dependence by HDAC inhibitor treatment. Int J Neuropsychopharmacol 2014; 17(2): 313-22.
[http://dx.doi.org/10.1017/S1461145713001144] [PMID: 24103311]

[128] Spencer JP. The impact of flavonoids on memory: physiological and molecular considerations. Chem Soc Rev 2009; 38(4): 1152-61.
[http://dx.doi.org/10.1039/b800422f] [PMID: 19421586]

[129] Lee BH, Choi SH, Shin TJ, *et al.* Effects of quercetin on α9α10 nicotinic acetylcholine receptor-mediated ion currents. Eur J Pharmacol 2011; 650(1): 79-85.
[http://dx.doi.org/10.1016/j.ejphar.2010.09.079] [PMID: 20950602]

[130] Chang Y, Lu CW, Lin TY, Huang SK, Wang SJ. Baicalein, a constituent of scutellaria baicalensis, reduces glutamate release and protects neuronal cell against kainic acid-induced excitotoxicity in rats. Am J Chin Med 2016; 44(5): 943-62.
[http://dx.doi.org/10.1142/S0192415X1650052X] [PMID: 27430911]

[131] Johnston GA. GABA(A) receptor channel pharmacology. Curr Pharm Des 2005; 11(15): 1867-85.
[http://dx.doi.org/10.2174/1381612054021024] [PMID: 15974965]

[132] Fernández S, Wasowski C, Paladini AC, Marder M. Sedative and sleep-enhancing properties of linarin, a flavonoid-isolated from Valeriana officinalis. Pharmacol Biochem Behav 2004; 77(2): 399-404.
[http://dx.doi.org/10.1016/j.pbb.2003.12.003] [PMID: 14751470]

[133] Nishida S, Satoh H. Possible involvement of Ca activated k channels, sk channel, in the quercetin-induced vasodilatation. Korean J Physiol Pharmacol 2009; 13(5): 361-5.
[http://dx.doi.org/10.4196/kjpp.2009.13.5.361] [PMID: 19915698]

[134] Hirsch EC, Hunot S, Hartmann A. Neuroinflammatory processes in Parkinson's disease. Parkinsonism Relat Disord 2005; 11 (Suppl. 1): S9-S15.
[http://dx.doi.org/10.1016/j.parkreldis.2004.10.013] [PMID: 15885630]

[135] McGeer EG, McGeer PL. Inflammatory processes in Alzheimer's disease. Prog Neuropsychopharmacol Biol Psychiatry 2003; 27(5): 741-9.
[http://dx.doi.org/10.1016/S0278-5846(03)00124-6] [PMID: 12921904]

[136] Adachi N, Tomonaga S, Tachibana T, Denbow DM, Furuse M. (-)-Epigallocatechin gallate attenuates acute stress responses through GABAergic system in the brain. Eur J Pharmacol 2006; 531(1-3): 171-5.
[http://dx.doi.org/10.1016/j.ejphar.2005.12.024] [PMID: 16457806]

[137] Nadkarni A, Endsley P, Bhatia U, *et al.* Community detoxification for alcohol dependence: A systematic review. Drug Alcohol Rev 2017; 36(3): 389-99.
[http://dx.doi.org/10.1111/dar.12440] [PMID: 27325204]

[138] Sperling W, Lesch OM. The reduction of alcohol consumption with novel pharmacological intervention. Eur Psychiatry 1996; 11(5): 217-26.
[http://dx.doi.org/10.1016/0924-9338(96)82327-3] [PMID: 19698456]

[139] Ryabinin AE. Role of hippocampus in alcohol-induced memory impairment: implications from behavioral and immediate early gene studies. Psychopharmacology (Berl) 1998; 139(1-2): 34-43. [http://dx.doi.org/10.1007/s002130050687] [PMID: 9768540]

[140] Lee H, Roh S, Kim DJ. Alcohol-induced blackout. Int J Environ Res Public Health 2009; 6(11): 2783-92. [http://dx.doi.org/10.3390/ijerph6112783] [PMID: 20049223]

[141] Oscar-Berman M. Function and dysfunction of prefrontal brain circuitry in alcoholic Korsakoff's syndrome. Neuropsychol Rev 2012; 22(2): 154-69. [http://dx.doi.org/10.1007/s11065-012-9198-x] [PMID: 22538385]

[142] Wetherill RR, Fromme K. Alcohol-induced blackouts: a review of recent clinical research with practical implications and recommendations for future studies. Alcohol Clin Exp Res 2016; 40(5): 922-35. [http://dx.doi.org/10.1111/acer.13051] [PMID: 27060868]

[143] Christmas D, Hood S, Nutt D. Potential novel anxiolytic drugs. Curr Pharm Des 2008; 14(33): 3534-46. [http://dx.doi.org/10.2174/138161208786848775] [PMID: 19075730]

[144] Dols A, Sienaert P, van Gerven H, *et al.* The prevalence and management of side effects of lithium and anticonvulsants as mood stabilizers in bipolar disorder from a clinical perspective: a review. Int Clin Psychopharmacol 2013; 28(6): 287-96. [http://dx.doi.org/10.1097/YIC.0b013e32836435e2] [PMID: 23873292]

[145] Atti AR, Ferrari Gozzi B, Zuliani G, *et al.* A systematic review of metabolic side effects related to the use of antipsychotic drugs in dementia. Int Psychogeriatr 2014; 26(1): 19-37. [http://dx.doi.org/10.1017/S1041610213001658] [PMID: 24103643]

[146] Gyllenhaal C, Merritt SL, Peterson SD, Block KI, Gochenour T. Efficacy and safety of herbal stimulants and sedatives in sleep disorders. Sleep Med Rev 2000; 4(3): 229-51. [http://dx.doi.org/10.1053/smrv.1999.0093] [PMID: 12531167]

[147] Abebe W. Herbal medication: potential for adverse interactions with analgesic drugs. J Clin Pharm Ther 2002; 27(6): 391-401. [http://dx.doi.org/10.1046/j.1365-2710.2002.00444.x] [PMID: 12472978]

[148] Ang-Lee MK, Moss J, Yuan CS. Herbal medicines and perioperative care. JAMA 2001; 286(2): 208-16. [http://dx.doi.org/10.1001/jama.286.2.208] [PMID: 11448284]

[149] Fong SY, Wong YC, Zuo Z. Alterations in the CNS effects of anti-epileptic drugs by Chinese herbal medicines. Expert Opin Drug Metab Toxicol 2014; 10(2): 249-67. [http://dx.doi.org/10.1517/17425255.2014.870554] [PMID: 24329405]

[150] Tutin TG, Heywood VH, Burges NA, *et al.* Flora Europaea, 3. United Kingdom: Cambridge University Press 1972; p. 256.

[151] Galishevskaya EE, Petrichenko VM. Phenolic compounds from two Melampyrum species 2010. [http://dx.doi.org/10.1007/s11094-010-0501-y]

[152] Vogl S, Atanasov AG, Binder M, *et al.* The herbal drug Melampyrum pratenseL. (Koch): isolation and identification of its bioactive compounds targeting mediators of inflammation. Evid Based Complement Alternat Med 2013; 2013395316 [http://dx.doi.org/10.1155/2013/395316] [PMID: 23533479]

[153] Sokolov PD. Plant Resources of USSR: Flowering Plants, Their Chemical Composition and the Use, Families: Caprifoliaceae–Plantaginaceae. Leningrad: Nauka 1990; pp. 147-50.

[154] Stajner D, Popović BM, Boza P, Kapor A. Antioxidant capacity of Melampyrum barbatum--weed and medicinal plant. Phytother Res 2009; 23(7): 1006-10.
[http://dx.doi.org/10.1002/ptr.2741] [PMID: 19140121]

[155] Damtoft S, Hansen SB, Jacobsen B, Jensen SR, Nelsen B. Iridoid glucosides from Melampyrum. Phytochemistry 1984; 23(10): 2387-9.
[http://dx.doi.org/10.1016/S0031-9422(00)80564-6]

[156] Roeder E, Bourauel T. Pyrrolizidine alkaloids from Melampyrum pratense. Nat Toxins 1992; 1(1): 35-7.
[http://dx.doi.org/10.1002/nt.2620010108] [PMID: 1344898]

[157] Munteanu MF, Vlase L. The determination of the iridoids from the Melampyrum species by modern chromatographic methods. Not Bot Horti Agrobot Cluj-Napoca 2011; 39(1): 79-83.
[http://dx.doi.org/10.15835/nbha3915803]

[158] Sun X, Sun GB, Wang M, Xiao J, Sun XB. Protective effects of cynaroside against H_2O_2-induced apoptosis in H9c2 cardiomyoblasts. J Cell Biochem 2011; 112(8): 2019-29.
[http://dx.doi.org/10.1002/jcb.23121] [PMID: 21445859]

[159] Xu J, Wang H, Ding K, *et al.* Luteolin provides neuroprotection in models of traumatic brain injury via the Nrf2-ARE pathway. Free Radic Biol Med 2014; 71: 186-95.
[http://dx.doi.org/10.1016/j.freeradbiomed.2014.03.009] [PMID: 24642087]

[160] Liu RL, Xiong QJ, Shu Q, *et al.* Hyperoside protects cortical neurons from oxygen-glucose deprivation-reperfusion induced injury *via* nitric oxide signal pathway. Brain Res 2012; 1469: 164-73.
[http://dx.doi.org/10.1016/j.brainres.2012.06.044] [PMID: 22771858]

[161] Sasaki K, El Omri A, Kondo S, Han J, Isoda H. Rosmarinus officinalis polyphenols produce anti-depressant like effect through monoaminergic and cholinergic functions modulation. Behav Brain Res 2013; 238: 86-94.
[http://dx.doi.org/10.1016/j.bbr.2012.10.010] [PMID: 23085339]

[162] Shaikh MF, Tan KN, Borges K. Anticonvulsant screening of luteolin in four mouse seizure models. Neurosci Lett 2013; 550: 195-9.
[http://dx.doi.org/10.1016/j.neulet.2013.06.065] [PMID: 23851253]

[163] Liu Y, Tian X, Gou L, Sun L, Ling X, Yin X. Luteolin attenuates diabetes-associated cognitive decline in rats. Brain Res Bull 2013; 94: 23-9.
[http://dx.doi.org/10.1016/j.brainresbull.2013.02.001] [PMID: 23415807]

[164] Zhao G, Qin GW, Wang J, Chu WJ, Guo LH. Functional activation of monoamine transporters by luteolin and apigenin isolated from the fruit of Perilla frutescens (L.) Britt. Neurochem Int 2010; 56(1): 168-76.
[http://dx.doi.org/10.1016/j.neuint.2009.09.015] [PMID: 19815045]

[165] Yi LT, Li JM, Li YC, Pan Y, Xu Q, Kong LD. Antidepressant-like behavioral and neurochemical effects of the citrus-associated chemical apigenin. Life Sci 2008; 82(13-14): 741-51.
[http://dx.doi.org/10.1016/j.lfs.2008.01.007] [PMID: 18308340]

[166] Viola H, Wasowski C, Levi de Stein M, *et al.* Apigenin, a component of Matricaria recutita flowers, is a central benzodiazepine receptors-ligand with anxiolytic effects. Planta Med 1995; 61(3): 213-6.
[http://dx.doi.org/10.1055/s-2006-958058] [PMID: 7617761]

[167] Han JH, Kim KJ, Jang HJ, *et al.* Effects of Apigenin on glutamate-induced $[Ca^{2+}]$(i) increases in cultured rat hippocampal neurons. Korean J Physiol Pharmacol 2008; 12(2): 43-9.
[http://dx.doi.org/10.4196/kjpp.2008.12.2.43] [PMID: 20157393]

[168] Kavvadias D, Sand P, Youdim KA, *et al.* The flavone hispidulin, a benzodiazepine receptor ligand with positive allosteric properties, traverses the blood-brain barrier and exhibits anticonvulsive effects. Br J Pharmacol 2004; 142(5): 811-20.
[http://dx.doi.org/10.1038/sj.bjp.0705828] [PMID: 15231642]

[169] Avallone R, Zanoli P, Puia G, Kleinschnitz M, Schreier P, Baraldi M. Pharmacological profile of apigenin, a flavonoid isolated from Matricaria chamomilla. Biochem Pharmacol 2000; 59(11): 1387-94.
[http://dx.doi.org/10.1016/S0006-2952(00)00264-1] [PMID: 10751547]

[170] Elsas SM, Rossi DJ, Raber J, *et al.* Passiflora incarnata L. (Passionflower) extracts elicit GABA currents in hippocampal neurons *in vitro*, and show anxiogenic and anticonvulsant effects *In vivo*, varying with extraction method. Phytomedicine 2010; 17(12): 940-9.
[http://dx.doi.org/10.1016/j.phymed.2010.03.002] [PMID: 20382514]

[171] Korkotian E, Botalova A, Odegova T, Galishevskaya E, Skryabina E, Segal M. Complex effects of aqueous extract of Melampyrum pratense and of its flavonoids on activity of primary cultured hippocampal neurons. J Ethnopharmacol 2015; 163: 220-8.
[http://dx.doi.org/10.1016/j.jep.2015.01.036] [PMID: 25656000]

[172] GRIN, Germplasm Resources Information Network (GRIN). 2017.https://npgsweb.ars-grin.gov/gringlobal/taxonomydetail.aspx?id=102290

[173] Cheriet T, Hanfer M, Boudjelal A, *et al.* Glycosyl flavonoid profile, *In vivo* antidiabetic and *in vitro* antioxidant properties of *Linaria* reflexa Desf. Nat Prod Res 2017; 31(17): 2042-8.
[http://dx.doi.org/10.1080/14786419.2016.1274889] [PMID: 28032514]

[174] Sutton DA. A revision of the tribe Antirrhineae. London: Oxford University press 1988; p. 575.

[175] Chater AO. Valdes B,Webb D A Linaria Mill Flora Europaea. New York: Cambridge University press 1972; Vol. 3: pp. 226-36.

[176] Miller P. Linaria Gard Dict. 8th. 1768; 16.

[177] Valdés B. Flavonoid pigments in flower and leaf of the genus *Linaria* (*Scrophulariaceae*). Phytochemistry 1970; 9: 1253-60.
[http://dx.doi.org/10.1016/S0031-9422(00)85316-9]

[178] Cheriet T, Mancini I, Seghiri R, Benayache F, Benayache S. Chemical constituents and biological activities of the genus *Linaria* (*Scrophulariaceae*). Nat Prod Res 2015; 29(17): 1589-613.
[http://dx.doi.org/10.1080/14786419.2014.999243] [PMID: 25674928]

[179] Klobb T. Two new glucosides: linarine and pectolinarine. CR (East Lansing Mich) 1907; 145: 331-4.

[180] Morita N, Shimizu M, Arisa WA. Studies on medical resources. Components of leavef of *Linaria* Japanica-miq and *Linaria* mill (*Scrophulariaceae*). Yakugaku Zasshi-Journal of the Parmaceutical Society of Japan 1974; 4(8): 913-6.
[http://dx.doi.org/10.1248/yakushi1947.94.8_913]

[181] Kuptsova LP, Ban'kovskii AI. New flavonoid from some species of *Linaria*. Chem Nat Compd 1970; 6: 128-9. [Russian.].
[http://dx.doi.org/10.1007/BF00564177]

[182] Smirnova LP, Glyzin VI, Patudin AV, Bankovskii AI. Acetyl-pectalinarine from several Salvia species 1974.

[183] Kiryanov A, Krivut B, Perelson M. Chromatospectrophotometric method of determining acetylpectolinarin in plant raw material, the finished product, and the medicinal form 1976.
[http://dx.doi.org/10.1007/BF00757988]

[184] Otsuka H. Isolation of isolinariins A and B, new flavonoid glycosides from *Linaria* japonica. J Nat Prod 1992; 55: 1252-5.
[http://dx.doi.org/10.1021/np50087a011]

[185] Patudin AB, Smirnova LG, Glizin VI, Bankovskii AI. Looking for pectalinarine and acetyl-pectalinarine in in *Linaria* Mill and *Saliria* L plants. Plant Resources. Leningrad: Nauka 1975; XI: pp. (2)204-10.

[186] Sing SE, Peterson RK. Assessing environmental risks for established invasive weeds: Dalmatian (*Linaria* dalmatica) and yellow (*L. vulgaris*) toadflax in North America. Int J Environ Res Public Health 2011; 8(7): 2828-53.
[http://dx.doi.org/10.3390/ijerph8072828] [PMID: 21845161]

[187] Jones F. Medicinal herb handbook: an herbal application guide for novice and clinician through simplified herbal remedy descriptions. USA: Lotus Press 1999.

[188] Hogan P, Huisinga K. An annotated catalog of the native and naturalized flora of Arizona. Flagstaff, Arizona: Arizona Ethnobotanical Research Association 1999.

[189] El'kina OV, Shramm NI, Molokhova EI, Petrichenko VM. Optimization of the process of extraction of biologically active substances from yellow toadflax (*Linaria vulgaris*) Herbs. Khimiko-farmatsevticheskii zhurnal 2014; 48(4): 32-4.

[190] Penn Y, Segal M, Moses E. Network synchronization in hippocampal neurons. Proc Natl Acad Sci USA 2016; 113(12): 3341-6.
[http://dx.doi.org/10.1073/pnas.1515105113] [PMID: 26961000]

[191] Aydoğdu I, Zihnioğlu F, Karayildirim T, Gülcemal D, Alankuş-Calişkan O, Bedir E. Alpha-glucosidase inhibitory constituents of *Linaria* kurdica subsp. eriocalyx. Nat Prod Commun 2010; 5(6): 841-4.
[PMID: 20614804]

Frontiers in Drug Design and Discovery, 2021, *Vol. 10*, 168-237

CHAPTER 5

Hybrid Smart Materials for Topical Drug Delivery: Application of Scaffolds

Talita Nascimento[1], **Henrique de Souza Picciani**[2], **K. Gyselle de Holanda e Silva**[1] and **Thaís Nogueira Barradas**[2,3,*]

[1] *Programa de Pós-graduação em Nanobiossistemas, Universidade Federal do Rio de Janeiro, Av. Carlos Chagas Filho, 373, Cidade Universitária, Ilha do Fundão – Rio de Janeiro – Brazil*

[2] *Instituto de Macromoléculas Professora Eloisa Mano, Universidade Federal do Rio de Janeiro (IMA/UFRJ), Centro de Tecnologia, Bl. J, Av. Horácio Macedo, 2030, Cidade Universitária, Ilha do Fundão – Rio de Janeiro – Brazil*

[3] *Universidade Federal de Juiz de Fora. Faculdade de Farmácia Departamento de Ciências Farmacêuticas. Rua José Lourenço Kelmer, s/n. Campus Universitário. São Pedro. Zip Code: 36036-900, Juiz de Fora - MG, Brazil*

Abstract: The recent advances in materials science have enabled great achievements in the development of polymer scaffolds, which can constitute innovative platforms for the development of novel topical drug delivery systems (TDDS) associated with site-specific or prolonged drug release. The application of polymer scaffolds as drug delivery systems often relies on their combination with many types of nanocarriers, such as liposomes, solid nanoparticles, micelles, nanogels and metallic nanoparticles. The combination of polymer scaffolds and drug nanocarriers and the association of controlled drug release properties provide novel materials, considered hybrid as they gather two therapeutic effects: scaffolding and drug delivery. Such hybrid scaffolds have been shown to be suitable for delivering drugs at controlled rates and site distribution. Many drug carriers are often associated with stability issues, drug leaking or considerable interaction with undesirable cells, hindering their clinical function. Hence, for topical application, drug nanocarriers are often introduced in conventional secondary vehicles such as creams and lotions in order to provide the viscosity, extended residence time and adhesiveness, properties necessary for the administration route. In addition, smart stimuli-responsive polymers can be used in the formulation of both scaffolds and nanocarriers, being promising approaches in the topical treatment of various diseases. In this context, hybrid smart polymer-based scaffolds are versatile platforms for the development of novel TDDS. Such smart materials, in addition to being able to combine the benefits of different structural components, can also respond to external stimuli such as temperature, pH, and redox status, which can increase the effectiveness of therapeutic agents and decrease harmful effects on the surrounding

* **Correspondent Author Thaís Nogueira Barradas:** Universidade Federal de Juiz de Fora. Faculdade de Farmácia Departamento de Ciências Farmacêuticas. Rua José Lourenço Kelmer, s/n. Campus Universitário. São Pedro. Zip Code: 36036-900, Juiz de Fora - MG, Brazil; Tel: (+55) 32 2102 3893/2102 3802; E-mail: thais.barradas@ifrj.edu.br

Atta-ur-Rehman and M. Iqbal Choudhary (Eds.)

tissue. In this chapter, the different polymer-based scaffolds, most nanocarriers and stimuli-responsive polymers are described as well as their most varied applications in the field of technological development of topical delivery systems for ideal drugs, which is still a challenge for formulation scientists.

Keywords: Hybrid systems, Nanoparticles, Polymer-based scaffolds, Polymers, Smart materials, Topical drug delivery.

INTRODUCTION

Lately, the main challenge of modern drug therapy is not finding more potent drugs but rather providing improved approaches to deliver those drugs to a specific place or target at the rate required inside the body [1]. To achieve this, great efforts have been made to develop novel drug delivery systems that can optimize drug absorption, distribution, half life time, release rate and site distribution. The research progress in nanotechnology and novel drug delivery systems allowed the development of novel pharmaceutical products, which bring several therapeutic advantages such as patient compliance and improvements in drug pharmacokinetics and pharmacodynamics.

Topical drug administration produces local effects, reducing the systemic drug circulation [2 - 4]. There are at least two relevant reasons for choosing topical drug delivery: (i) when systemic administration causes toxic side effects due to drug interaction with other biological compartments; (ii) when the affected tissue is difficult to be reached at sufficient drug concentration, or perfusion rate is reduced [5, 6].

Many drug carriers are used for topical and controlled drug delivery. Most of them are nano-sized carriers such as nanoparticles, micelles, liposomes and other lipid-based nanoparticles. Drug encapsulation into nanocarriers enables the production of tailor-made drug release rate, depending on the physicochemical properties of both drug and polymer matrix composition, whether polymeric or lipid [6].

Polymer-based scaffolds have been optimized over the last decade, in order to improve biocompatibility, cell proliferation capacity and incorporate more functionalities to local treatment. They are mostly constituted by biopolymers that arise as interesting materials due to their biocompatibility and biodegradability [7, 8].

Some examples of biocompatible polymers applied as scaffolds for drug delivery are: collagen, chitosan, alginate, poly (lactic acid) (PLA), poly (glycolic acid)

(PGA), poly (co-glycolic lactic acid) (PLGA), polystyrene (PS), poly (l-lactic acid) (PLLA), polydioxinone (PDO), poly (ε-caprolactone-co-lactic) (PCLA) and poly (ε-caprolactone) (PCL) [9, 10]. Polymers are be widely used for scaffolds production by the techniques as phase separation, self-assembly, electrospinning *etc.* Among those techniques, electrospinning is one of the most studied and applied in recent years [8, 11].

The selection of the proper fabrication method can provide the development of porous materials with high drug diffusivity, being favorable to originate novel drug delivery systems. The therapeutic potential of scaffolds can be enhanced when combined with drug delivery vehicles as nanocarriers. Such combination can overcome some of the main drawbacks in TDDS and enables novel applications for scaffolding materials, opening a new window of opportunities for these hybrid materials. Moreover, the application of stimuli-responsive smart polymers that can change their macrostructure of self-assemble with external stimuli such as polarity, pH, temperature and redox potential or yet, sensible to enzymatic/hydrolytic degradation can provide novel materials with different and interesting drug release properties [12 - 14].

Hybrid smart systems that therefore combine drug nanocarriers with polymeric stimuli-responsive scaffolds can represent a new concept of rational and versatile therapy by providing multifunctionality and the development of more complex drug delivery systems capable of treating different conditions of human health more effectively. In a general aspect, these materials can be classified as nanocomposites, being formed by two phases: one dispersed composed by the nanocarriers and the other, continuous, composed by the polymeric scaffolds matrix. The development of nanostructured polymeric hybrid smart scaffolds can be seen as a multidisciplinary area, due to its enormous potential in various branches of science and technology. In this chapter, various nanocarriers associated to polymeric scaffolds and stimuli-responsive polymers are described and their applications are presented. The numerous possibilities for developing innovative and advanced materials in the field of pharmaceutical technology for new TDDS will be addressed. In this way, Fig. (**1**) shows the summary chart containing the types of polymer-based scaffold that can be applied into some tissues such as bone, topical (skin, eyes, gastrointestinal tract and vagina), neuronal and vascular. Also, examples of biomolecules and nanoparticles that can be incorporated into the scaffolds are mentioned in Fig. (**1**).

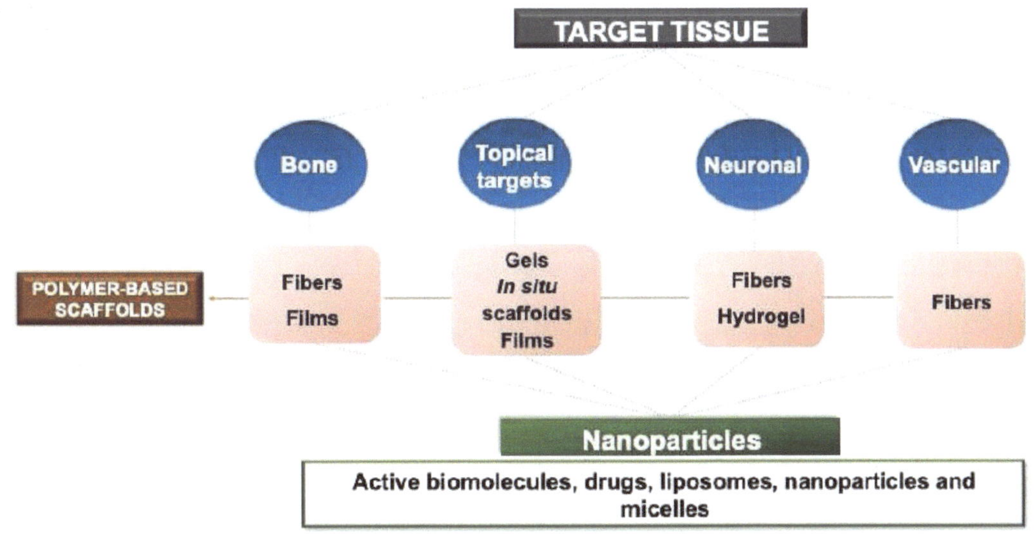

Fig. (1). Summary chart of examples from polymer-based scaffolds and their tissue targets.

TOPICAL DRUG DELIVERY: GENERAL ASPECTS

In the last decades, the demand for novel therapies with reduced side effects and enhanced patient compliance has been increased. Conventional approaches often rely on oral or systemic administration of drugs in a single-dose drug delivery system. The severity of the adverse effects depends on the drug pharmacokinetics and pharmacodynamics and can be especially serious for drugs with small therapeutic index [15]. In this context, topical approaches in replacement of systemic drug delivery systems can be preferable.

Topical drug delivery is often used to refer to dermal drug delivery. Indeed, every dermal drug delivery system intended to treat a local skin infection provides a topical drug delivery. Besides, skin constitutes the most readily accessible organ for topical application of drug delivery systems, which explains why dermatological TDDS are the most commonly studied and developed [16 - 18]. However, the expression "topical drug delivery" should not to be considered a synonym of dermal drug delivery, once it can be applied to other anatomical sites, such as in the gastrointestinal tract, ophthalmic, buccal, ear, vaginal, periodontal and rectal routes, or as implants in several anatomical sites [19 - 22].

TDDS enable avoiding of hepatic first-pass metabolism and other gastro-intestinal incompatibility or inactivation, achieving high drug concentration at the target site. They are convenient to use and of easy application even to unconscious patients and also offer fast and easy treatment suspension. Topical drug delivery provides direct access to the affected tissue and drugs can be released in a very controlled pattern, which allows treatment with drugs with short half-life and narrows therapeutic window. Moreover, topical pharmaceutical products can reduce the total amount of drug administered, as they improve drug local bioavailability, being also interesting from the economical point of view. Those advantages are responsible for a better patient compliance to the treatment with reduced toxicity and, more importantly, higher effectiveness avoiding major fluctuation of drug plasma levels and reducing side effects [16, 23 - 25].

Several dosage forms are often applied to TDDS. The most commonly used are: gels, creams, lotions, foams, ointments or sprays, as summarized in Fig. (**2**) [26]. Creams, ointments, and gels are probably the most commercially available as topical pharmaceutical dosage forms.

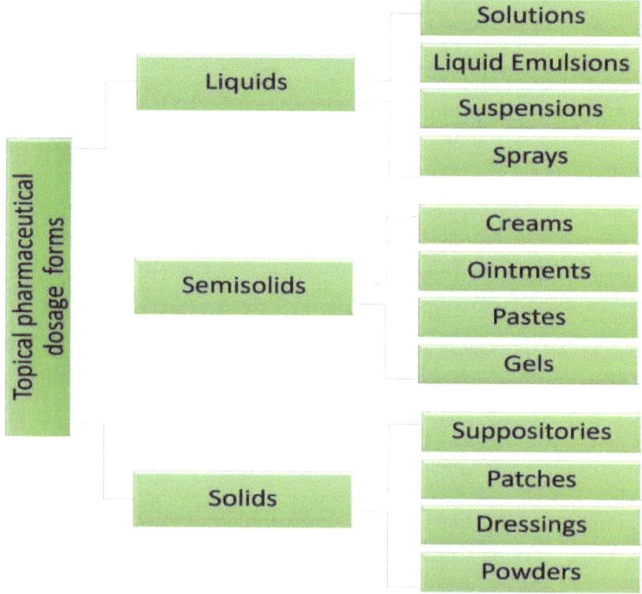

Fig. (2). Most common pharmaceutical dosage forms for topical drug delivery.

Topical Formulation Main Aspects

Paul Elrich first introduced, in 1909, the concept of "magic bullet" to refer to site-specific drug delivery intended to achieve increased therapeutic efficacy and patient compliance. The concept of "magic bullet" aims to reduce systemic toxicity as it increases site selectivity, since the formulation should delivery the active molecule to the desired tissue without interacting to surrounding tissues or organs [27].

Several pharmacokinetics events are involved once a topical drug release formulation is administrated. They follow a well-known sequence that includes drug initial release, absorption, distribution, metabolism and, eventually, elimination [21]. It is mandatory, therefore, that the formulation enables the diffusion of drug from inside out to reach the target tissue in a suitable therapeutic concentration. Drug release is the most critical phenomenon, as it is essential to the therapeutic effects, and constitutes the diffusion of the bioactive molecule from the original dosage form, reaching the target tissue.

The selection of the best-suited topical formulation relies on its purpose, application site and the extent and rate of drug release, which should be well defined and predictable. Thus, *In vitro* drug release rates are important tools to screen the most adequate formulation during pre-formulation studies and serve as a target quality parameter to be monitored. The formulation must ensure that the drug is capable of leaving its initial condition to reach the affected tissue or site of action at a therapeutic concentration. Moreover, the formulation should provide reasonable shelf life and also physical and chemical stability of both drug and the formulation itself, without any incompatibility among all components.

Topical Controlled Drug Delivery

Temporal controlled drug release formulations are able to maintain drug concentration within the therapeutic window during an increased and extended amount of time. Spatial distribution controlled topical drug release formulations aim to selectively accumulate in a precise target tissue based on particular conditions such as abnormal vasculature, pH, temperature, redox conditions, *etc.* [28 - 32]. Drug release is highly influenced by the composition of the formulation, drug content, the presence of polymers and other excipients, their concentrations and interactions [28].

Langer and Peppas classified controlled drug release polymeric systems based on their mechanism of drug release [33]. According to Langer and Peppas, drug release phenomena can be classified as: i) diffusion controlled, ii) erosion controlled iii) swelling controlled or iv) stimuli-controlled (Fig. **3**) [33]. Depending on the type of controlled drug release system, a mathematical kinetic model for drug release kinetic can be established. The most common are Zero order model, first order model, Higuchi, Hixson-Crowell, Korsmeyer-Peppas, among others [34, 35].

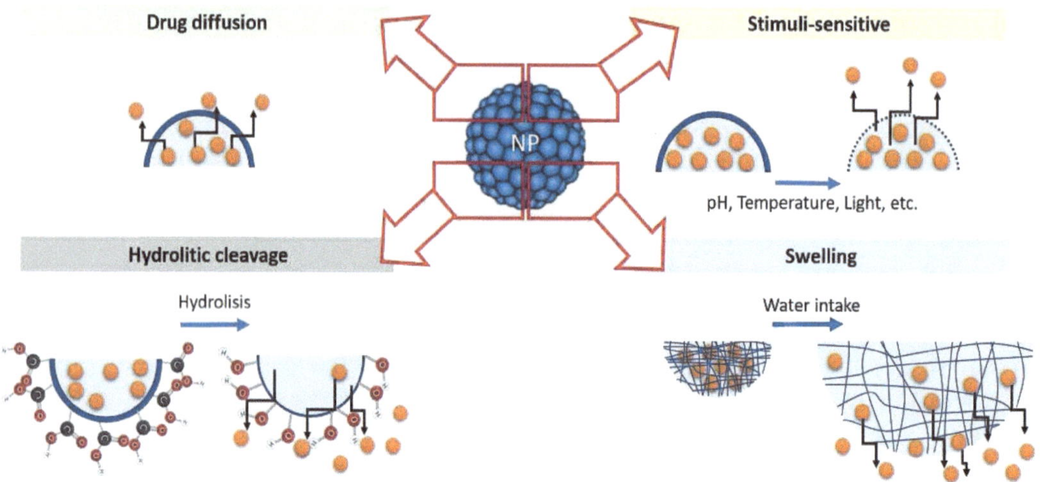

Fig. (3). Representation of the common phenomena involved in drug release.

Diffusion-controlled drug release is triggered by the difference of concentration between the formulation and the surrounding tissue. Such phenomenon usually is depicted as a high initial release, followed by a steady state achieved as drug release rate decreases. Swelling-controlled drug release systems are capable of adsorb high amounts of water when placed in an aqueous environment, like body fluids for example. As water diffused into the formulation, the polymeric matrix swallows and polymer chain relaxation provides drug diffusion from the formulation to the target tissues [36]. Hydrogels are common polymer formulations constituted of a three-dimensional network of cross-linked hydrophilic polymer chains. Crosslink degree normally dictates the mesh size, which control of drug diffusion [37, 38].

Erodible drug release formulations comprise biodegradable polymer matrixes that undergo erosion in biological environments by hydrolytic or enzymatic degradation. Both bulk and surface degradation are well-known phenomena that can occur depending on the polymer chain characteristics, such as molecular weight, end groups and crystallinity [28].

Stimuli-responsive materials are mostly based on specific polymers with particular characteristics such as pH or temperature-dependent solubility, as is the case of chitosan and poly- (propylene oxide)-poly (ethylene oxide) block copolymers, respectively [39, 40]. Stimuli-controlled drug release systems can be considered "smart" drug delivery systems, once they respond to the change of external particular conditions, such as temperature, pH, ionic strength, electric or magnetic fields [12, 41]. Such particular conditions are often found as unique characteristics of certain tissues and biological compartments, which allow the development of novel smart drug delivery systems for target-specific drug therapy.

Generally, more than one release mechanism can take place at the same time, affecting the drug release phenomena. Nevertheless, often one mechanism can be more dominant than the others. Thus, formulations can be tailored to provide great drug release control, modulation of drug release kinetics and rate [42].

Nanostructured Drug Carriers

In the last decades, several drug carriers have been developed and applied to improve topical drug delivery regarding many aspects as drug stability, drug absorption without systemic side effects. Fig. (**4**) summarizes the main nanostructured drug carriers. Nanostructured drug carriers as liposomes, nanoemulsions, lipid nanoparticles, ethosomes, nanogels and polymer nanoparticles constitute a primary drug vehicle, which can be administered alone or combined to a secondary formulation as creams, gels, lotions, films, *etc*. [5, 43, 44]. The combination of drug nanocarriers with a secondary pharmaceutical dosage form opens a wide range of opportunities of topical drug delivery products, being able to control drug release profile for many desirables therapeutic effects. These formulations can be tailored to act both as drug transporters and reservoirs in controlling drug release rate and site.

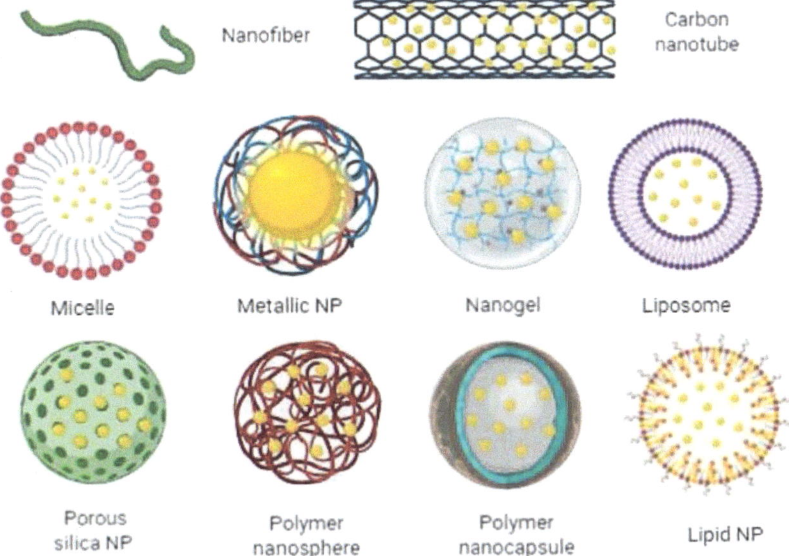

Fig. (4). Graphical representations of the main nanostructured drug carriers Adapted from Lee *et al*. [28].

Liposomes have been extensively studied and the most common nanocarriers to topical drug delivery [26, 28, 45]. Liposomes are uni- or multi- vesicular structures constituted by phospholipid bilayers and cholesterol that can entrap hydrophilic drugs in its inner compartment or hydrophobic drugs in the lipid bilayer [26, 46]. Liposomes provide the unique opportunity of surface modification, which has been widely explored to the development of target-specific drug delivery systems or prolong drug circulation half-life [28, 47].

However, since liposomes are known as thermodynamic unstable systems, novel lipid nanocarriers have been developed to overcome instability drawbacks, such as aggregation and drug leaking [48, 49]. Both liposomes and lipid nanoparticles are vesicle-like lipid nanocarriers, but slightly different from the composition and structural point of view. Lipid nanoparticles comprise two major classes of different nanocarriers: Solid lipid nanoparticles (SLN) and nanostructured lipid carriers (NLC). As traditional liposomes comprise one or more layers of lipid bilayer, SLN presents a continuous micelle-like structure, which encapsulate lipophilic drugs in a solid lipid core [50]. SLNs are advantageous such as improved formulation stability, increased bioavailability of lipophilic drugs and high loading capacity [49]. Their solid lipid matrix core are stabilized by surfactants and, possibly, co-surfactants. Different types of lipids can be used as core materials such as anionic, non-ionic and cationic lipids, which make SLN highly explored for DNA and RNA encapsulation [47, 51]. However, as they are composed of a solid core, SLN feature classical stability issues, with the decrease of drug loading capacity over time. In this context, NLC are considered the second generation of lipid nanoparticles, as they provide the incorporation of liquid lipids into the solid lipid core, increasing the drug loading, and preventing drug expulsion during storage [52, 53].

Polymeric micelles are produced from amphiphilic block copolymers composed by blocks with segments with different polarities that can self-assemble into vesicles in aqueous solutions under certain environmental conditions such as temperature, ionic strength, providing a core-shell nanocarrier [54, 55]. Polymeric micelles are often used to encapsulate hydrophobic drugs, constituting colloidal nanocarriers with relatively small sizes and narrow size distribution and with the unique characteristic of providing liquid-liquid dispersions, often referred as nanoemulsions [54, 56 - 58]. As polymers play the role of surfactants for polymeric micelles, their interaction with the oil core and the entrapped drug can influence drug release. Polymer chain size and polarity are responsible for the strength of water-oil interface, which provide physicochemical stability for nanoemulsions.

Polymeric nanoparticles are solid particles that encapsulate the drug in a polymer matrix. Polymer nanoparticles can be classified as nanocapsules or core-shell nanospheres depending on the composition of the core material, its affinity with polymer matrix and the preparation method [59 - 61]. Drug release from polymer nanoparticles is strongly dependent on the type of polymer used as either core material or matrix. For instance, stimuli-responsive, erodible, cross-linked and both hydrophilic and lipophilic polymers can be used in order to achieve site-specific and temporal controlled drug release.

Nanogels comprise nanoparticles made of three dimensional cross-linked polymer networks, as hydrogels, which can encapsulate either hydrophilic or lipophilic drugs [62, 63]. Nanogels are versatile materials and offer chemical flexibility, which provide the unique opportunity to gather different release mechanism in a single material. Swelling, erosion and diffusion are the most important mechanisms involved in drug release from nanogels [28]. Network properties, such as hydrogel mesh size, polymer chain structure, water uptake capacity, swelling degree and the type of crosslink bonds directly influence drug release profile. Moreover, covalent crosslinks lead to erosion-controlled drug release, since swelling and chain relaxation are hindered phenomena, once covalent bonds among polymer macromolecules exist. On the other hand, physical entanglements among polymer chains provide physically cross-linked hydrogels, which are more dependent on swelling and polymer chain relaxation phenomena for drug delivery to take place [59, 63].

Inorganic drug nanocarriers comprise both metallic and silica nanoparticles. Metallic nanoparticles feature a unique combination of interesting physical, chemical, optical and even electronic properties that can be explored for the development of stimuli-responsive drug delivery systems [64]. They offer easy preparation and can be biocompatible when combined or coated with biocompatible polymers and other biomolecules. A wide range of metallic nanoparticles, especially silver nanoparticles, has been explored due to their antimicrobial activity [65, 66]. Both titanium dioxide (TiO_2) and zinc oxide (ZnO) nanoparticles are widely used in cosmetics formulations due to their protective property against ultraviolet radiation [64]. Magnetically-responsive nanoparticles can be obtained from a magnetic core of magnetite (Fe_3O_4) or maghemite (Fe_2O_3) nanoparticles covered with biocompatible polymers [12, 64, 67]. Magnetic guidance or permanent magnetic fields can be used to trigger drug release due to conformational changes that take place as consequence of Brownian motion and rotational motion in the magnetic particles. Superparamagnetism is particularly explored for target hyperthermia and selective heat damage to localized tumors [14, 68].

Silica nanoparticles are biocompatible, present low toxicity, inert upon pH changes and often degradable. They offer a broad range of sizes and easy obtaining methods [69]. Silica matrixes are often mesoporous, which allows the encapsulation of small molecules as drugs and other bioactive molecules. Pore size and distribution can influence and control drug release rates. Besides, the surface of silica nanoparticles are composed by a high concentration of functional groups that can be easily functionalized by silane technology, revealing uncountable possibilities for developing site-specific targeting strategies [69 - 71]. The recent advances in polymer electrospinning technique allowed obtaining nanofibers with a wide range of morphologies that can be applied for several purposes. Electrospun nanofibers are considered drug carriers, since they can entrap several bioactive molecules such as vitamins, drug, growth factors and proteins [64, 72]. The encapsulated bioactive molecules can be protected from rapid decomposition or deactivation in biological environments. Moreover, nanofibers allow controlled drug release, encapsulation of poorly soluble drug with low bioavailability [72]. Polymeric nanofibers are sophisticated topical drug delivery templates used in bandages or sutures that can eventually dissolve or be absorbed in the human body. Their fibrous-like morphology provides bioadhesive properties due to nano-sized porous structures that can absorb moisture from the biological environment [64, 73]. Moreover, the high surface-to-volume ratio of nanofibers allows cell attachment, in a scaffolding role, which makes them interesting carriers for local release of growth factors [7, 11]. Erosion and diffusion phenomena are often observed as the main drug release mechanisms related to polymeric nanofibers [72].

Finally, is worth noting that the selection of the most adequate nanocarrier and dosage form should be based on the physicochemical properties of the drug, the affected site to be treated, scale up capacity and the desired product profile, which can vary depending on the ultimate purpose of the topical product.

POLYMER BASED SCAFFOLDS

Polymer-based scaffolds are porous biomaterials composed of polymer matrices that provide a three dimensional mechanical support, allowing numerous applications especially in regenerative medicine and tissue engineering. Compared to natural polymers, synthetic polymers offer the possibility to better adapt to more specific functions, and allow better control of the scaffold properties [74]. Thus, the scaffolds formulations and fabrication methods have been improved over the years. Overall, polymer-based scaffolds consist of biomaterials, they have been used to develop different devices, which replace and mimic often-compromised tissues [10].

Several natural polymers such as hyaluronic acid, alginate and cellulose feature interesting properties to a wide range of biomedical applications, such as tissue engineering, wound dressings and drug delivery, as reviewed by Lee *et al.* [75]. On the other hand, synthetic biodegradable polymers are widely used due to the possibility of avoiding invasive procedures to remove implanted scaffolds [11].

Both natural and synthetic polymers designed to tissue engineering can provide biomaterials, as scaffolds used to treat, improve or replace any tissue or organ, while maintaining its functionality [76 - 78]. The biodegradation rate can be tailored by producing polymer blends or changing polymer properties, such as molecular weight, crystallinity and hydrophobicity [11, 79, 80]. Table **1** shows some examples of commercially available materials applied to the biomedical area.

The use of polymer blends with both synthetic and natural polymers is useful since they provide structure and cell attachment, respectively [11]. Stitzel *et al.* produced vascular grafts scaffolds using polymer blends with Type I collagen (45%), elastin (15%), which are natural components of blood vessel walls, and PLGA (40%). The increase of PLGA concentration improved mechanical properties such as burst strength and compliance, compared to grafts composed by collagen and elastin blends [79].

Kim *et al.* reported the control of degradation rate and hydrophilicity in PLA-based scaffolds by producing blends with PLGA random copolymers, poly (lactide-b-ethylene glycol-b-lactide) (PLA-b-PEG-b-PLA) triblock copolymers and lactide. Electrospun scaffolds based on the multi-component polymer blends were constituted of randomly interconnected webs of sub-micron sized fibers. Their results showed that electrospun scaffold with 40 wt.% of PLA, 25 wt.% PLGA (LA/GA=50/50), 20 wt.% PLA-b-PEG-b-PLA, and 15 wt.% lactide provided a rapid 65% weight loss in approximately 7 weeks and showed reduced hydrophilicity in approximately 50%. The polymer blend provided suitable scaffolds for cell storage with adequate porosity, mechanical flexibility and tunable biodegradability [81].

Post-drawing treatments like thermal treatments can affect scaffold degradation rate and mechanical properties. Zong *et al.* performed post-drawing thermal treatment of PLGA (GA/LA 90:10) scaffolds and observed significant alterations in microstructure, morphology and texture of scaffolds. Those are important properties and they directly affect the degradation rate and mechanical properties of scaffold materials. Moreover, annealing at high temperatures with no posterior drawing provided high crystallinity materials with lamellar structure, however with no overall orientation. Annealing followed by drawing treatment provided an evident crystal orientation, which improved mechanical properties, such as stretching and tensile strength. *In vitro* biodegration significantly increased from 2 to 12 days [80].

To be used for tissue engineering, implants or drug delivery purposes, polymers are required to maintain certain essential characteristics described in Table **2**. The scaffolds should feature a suitable surface chemistry to allow cell proliferation and rearrangement of a functional tissue. To achieve that, it is necessary the polymer matrix to meet some important requirements such as biocompatibility, proper mechanical properties, porosity, biodegradability and bioreabsorption [82].

Table 1. List of the main scaffolds commercially available for biomedical applications.

Polymer	Main properties	Biomedical Application	Commercial Nomenclature
PGA	Regeneration of biological tissue and adequate mechanical properties	Internal bone fixation device	Biofix® and DEXON®
PLGA	Mesh-forming capacity and high biodegradation rate	Skin graft	VicrylMesh®
PLLA	Adequate tensile strength and non-degradable fibers	Replacement of ligaments, blood vessels and orthopedic fixation devices	DEXON® and Dacron®
PCA	Synthetic surgical glue, skin adhesive, and drug encapsulation	Topical dressings and adhesives	Biobrane & Alloderm® and Dermabond®
Collagen	Matrix for fibroblasts and keratinocytes seeding	Artificial skin substitute for dermal application	Apligraf®
Collagen	Guided bone regeneration with barrier to prevent cell migration and passage just for essential nutrients	Periodontal tissue regeneration	Biomend®
Alginate	Exudate absorption and wound protection from contamination.	Wound healing inflicted by skin trauma	Kaltostat®

Adapted from Dhandayuthapani *et al.* [83] and Bakhshayesh *et al.*[84].

Table 2. The main requirements of polymeric scaffolds for application in tissue engineering.

Biotechnological Requirement	Scaffold Properties
Ability to carry biomolecular signals	Pore size adjusted to reconstituting cell
Mechanical properties that prevent cellular stress	High permeability for diffusion
Ability to be remolded	Promotion of cellular functions
Surface capable of cell attachment	High porosity

Adapted from Cui *et al.* [86] and Ravichandran *et al.* [87].

Considering that, a TDDS refers to formulations applied to superficial areas such as skin, eyes, nose, and vagina to improve the topical healing process, scaffolds-like devices should present similar mechanical properties to soft tissues like elasticity and plasticity, typical of viscoelastic materials such as polymers [85]. The most critical mechanical properties to be considered for scaffold development are: tensile strength, shear strength, elasticity, hardness, surface rigidity, fatigue resistance, ductility and compression. The application of the polymer-based scaffolds in the regeneration of bone tissue requires a polymer with elasticity and resistance to compression comparable to bone tissue, in order to avoid fractures. Moreover, surface roughness should be adequate to enable cells attachment and adherence.

Some essential polymer properties to producing scaffolds are: bioreabsorption, capacity of sterilization to prevent infections and similarity to the endogenous macromolecules. Biocompatibility and low toxicity are essential polymer properties so that the rejection process does not occur during scaffold use. Biodegradability enables the human cells to form their own matrix while polymer chains are degraded. The biodegradation process occurs according to polymer molecular characteristics like degree of crystallinity, molecular weight, chemical composition and molecular structure. It is noteworthy that some polymer properties can directly alter the physiology of biological tissues and organs. For example, the use of non-degradable polymers requires that their molecules should be small enough to not affect renal clearance, avoiding accumulation of polymer particles in human organs such as the kidneys [87].

On the other hand, scaffolds characteristics as porosity, roughness and surface properties, and presence of additives, in addition to the size, geometry and administration site directly affect both biodegradation and biocompatibility of scaffolds [10].

The ability to bioreabsorption is one of the main requirements that the scaffolds used as grafts must present. *In vivo* polymer scaffolds degradation enables cell proliferation and attachment, as a new tissue is being formed [10]. The degradation process occurs according to the nature of the polymer and is influenced by polymer scaffolds morphological properties.

Types of Polymer-based Scaffolds

The morphology of scaffolds may vary according to their final purpose or application, being also important to consider type of treatment needed for long or short residence time. Among the scaffolds structures, a wide range of possible morphologies can be listed, such as: nanotubes, fibers, nanofibers, foams, sponges, hydrogel and spheres. Some of them are shown in Fig. (**5**).

When scaffolds are designed for drug delivery purposes, the ideal morphology comprises porous structures such as hydrogels, nanofibers and films, which allow drug encapsulation and diffusion. Moreover, high porosity is desirable, since they improve bioadhesivity [88].

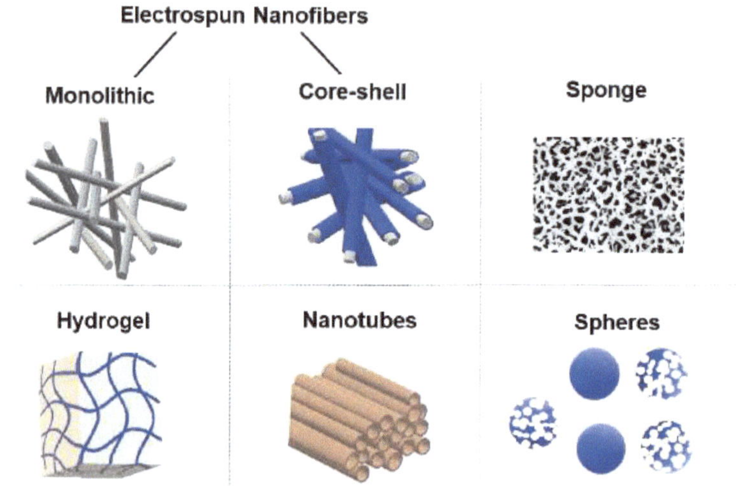

Fig. (5). Examples of polymer scaffolds and structures for biomedical applications.

SCAFFOLDS OBTENTION METHODS

The obtention method can dictate the morphologic characteristics observed as final results in the scaffolds. Hence, the right selection of the proper methodology allows achieving critical parameters such as drug solubility and the drug release rates. The most studied techniques to scaffold production are: phase separation induced by immiscible or thermal solvent, emulsion by lyophilization, leaching, 3D printing, and electrospinning.

In order to choose the most suitable scaffold production technique, it is necessary to consider that each method feature particular characteristics and specific parameters such as: processing temperature, which can trigger degradation phenomena for both polymer and drug molecules; the use of organic solvent during preparation that rises serious toxicity concerns; the shape of the pores; the cost of production and manufacturing time. Fig. (**6**) shows the different materials morphologies that can be obtained by each possible technique applied.

Phase Separation Method

Phase separation is a simple and inexpensive approach to produce scaffolds [89]. Phase separation can be induced by different approaches, using temperature, vapor or mixing non-miscible solvents, depending on the type of scaffolds required. It is necessary to consider that the use of higher temperatures could rupture polymer chemical bonds, affecting scaffold morphology. Nevertheless, the use of organic solvents should consider that their residues might affect tissue recovery by triggering protein structural alterations and immunogenic responses [90].

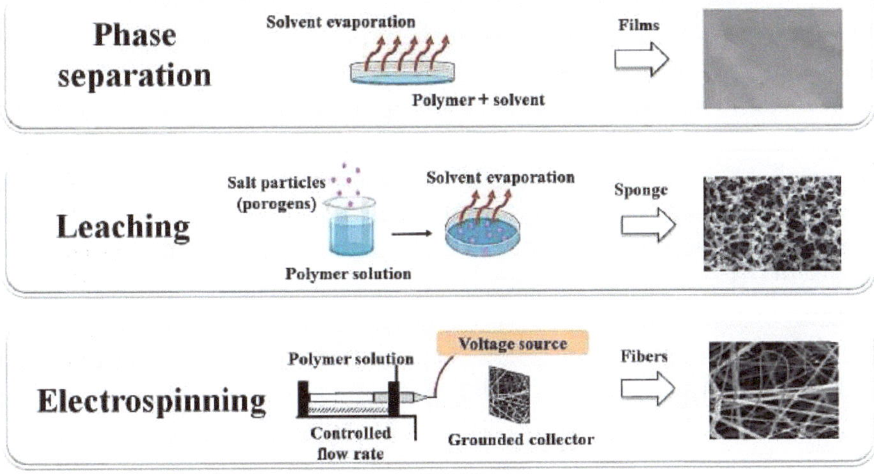

Fig. (6). Examples of techniques and types of polymer scaffolds.

Different morphologies of topical dosage forms, such as films or fibers can be obtained upon *in situ* solvent evaporation. In these cases, the drug is dissolved or suspended as nanocarriers in a polymer solution. The polymer network of the film/fiber constitutes an external reservoir and control drug release by using a secondary drug vehicle [91]. The solvent evaporation rate affects scaffold formation, and it can be controlled by polymer concentration, solvent volatility, temperature, pressure and the use of cosolvents. In solvent evaporation methodologies, the polymer colloidal suspension is first poured on a surface, for example, a glass plate or a petri dish. Subsequently, the solvent can evaporate with ambient temperature or under controlled temperature in an oven for a certain time. Morphologic aspects such as porosity, roughness and elasticity are commonly influenced by the drying step.

Solid–liquid phase separation occurs when the solvent forms crystals at lower temperatures before the phase separation takes place between the solvent and polymer. Solvent sublimation leads to ladder-like porous structure in the scaffolds. Liquid–liquid phase separation, on the other hand, generates polymer-rich and polymer-lean liquid phases [92].

The phase separation method can be also applied by thermally induced phase separation (TIPS). TIPS involves the solvent evaporation followed by a decrease in temperature, resulting in a porous structure with complete solvent evaporation [92]. As a result of temperature decrease, the homogeneous polymer solution is replaced by a polymer-rich phase and a solvent-rich phase, reflecting the phase separation phenomenon [93]. TIPS uses the thermal energy as a driving force to induce phase separation, which can occur by exposing the polymer solution low temperatures solution below its solubility temperature [94].

Remarkably, TIPS process involves other parameters, such polymer nature, polymer concentration and solvent/nonsolvent ratio [95]. Each parameter can influence the scaffold appearance, morphology, porosity, and the amorphous and crystalline proportions. Among the various methods available to fabricate porous scaffold, TIPS had received attention due to its simplicity and versatility, allowing the production a wide range of pores type, size, shape, and interconnections [96]. Guo *et al.* (2016) [97] reported how TIPS parameters can influence the porous scaffold morphology. In their work, the effect of copolymer concentration and solvent ratio were evaluated to generate scaffolds suitable to tissue engineering. For instance, their results showed that the decrease of temperature allowed the fabrication of scaffolds with interconnected porous.

The solvents used in TIPS are important factors, since polymer/solvent compatibility directly affects thermodynamic properties such as crystallization temperature [98]. Jing *et al.* [99], investigated different solvents to produce scaffolds suitable for tissue engineering. The authors pointed that the scaffolds morphologies changed according to thermodynamics of the phase separation of each solvent. Moreover, phase separation can be also modified according to polymer molecular weight.

Gay *et al.* (2018) [100] showed that polymer concentration, molecular weight, and type of organic solvent were essential parameters to determine the scaffold characteristics and their relation to the tissue engineering application. In this work, the scaffolds were obtained from PLLA with different molecular weights. The scaffolds obtained with higher PLLA molecular weight showed more stiffness, leading to a modulation in their mechanical properties, which make them suitable to bone and cartilage regeneration. Additionally, Onder *et al.* [101]. presented the influence of polymer concentration to control pore size and porosity in a scaffold for biomedical applications. A mixture of solvent and nonsolvent was used as a strategy to control polymer-solvent compatibility, generating a foam-like morphology due to the large amounts of nonsolvent used in the scaffold preparation. Therefore, using different TIPS methods and controlling their parameters can affect scaffold properties and influence their application.

Although TIPS can generate tailored membranes, the nonsolvent induced phase separation (NIPS) is more versatile and scalable method [102]. NIPS consists of a biphasic system: one is a polymer-rich solution that provides the polymer matrix after the precipitation and the other one is a polymer-poor phase that forms membrane pores after it is removed from the precipitated polymer solution [103]. The solvent-nonsolvent system must be miscible, as the polymer film solidifies through the exchange of the solvent and non-solvent [104]. NIPS is often used for the fabrication of porous membranes and it is considered a very easy and clean process [105]. Furthermore, it also is possible to obtain an average pore size that varies between the micrometric and nanometric scale [106].

The vapor-induced phase separation (VIPS) technique can be applied to obtain polymer membranes. In VIPS methodology, the polymer solution is cast on an appropriate substrate and the phase separation occurs after the exposition to a gas, which allows solvent evaporation from the solution [107]. In VIPS, membranes can present porous on their top surface by adjusting the vapor-induced time. The time of exposure to vapor also regulates the pore size. However, to provide easier porous formation in the scaffold surface with VIPS method, the use of a low polymer concentration is more favorable [108]. Although low polymer concentration can provide a membrane with poor mechanical properties, VIPS presents the ability to better control phase inversion rate than other methods, providing controlled tailored morphology [109].

All solvent evaporation techniques are based essentially on the same principle in which the phase separation occurs before the polymer matrix solidification [102]. These phase separations are promoted by a non-solvent (NIPS) or temperature alteration (TIPS) or vapor induced by a moisture environment (VIPS). Fig. (**7**) depicts the schematic representation of each method.

The main parameter of solvent evaporation-based techniques is the polymer-solvent interaction. The slow solvent evaporation can originate over wet substrates. On the other hand, the fast solvent evaporation leads to the formation of polymer-containing droplets dried before either affecting on the substrate surface with a spray drying effect [110]. Besides, the physicochemical properties of polymer solution and the use of cosolvents or other types of additives can influence on final membrane morphology, as previously stated [111]. As an example, the formation of either porous top layer or dense film layer depends on the diffusion rate ratio of solvent to non-solvent [112]. Table **3** shows some of the experimental parameters of solvent evaporation methods.

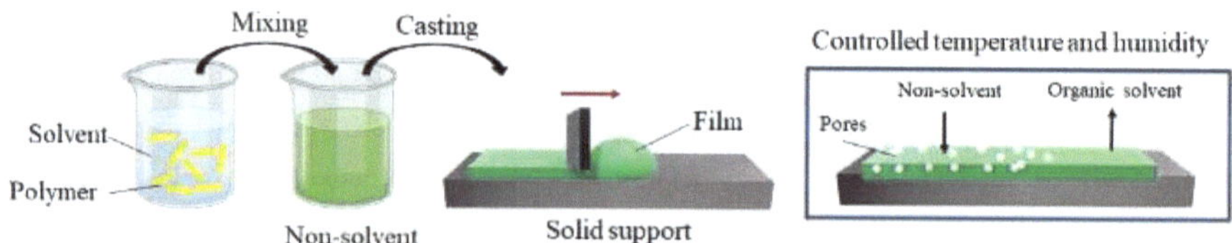

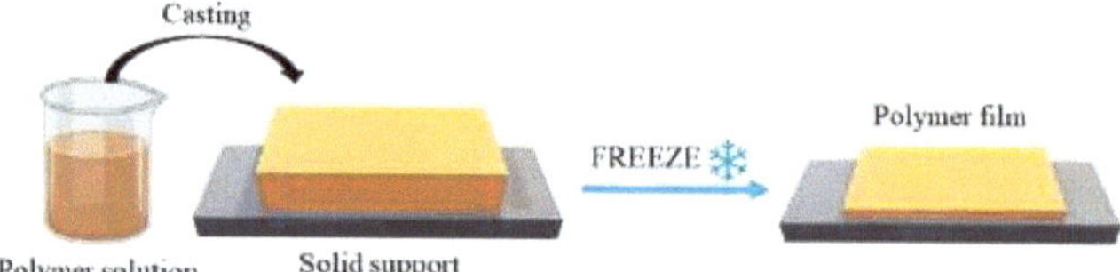

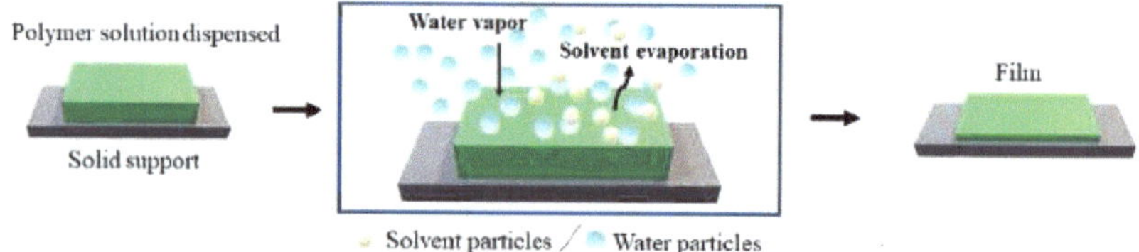

Fig. (7). Schematic representation of solvent evaporation methods: NIPS (A), TIPS (B) and VIPS (C). Adapted from Kim, J. F [102].

Table 3. Examples of experimental parameters of solvent evaporation methods. Adapted from Holda *et al.* [111] and Soroko *et al.* [112].

Solvent Evaporation Parameters	
Polymer solution	Polymer concentration Type of solvent/non-solvent Cosolvent/solvent ratio Speed of casting
Types of support material	Glass Polymer Metal
Environmental parameters	Temperature of the evaporation Relative humidity
Other parameters	Atmospheric conditions during and after casting Composition of the coagulation bath Post-treatment of the polymer membrane

Although solvent evaporation methods are simple approaches to obtain polymer scaffolds, they present considerable disadvantages. For instance, often a large amount of organic solvents such as dimethylformamide (DMF), dimethyl sulfoxide (DMSO) and tetrahydrofuran (THF) remain trapped within the scaffolds, which can lead to negative impacts on operational safety, economic costs, the environment and human health [113]. Another disadvantage, particularly for NIPS is that it generates significant amounts of solvent-contaminated wastewater, thus it is essential to search for green alternative methods [102].

In general, phase separation techniques provide membranes with asymmetric structures [103, 104]. Once polymer blends are used, phase separation can lead to a wide range of morphologies such as bicontinuous structure, clusters, or pores, which can be modified with the substrate, pressure, temperature, and environmental conditions [114].

Leaching Method

Leaching technique involves mixing water-soluble salt particles in a polymer solution. The solution is cast into the desired shape mold, followed by solvent elimination, allowing salt particles to be leached out with water [115]. Therefore, as the salt particles are leached out with water removal, a porous structure is formed.

Leaching technique produces materials with high porosity rate and larger pore range in comparison with phase separation techniques, *i.e.*, between 100-500 micrometers [116]. Additionally, polymer leaching is a cost-effective method that can produce porous scaffolds with fully interconnected networks in cylinder shape, providing larger pores [117]. Highly open porous and sponge-like structures are essentially required to improve tissue regeneration by enhancing communication between cells and inducing their cytoskeletal organization [118]. Due to this high porosity, in comparison with other methods, leaching is often more appropriated to induce cell proliferation and tissue recovery.

Experimental combinations of polymers are also applied in the leaching process to improve the development of polymer scaffolds membranes. Thadavirul *et al.* [119] used PEG as an additive to provide pores in a PCL membrane. Thus, a porous structure is obtained not by conventional salt leaching, but by leaching out an aqueous PEG solution. PCL can also be seen in recent works as Sempertegui *et al.* [120], using the same production method to produce polymer scaffolds membranes for tissue recovery.

Bone tissues are complex structures to replace or recover. Therefore, polymer scaffolds are used as a platform of protein delivery such as morphogenetic proteins. The combination of these proteins with the high porous salt-leached membrane scaffolds enhances cell proliferation. Song *et al.* [121] fabricated PCL biphasic composite scaffolds to immobilize collagen and bone morphogenetic protein (BMP) controlled local release. Their results showed that combined layer-by-layer leaching techniques produced PCL-based scaffolds, which provided BMP controlled release for 4 weeks, suggesting greater bone regeneration in critical size defect. This work highlighted that polymer scaffold obtained by leaching can be used not only in tissue engineering but also as a drug delivery platform.

Recently, Varshney *et al.* [122] developed three-dimensional macroporous scaffolds for cell culture in skin tissue scaffolds. The fabrication included the salt leaching method of polydimethylsiloxane (PDMS). After scaffold formation, collagen was used as a coating to enable cell adhesion. Experimental results showed skin cell adhesion, infiltration and viability improvements.

In Situ Polymerization Methods

Polymers that respond to external stimulation as pH, temperature or ionic strength are considered “smart” or stimuli-responsive materials and they provide networks as nanogels, dendrimers and cross-linked hydrogels [123]. Stimuli-responsive hydrogels can be formed by *in situ* methods through chemical reactions or electrostatic interactions, with the addition of the polymer followed by its immediate gelation [116]. These smart hydrogels could change their matrix structure to adapt to the target tissue and its environmental conditions. For example, acid pH values could lead to polymer chain modification or polymer matrix relaxation.

Specifically, *in situ* produced hydrogels formed by physical entanglements include spontaneous hydrogel bonds between water-soluble polymer chains or chemical methods as Michael addition reaction, photo polymerization or enzymatic reactions [124]. In this way, solvent exchange, *in situ* crosslinks, pH or temperature changes are transformations that lead the transformation of liquid polymer solution or dispersions into a solid-state or semi-solid polymer matrix. Polymer precipitation provides a solid polymer scaffold that allows drug molecules to be trapped, enabling slow controlled drug release [125].

Wei *et al.* [126] obtained a hydrogel by *in situ* polymerization of a polysaccharide-based scaffolds from dimethylaminoethyl methacrylate monomers using a crosslinking agent, N,N′-methylenebis (acrylamide). After the incorporation of the catalyst agent, the polymerization reaction was carried overnight at room temperature. The end of the *In situ* polymerization reaction produced a stimuli-responsive hydrogel capable to present an increased drug release rate in acid pH values produced, as polymer amine groups are protonated at low pH values, being more soluble in water.

In situ polymerization has been also applied to the production of films with a layer-by-layer (LbL) method. The LbL assembly has been widely used to fabricate stimuli-responsive films and it involves altering the deposition of different interacting materials, which allows simple control over film thickness [127]. The method is based on electrostatic adsorption between layers. During film production, the charged top layer must be insoluble, but the bottom layer should become fully soluble at physiological pH [128].

Park *et al.* [129] applied the LbL method to provide multilayer polyelectrolyte films incorporated poly (ethylene glycol)-block-poly (ε-caprolactone) (PEG---PCL) block copolymer- based micelles as drug carriers for dexamethasone encapsulation, a well-known osteogenisis-inducing drug. For layers assembly, the authors used different polyelectrolyte solutions such as alginate-micelle blends, with pH 2.0, poly (acrylic acid) with pH 4.0 and poly (allylamine hydrochloride) with pH 8.0. First, a silicon wafer was dipped in a cationic polyelectrolyte solution, washed and then dipped in a negatively charged solution containing micelles. To each layer, a hydrophilic charged polymer, alginate or chitosan was applied. The results showed that brushing layer-by-layer assembly method was simple and faster compared to the conventional surface coating method, especially for dentistry applications.

Polymer gel *in situ* formation is usually considered as a technique to topical mucosal routes as oral, ocular, rectal and vaginal routes [130]. Since each tissue presents different aspects like pH and temperature, such environmental aspects are often relevant to choose formulation components. Polymers as pectin, xyloglucan, and gellan gum are suitable for oral drug delivery systems. Divalent ions like calcium ions might be used to form ionic complex with such polymer, promoting gelation [131].

In situ microparticle (ISM) method is based on a biphasic system. In this context, two immiscible phases are put into contact, one containing the polymer-solvent phase that is emulsified into another phase, an outer phase [132]. Although this technique does not provide a proper membrane, microparticles contribute to enhance drug encapsulation efficiency and provide slow drug release as shown by recent works as Chauhan *et al.* [133] and Amini-Fazl *et al.* [134].

Electrospinning

Unlike the techniques mentioned above, electrospinning features many controllable parameters that optimize the scaffold production. This technique consists of applying an electric field to a polymeric solution in a grounded system [135]. The nanofibers produced by this method may present different morphology, porosity, malleability, shape, and size, all of which are dependent on the parameters used.

Electrospinning was first proposed by Formhal and later revisited by Reneker and Doshi [136]. However, the electrodynamics phenomenon, known as electrospinning began to be applied to the production of nanofibers for scientific and nanotechnology fields between 1990 and 2000 [137]. Electrospinning technique basically consists of applying an electric field into a polymeric solution in a grounded system. Fig. (**8**) schematically shows the electrospinning process in which a syringe containing a polymeric solution is coupled to a flow pump. The pump is responsible for controlling the flow through the needle and it is connected to a high voltage source with negative or positive polarity.

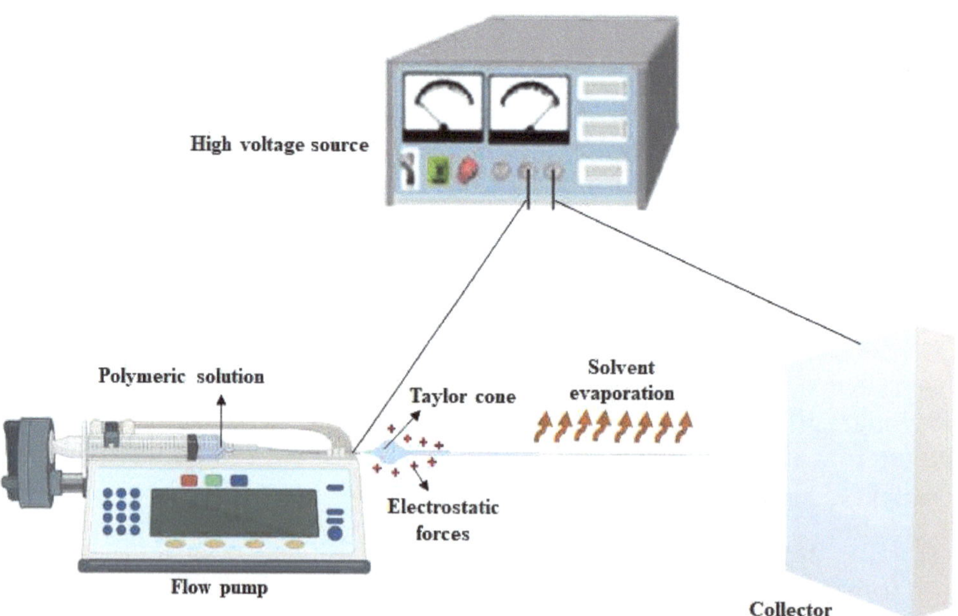

Fig. (8). Schematic representation of electrospinning technique with emphasis on the formation of the Taylor cone.

According to Sir Geoffrey Ingram Taylor, the droplet formed at the end of the needle stretches when a tension is applied, proving a cone, which was later called as Taylor's cone [137]. Still in this study, it was observed that the jet of the solution is generated at the vertex, so the electrospinning can generate fibers of dimensions smaller than the diameter of the needle used [138]. The droplet of the polymeric solution is stretched due to the high intensity electric fields applied (~ 100 KV / cm), leading to the formation of the Taylor's cone also represented by Fig. (**8**). The Taylor cone forms when the applied voltage allows the electrostatic forces to overcome the surface tension of the solution. Right after the cone is formed, the jet stretches.

The fiber morphology generated by the electrospinning technique depends on several aspects, such as: the chemistry of polymer used, the volume of solution, the viscosity of the polymeric solution, the solvents used, process temperature, among others [139]. Depending on the purpose of the scaffolds, they are required to present different morphologies, which is achievable due to the different the methods used during electrospinning, enabling to change several aspects of the support. Electrospun fibrous scaffolds feature high surface area, which improve cell adhesion, migration, and proliferation and maintain nutrient transport through porosity [140]. Due to these characteristics, there are many researches efforts focused on this type of material for engineering vascular, bone and nervous tissues.

In this way, electrospinning is considered a method that has been extensively studied in recent years due to its ease of use and application in tissue engineering. The obtained scaffolds can present fibers with different surfaces aspects, which depend on the process parameters. Also, depending on the purpose, the most relevant parameters should be optimized in order to obtain tailored structures. The main electrospinning parameters are divided into three categories: solution parameters, process parameters and factors related to the environment [141].

Examples of solution main parameters include conductivity, surface tension and viscosity; meanwhile process parameters consist of voltage, collector distance and flow rate [72]. Some of them directly affect the fiber diameter, for example: rheological properties of the polymer solution used; speed of rotation of the rotational collector; applied voltage and environmental conditions. The size and number of pores in the scaffold can also be controlled through the process. Table **4** summarizes electrospinning parameters and their impact morphological aspects of scaffolds.

Table 4. Electrospinning parameters and morphological aspects of scaffolds.

Parameter	Morphological Aspect	References
Process-related parameters		
Applied voltage		
Distance between tip and jet collector	Fiber morphology and diameter.	[135,142]
Flow rate	Increase in flow rate leads to larger fiber diameter and pore sizes. High flow rates produce fibers with non-uniform dimensions	[72,135,142,143]
Ambient-related parameters		
Temperature	Higher temperature reduces both solution viscosity and fiber diameter	[144]
Humidity	High humidity levels lead to circular pores and larger diameter fibers	[145]
Solution-related parameters		
Polymer Molecular weight	Higher polymer molecular weight produces uniform fiber morphology and increased mechanical strength	[135,146]
Viscosity and polymer concentration	Both low polymer concentration and viscosity leads to beady morphology. Higher viscosity and polymer concentration produces larger fiber diameter	[143,146]
Conductivity/charge density	Increased conductivity leads to uniform fibers hindering the formation of beads	[135]

In order to properly choose a specific electrospinning solvent, its vapor pressure under the processing conditions needs to be considered, as this selection is essential to achieve porous morphology [147]. Solutions with low polymer concentrations are low viscous and enable to obtain a mixture of polymer granules and fibers. Low viscous solutions lead to the generation of unstable jets, resulting in the dispersion of polymer droplets in the collector [148]. On the other hand, as polymer concentration increases, the granules become spindle fibers [149 - 152]. A slight increase in viscosity can lead to an increase in fiber diameter and disappearance of polymer granules. The presence of ionic species provides a considerable increase in conductivity, reducing critical voltage, enhancing jet deposition on the collector and enabling to obtain fibers with smaller diameters [135, 138].

Besides polymer solution parameters, electrospinning often rely on process-related parameters, which are mainly the applied voltage, flow rate, type of collector, and distance between the syringe and the collector. The modulation of such parameters directly affects the morphology of electrospun fibers. Applied voltage is considered the main factor in electrospinning during jet formation.

When the electric field reaches a critical voltage, the droplet at the cone tip overcomes its surface tension and a solution jet is generated. After the formation of the Taylor cone, the jet is electrified and stretched towards the collector. The critical voltage value for electrospinning is increased when the concentration of the solution is increased. On the contrary, increasing temperature induces to a reduced viscosity and increased mobility of polymer molecules; therefore the critical voltage required for the electrospinning is decreased.

The increase in electric tension is reported to lead to electrostatic repulsion, favoring the obtention of narrow fibers, with reduced diameter [135]. This theoretical proposal is illustrated in Equation 1, which shows the reduction in fiber diameter with the increase of the applied tension. The equation shows that there is a relationship between the voltage and the diameter of the fiber.

Equation 1 - Relation between fiber diameter and applied voltage. Where: h is the jet radius [m]; r_s is resistivity of the solution [Ω.m]; ρ is the density [kg/m^3]; Q is the flow rate [m^3/s]; Z is the distance from the nozzle to the collector [m]; U is voltage [kV]. Adapted from Cramariuc *et al.* [153].

$$h = \left(\frac{2 r_s \rho Q^3}{\pi^3} \; \frac{Z}{U^2} \right)^{1/6}$$

Flow rate is an important parameter that can be adequately controlled so that there is enough time to allow solvent evaporation [154]. The flow can favor the formation of pores with uniformity in size and can also lead to the formation of crimped fibers with strand shapes instead of smooth fibers. Meanwhile, the collector, regardless of the type, it is always connected to a grounding system or with an opposite charged apparatus, so that electrospun fibers can reach the collector more quickly during the electrospinning process [138]. Thus, the collectors that can be used in electrospinning are fixed, mobile such as swiveling rods or wheels, liquid bath, wire mesh, grid or roller and parallel bars.

The distance between the collector and the syringe is considered an important factor, as the intensity of the electric field varies with both the voltage and the applied distance [153]. The distance between the tip of the nozzle and the collector must have a minimum value to guarantee the total solvent evaporation, and a maximum value for the electric field to be effective in stabilizing the Taylor cone.

Several environment-related parameters also affect the result of electrospinning, being both temperature and humidity those considered the most important. Temperature variation directly changes the fiber diameter, as there is an inverse relationship between polymer solution viscosity and temperature. Thus, by increasing temperature, there is a reduction in the viscosity of the polymeric solution [135], which may result in a decrease of fiber diameter previously stated.

Humidity can directly affect the formation of porous fibers, as an increase in moisture leads to an increase in the number, diameter and distribution of pores [135, 139, 155]. The vapor originated from moisture evaporation, promotes phase separation, leading to the formation of pores on the fiber surface of hydrophobic polymer [156]. Moreover, with the increase of the pore size and numbers, coalescence can occur providing the development of larger pores [155].

Even though electrospinning features many advantages such as simplicity, obtention of nanoscale fibers, high surface-to-volume ratio fibers, wide variety of scaffolds sizes and shapes [135, 146], some limitations have been pointed [157]. The most cited limitations are, the low production rate and presence of cytotoxic solvents. In addition, for application for drug release or growth factors encapsulation, the electrospun nanofibers show limitations regarding drug incorporation. Moreover, the rapid solvent evaporation may result in amorphous dispersions [158].

Despite the disadvantages mentioned, the electrospinning offers a simple and robust process that provides controllable micro/nano-sized fibers and it creates nanofibers with high quality stability to mimic the native ECM structure [159]. For this reason, electrospinning continues to be studied in order to improve and find the proper materials and process conditions for more suitable and specific applications [11, 135].

Three Dimension (3D) Printing

Among all techniques previously described, 3D printing is the most recently developed. 3D printing, also called as additive manufacturing, has emerged as a versatile production method, being applied in a wide range of fields [8, 160]. Regarding to tissue engineering, 3D printing allowed a simple and fast method to incorporate drugs and other bioactive molecules, as cytokines and growth factors into scaffolds, providing hybrid materials that combine scaffolding and drug delivery properties.

Printing process occurs by the use of a computer-scanned image that is able to provide more detailed parts with well-defined micro and nanostructures [161]. 3D printing is fast production and cost-effectiveness so that it is capable to be applied to personalize medical prosthetics or devices obtained through a digital 3D file using computer-aided design software or imaging techniques [162].

The 3D printing technique includes more than 40 different printing processes such as inkjet printing, stereolithography (SLA), selective laser sintering (SLS), fused filament deposition (FDM) and three-dimensional printing (3DP) [163, 164]. In all 3D printing methods, the scaffolds is created according to a 3D computer-aided model, which provides a 3D model and printed into layers. Among all 3D printing processes, FDM is the most widely used in pharmaceuticals, being extremely versatile in the development of drug delivery systems [165].

Prior to the printing step, FDM requires the production of extruded filaments by hot-melt extrusion technology often composed by thermoplastic polymers blended with drugs [166]. FDM method relies on the use of computer aid designs (CAD) software to provide the design that is downloaded to the 3D printer software using stereolithography. Then, the filament is melted and deposited by a moving nozzle in an x-y noddle movement on the printer platform [167]. During FDM 3D printing, the filaments are deposited as layers that benefit the design of dosage forms, providing the unique opportunity to control the spatial distribution of an active pharmaceutical ingredient (Fig. **9**) [168].

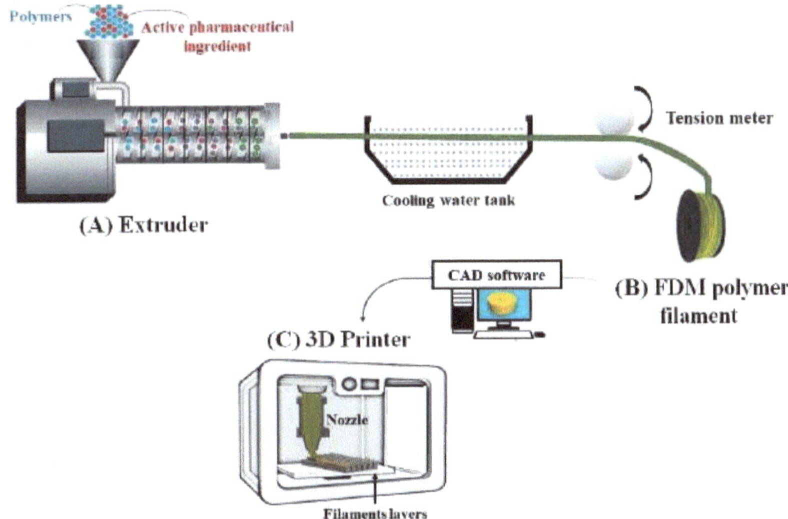

Fig. (9). Example of FDM-3D printing method. First the extrusion of polymers and addition of active pharmaceutical ingredients as drugs (A) to form the FDM polymer filament (B). After polymer filament formation, the CAD software is used to set morphology of the biomedical device that is printed (C). Adapted from Tan *et al*. [166].

Although FDM has been a popular and widely used method, it is a limited for the incorporation of biomolecules such as cellular growth factors due to high temperatures required to produce hot-melt extruded filaments [88]. In this way, to overcome FDM limitations, it is possible to incorporate active pharmaceutical ingredients after filament printing. For example, Beck *et al.* [169] soaked 3D printed devices in a liquid suspension containing drug nanoparticles. Liquid frozen deposition manufacturing (LFDM) which is also known as frozen-form method (FFM) is also a very exploited technique for the incorporation of drugs and bioactive molecules in 3D printed devices [160].

Different from FDM, in frozen-form method (FFM) polymer is dissolved in a solvent into a low-temperature cooling platform below solvent crystallization temperature, which promotes polymer solution freezing and thermally induced phase separation [170]. For instance, Liao *et al.* [171] used FFM to fabricate polymer scaffolds as potential biomedical devices in square and tubular morphologies. Also, polyurethane was used in scaffold fabrication without the use of organic solvents, which is beneficial for both environment and human tissues.

Other example of 3D printing process for drug delivery is stereolithography (SLS) or photopolymerization. This process involves exposing liquid resins to ultraviolet or other high-energy light source to induce polymerization reaction, which is considered one of most fast methods among 3D printing [172]. Photopolymers are submitted to ultraviolet (UV) laser and dispersed into layered multiple times to achieve the desired design, which can be advanced therapeutic drug carrier devices such as microneedles or painless needles [173]. In addition, SLS 3D printing presents the possibility to combine multiple drugs or bioactive molecules with distinct release properties in a single dosage form [174].

Despite leaching, freeze-drying, and electrospinning are methods that produce porous scaffolds, 3D printing provides a more controlled architecture without shape or geometry limitations [175]. In general, 3D printing has many advantages in drug delivery, such as easy designed product modification, development of personalized therapeutic devices, multidrug incorporation, and modulation of drug delivery profile with shape and density [169, 176]. 3D printing medicine emerges as a new research field with potential to expand drug delivery with devices in freeform geometries [176].

The desired biomedical application of scaffolds can influence the choice of the best production technology without compromising polymer properties. Although biodegradable and biocompatible properties are crucial for biomedical applications of polymer-based scaffolds, it is necessary to consider if the chosen method requires a great amount of solvent that could be toxic. Other criteria include drugs' physical-chemical characteristics, which are relevant to choose the method without compromising the drug bioavailability and pharmacological activity. Table **5** gathers the main information and shows some examples of all obtention techniques of polymer-based scaffolds and their biomedical application.

As shown in Table **5**, a wide range of scaffolds types and morphologies can be produced with the same obtention method, which reflects their versatility. Besides, the type of polymer, additives, and the applied method directly influence the morphology, amorphous, and crystal phases of polymer-based scaffolds. Each characteristic can influence the aftermost results such as drug/protein release and cell culture.

Table 5. Examples of techniques, the obtained dosage form with active pharmaceutical ingredients, their applications, and advantages.

Technique	Dosage Form	Active Pharmaceutical Ingredients	Biomedical Application and Advantages
Solvent evaporation	Film	Betamethasone-17-valerate	Prolonged dermal drug delivery [91]
	Blended polymer film	Rhodamine B (model drug)	Improvement of film stability for drug control release [177]
	Hydrogel film	Metformin hydrochloride	Improvement drug effectiveness with pH sensitive formulation [178]
	Hydrogel	Doxorubicin micelles	Improvement of drug solubility and enhancing cell targeting [179]
Leaching	Porous scaffold	-	Bone tissue engineering and a scaffold with long degradation period [180]
	Scaffold	Bone morphogenetic protein-2	Facilitates periodontal wound healing [181]
	Wound dressing	Collagen	Accelerate skin healing process [122]
Electrospinning	Nanofibers	Naproxen	Topical administration and local pain treatments [182]
	Core-shell fibers	Tamoxifen citrate	Enhancing fast dissolution of poorly water-soluble drugs [183]
	Nanofiber	Salicylic acid	Drug controlled release for wound treatments [184]
	Core-shell fibers	Bone morphogenetic protein-2	Drug controlled release for bone tissue engineering [185]

(Table 5) cont.....

In situ	Implant	Dexamethasone	Intraocular delivery of a limited soluble drug [125]
	Film	Dexamethasone	Clinical and non-immunogenic for hydrophobic drug carrier [129]
	Hydrogel	5-fluorouracil (5-FU)	Controlled drug release and wound healing applications [186]
3D printing	Microneedles	Insulin	Transdermal patch for diabetes [187]
	Pellets	Paracetamol and Ibuprofen	Multidrug oral dispense for pediatric and geriatric patients [188]
	Film	Aripiprazol	Oral fast dissolve films for patients with swallowing problems [176]
	Tablets	5-aminosalicylic acid and 4-aminosalicylic acid	Low-cost alternative for tailored oral drug dosage and modified release [188]

CHARACTERIZATION

Polymer-based scaffolds for topical applications are often characterized in terms of morphology, thermal behavior, crystallinity, and drug release profile. The most applied thermal techniques are Thermogravimetric Analysis (TGA) and Differential Scanning Calorimetry (DSC), the latter often used to correlate with the degree of crystallinity (Xc) of the material according to X-ray Diffractometry (XRD), which is vastly used to characterize the materials microstructure. Modern electron microscopies allow the material to be evaluated at its nanoscale. Scanning electron microscopy (SEM) is an example of an analysis that provides images, allowing evaluating aspects of the material such as porosity, uniformity and possible modifications according to the applied parameters.

Thermal Analysis (TGA, DSC and DMTA) and Crystallinity Evaluation (XRD)

Thermogravimetric Analysis (TGA) measures the mass loss as a function of temperature over time in a controlled atmosphere. Generally, polymer-based materials undergo degradation processes as temperature is raised, which can be related to ruptures of intramolecular chemical bonds. TGA also reflects bulk properties such as composition, purity, absorbed moisture contents and decomposition reactions [189]. In this way, it is possible to evaluate polymer structure and the thermal effects of nanostructures added to hybrid scaffolds.

El-Newehya *et al.* [190] reported the influence of different polymer blends compositions of scaffolding materials on TGA results. In this work, electrospun nanofibers loaded with sodium diclofenac were obtained by blending different ratios of PVA and carboxymethyl cellulose (CMC). As a result of the blends, fibers presented higher thermal stabilities observed as higher decomposition temperatures. Singh *et al.* [191] designed hydrogels obtained by copolymerization of PVP and acacia gum (GA). Their TGA results revealed the influence of grafting two different materials in achieving higher degradation temperatures. For instance, PVP/GA grafted hydrogels showed that GA decomposition occurred in two distinct temperatures, 137°C and 455°C, which was attributed to the grafting between PVP and GA.

Recently, Abilova *et al.* [192] designed scaffold films of poly (2-ethyl-2-oxazoline) (POZ) and chitosan obtained by aqueous solutions casting for ocular drug delivery. Although POZ is a promising polymer for biomedical applications, it does not exhibit mucoadhesion. Therefore, chitosan, a well-known mucoadhesive polymer, was added into film formulation. Also, chitosan provided a higher film thermal stability due to hydrogen bonds with POZ. Hence, TGA results revealed that POZ-based films presented higher degradation temperatures when chitosan was added to the scaffold formulation.

Although TGA is widely found as standard thermal characterization, this technique is incapable of detecting phase transitions, polymorphic transformations or a reactions for which mass is not variable [193]. For this reason, DSC assays are considered more appropriated, as they can expose relevant phase transitions in polymers such as glass transition (T_g) and crystal melting transition (T_m), closely related to crystallinity degree of most materials.

In DSC thermograms some phase transitions can be visualized in the curve of heat flow (W/g) as a function of temperature or time, allowing the investigation of amorphous phase, exothermic events and endothermic transitions [194]. Initially, the amorphous phase is associated with Tg, which represents the transition from the glassy to the rubbery state. On the other hand, the exothermic event is represented by a cold crystallization temperature (Tcc), which occurs when the material absorbs energy by heating, allowing the formation of crystals in the polymer matrix. The thermograms present endothermic transitions in higher temperatures represented by Tm, which is associated with the melting of the crystal phase.

Hollander *et al.* [195] reports how DSC could reveal transitions as a consequence of drug incorporation in a 3D printed intrauterine scaffold fabricated with a PCL matrix containing Indomethacin. In this way, polymer filaments were produced at

100°C, which is above Tm of PCL, but below than drug melting point temperature. According to DSC results, the thermograms for 3D printing scaffold did not show a maximum single peak of endothermic events related to Indomethacin. As a result, it could be considered that indomethacin was properly incorporated and dissolved in the polymer matrix.

Other types of scaffolds for drug delivery have been also characterized by means of DSC in order to evaluate drug incorporation in a different methodology. For instance, Dalton *et al.* [196] synthesized a hydrogel scaffold by photopolymerization of hydrophilic acetic acid (AA) with thermosensitive N–vinylcaprolactam (NVCL) monomer at different ratios for drug delivery purposes. Hydrogels were design to have lower critical solution temperature (LCST) close to physiological temperature by tuning phase transition temperature of NVCL. These transitions were analyzed using DSC, which showed that the LCST of the PNVCL/AA solutions increased slightly with increasing concentration of AA. The hydrogels prepared were thermoreversible and transparent indicating that NVCL presented amorphous phase confirmed by Tg in DSC without any remarked Tm peak and crystallization.

Polymer-drug interactions are also reported in recent works as Moydeen *et al.* [197]. A PVP electrospun scaffold containing ciprofloxacin and dexamethasone for wound healing were developed and characterized. Polymer-drug interactions were studied by DSC. The obtained thermograms exhibited the increase in Tg from pure PVP nanofibers to the dexamethasone-loaded nanofibers, indicating that the drug could establish hydrogen bonds with the polymer matrix. Moreover, the single Tg peak obtained for nanofibers suggested the miscible mixture from all components was obtained.

Thermal transitions results can be corroborated and further understood with the help of X-ray diffractions (XRD) experiments, which can display sharp peaks related to crystal formation and large amorphous peaks. XRD results provide the obtention of many microstructural parameters as, for example, the relative area of the diffraction peaks and the amorphous region, which can be associated to the crystallinity degree (Xc). Hence, XRD exhibits results from polymer-based material and its eventual changes upon drug incorporation or drug release.

Crystalline and amorphous phase ratios are useful for drug delivery applications, as it is possible to relate some chemical-physical properties with important target attributes like biocompatibility, burst effect or a controlled release. For example, Feng *et al.* [198] synthesized a triblock PCL-PEG-PCL copolymer scaffold incorporated with tetracycline, an antibiotic drug. Polyurethane acrylates (PUA) were added as crosslinker to improve scaffolds properties and provide further control of the drug release. According the increase of PCL molecular weight (in copolymer composition), lead to an increase in scaffolds crystallinity, as revealed by XRD results. Thus, the higher crystallinity of PCL-PEG-PCL scaffold cross-linked with PUA allowed reducing swelling in water, maintaining the drug reservoir and consequently controlling tetracycline release.

Besides control release, improving solubility and targeting drugs delivery are one of the usual goals of cancer chemotherapy. In this context, Ullah *et al.* [199] used gelatin smart hydrogels to overcome unspecific target and toxicity of intravenous oxaliplatin (OXP). The gelatin smart hydrogel diffractogram presented a broad peak around 30°, which is usually related to amorphous materials. Moreover this, OXP sharp peaks were not observed, suggesting a significant reduction of OXP crystallinity with drug incorporation into hydrogels. As a result, the amorphous hydrogel matrix facilitated OXP dispersion due to the amorphization phenomenon.

Recently, Alagha *et al.* [200] demonstrated how polymer crystallinity directly affects the drug release. A chitosan-collagen biosponge-like scaffold loaded with dexamethasone was designed to promote oral wound healing. Collagen was previously mixed with chitosan, which impaired the formation of chitosan crystals. Consequently, the biosponge-like scaffolds did not exhibit sharped peaks on XRD diffractograms. *In vitro* release tests proved that semi-crystallized matrix allowed water uptake, followed by swelling, and facile drug diffusion.

Microscopy and Microanalysis

Microscopy is widely used as a tool to analyze polymer surfaces. Although microscopic images are not conclusive alone, these characterizations techniques corroborate with DSC, XRD and *in vitro* release results. A wide range of different microscopies can be applied, depending on the type of structure to be characterized. It is known that optical light microscopy can only provide images with micrometer resolution, for more detailed characterization of nano-sized structures, electron microscopy techniques are further suitable [201]. Among them, scanning electron microscope (SEM) and transmission electron microscopy (TEM) are commonly used in micro and nanostructured scaffolds.

In general surface morphology, drug particles, crystallinity, amorphous and component sizes characterization can be observed with electron microscopy. Yadollahi *et al.* [202], for example, incorporated nanoparticles in chitosan hydrogels and SEM micrographs revealed particles with a size range of 10-25 nm. Ye and Hu (2016) [203] produced nanoparticles of 209 nm and measuring them with SEM, which displayed them in a PVA hydrogel scaffold matrix.

When investigating the polymer matrix through SEM, Ribeiro *et al.* [204] confirmed porous with diverse shapes on cellulose films and a homogeneous surface due to film cast technique. In this work, the authors used SEM to determine film thickness of films formulated with different amounts of polymer and solvents. Latter, Sarwar *et al.* [205] demonstrated through SEM the dispersion of the particles in a chitosan-methoxy polyethylene glycol blended film. Both groups remarked that films presented surface homogeneity owing to miscibility of all components.

In addition to hydrogels and films, electrospun fibers are often submitted to SEM and TEM, being the latter one more applied to core-shell fibers. Considering coaxial structures, Yu *et al.* [206] designed a long-term antibacterial scaffold where amoxicillin-loaded nanomicelles were incorporated into PCL-PVA core-shell fibers. SEM images presented the size of nanomicelles and nanofibers highlighting fibers surfaces smoothness. On the other hand, TEM confirmed the core-shell structure with the electrospinning parameters and the micelles spread in the core-fiber.

Silva *et al.* [185] evaluated coaxial electrospun fibers of PLA-PVA through SEM and TEM. In TEM analysis, fibers were produced containing iron in core-solution, which promotes differences between areas based on their electron density. TEM images of the obtained fibers showed a darker interior, as a consequence of higher iron electron density. Shell fibers with low electron density were more lightened, confirming coaxial obtention. Overall, their electron microscopy results evidenced how optimization of parameters in electrospinning can change surfaces of fibers along with range of diameters and porosity.

HYBRID SCAFFOLDS

Novel therapeutic devices that combine scaffolding and drug delivery properties can be considered as hybrid materials. The development of formulations based on these hybrid materials for topical use aims at the optimization of pharmacokinetic and pharmacodynamic parameters since they can provide increased solubility, permeability, absorption, biocompatibility, bioadhesivity, as well as the control of release rate and targeted drug delivery, increased stability and decrease in adverse effects by favoring a decrease in the concentration of drugs to obtain the therapeutic effect.

In general, in such hybrid materials, drugs can be loaded into nanostructured vesicular carriers, as nanoparticles or into nanofibers, that compose the scaffold it self. These drug nanocarriers can have different compositions, which directly influences their applicability and choice for each type of drug, required permeability level and desired activity. Nanoparticulate systems comprehend a wide range of different nanocarriers between systems based on surfactants, lipid, inorganic components and those consisting of polymers as a coating material. They are promising and versatile systems for controlled topical drug release.

All of these systems can be modified to meet therapeutic properties with the introduction of functional groups or chemical modifications that can (i) increase the drug retention time at the target site, (ii) prevent early leakage of the drug, increase the stability of its content, (iii) introducing ligands, such as antibodies, for the vectorization of the release to a specific type of cells, (iv) promoting the release according to external stimuli.

However, many of these drug carriers are often associated with problems, especially with stability drawbacks. In addition, for topical application, these systems must be introduced in conventional vehicles to provide the viscosity, extended residence time and adhesiveness, mechanical properties that are required for the topical administration route.

On the other hand, the introduction of drug nanocarriers in polymer-based scaffolds opens a window of new opportunities to develop innovative and multifunctional formulations since it combines the interesting characteristics related to nanotechnology with the properties of such polymer-based scaffolds, as biocompatibility and bioabsorption. Other evident advantages are the possibility of incorporating both hydrophilic and lipophilic or incompatible substances; wide-ranging nature and composition of vehicles (without predominance of instability and degradation mechanisms of the drug); targeting specific targets, *etc.* In addition, several biopolymers can be used as adjuvants in the topical treatment of several diseases because they feature anti-inflammatory or antimicrobial pharmacological activity [76, 207, 208].

The dispersion of nanocarriers in a polymer-based scaffold matrix constitutes systems that can be considered composite or hybrid scaffolds, since they are often composed of nanometric structures entrapped in a polymer-based matrix, as in a “plum pudding”, also called soft nanocomposite materials [209 - 212]. These materials emerge as novel materials for biomedical use. In composite scaffolds, nanocarriers are immobilized either covalently or noncovalently in polymeric matrix. From the interaction of nanocarriers with polymer chains, novel physical properties arise, which are not observed for the components separately. Such as higher mechanical performance, changes in swelling and sensibility to external stimuli [213].

The formation of a nanocomposite material increases biocompatibility of nanocarriers and may prevent their diffusion to other tissues *in vivo* [213].

Moreover, scaffolds can also impact in the drug release kinetic profile as they represent an additional vehicle, acting as a diffusional barrier, preventing the burst release effect, often related to nanostructured drug carriers [213, 214]. Fig. (**10**) presents these systems in a simplified manner, where D1 and D2 represent the diffusion coefficients of the drug from the secondary release vehicle and the hydrogel, respectively.

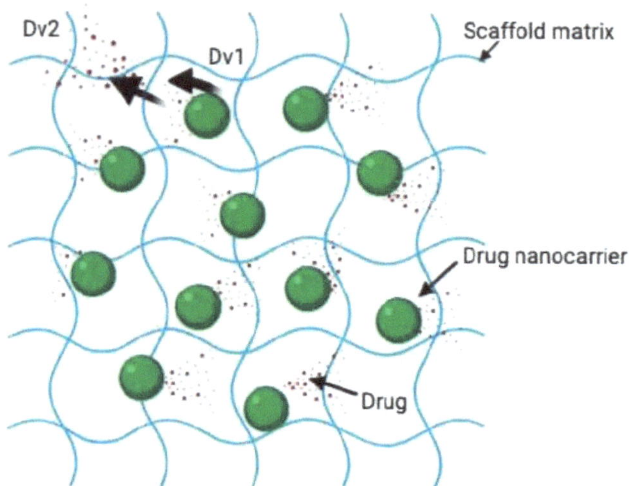

Fig. (10). "Plum pudding" model for composite scaffold with drugs compounds encapsulated in a secondary release vehicle such as nanoparticles. Dv1 and Dv2 stand for diffusion coefficient from the first drug vehicle (nanocarrier) and from the second drug vehicle (hydrogel). Adapted from Hoare *et al.* [213].

In such systems, nanocarriers are often trapped into a three-dimensional hydrogel network. The introduction of nanocarriers in a polymer matrix increases their stability against the formation of supramolecular aggregates. Additionally, composite scaffolds are able to control the rate and time of drug release, optimizing the therapeutic effects [209, 215]. Such therapeutic improvement is also related to adhesive properties provided by hydrogel-forming polymers, which increases drug residence time at the therapeutic site. This phenomenon favors pharmacological activity of the active principle by ensuring the intimate contact of the particles with the target tissue [213].

The scaffold polymeric matrix is important for the controlled release of bioactive ingredients, which occurs through aqueous channels and porous structures present in the polymer-based scaffolds. Hybrid scaffold-based drug delivery materials can be design to spatially and temporally control the release of bioactive agents by tuning their physico-chemical properties [82, 213].

For most non-biodegradable polymer-based scaffolds, diffusion plays a leading role for drug release profile. The combination with biodegradable drug nanocarriers can provide complex release behavior. Hence, the diffusion from drug molecules and biodegradation should be taken into consideration when designing hybrid scaffolds [11].

Hybrid scaffolds feature the advantage of combining the favorable therapeutic efficacy characteristics and enhanced penetration attributed to nanocarriers with physical stability related to scaffolds, which can prevent migration of nanocarriers to other biological compartments and provide an additional diffuse barrier for drug release [213, 216]. In addition, fibrous surface as the ones present in electrospun nanofibers scaffolds has been related to high mucoadhesiveness, improving therapeutic efficacy, which make such scaffolds an ideal candidate for topical drug delivery [145, 217].

Burst release can be observed for drug-loaded nanofibers or nanoparticle-loaded scaffolds can be often observed, which is an indicative of a non-homogeneous drug distribution in the systems. In general, hydrophobic drugs should be loaded into hydrophobic polymers and hydrophilic drugs should be loaded into hydrophilic polymers [11]. In this context, it can be said that, polymer-drug compatibility, physicochemical properties of polymers and drug and drug distribution state can greatly influence drug release kinetics and should be greatly considered.

On the other hand, the initial fast drug release can originate biphasic delivery systems to better adapt to some clinical needs. A biphasic drug release system contains a fast release compartment that shows a rapid increase in drug release for prompt therapeutic effect. A second compartment provides a sustained release, which prevents repeated administrations.

Bioengineered liposome-based hybrid scaffolds can be developed to optimize the therapeutic potential of liposomes by enabling enhanced drug release properties, environmental responsiveness and potency. The introduction of liposomes increases mechanical strength, rheological properties and biocompatibility of polymer scaffolds. Moreover, several applications can be explored using different scaffolds, polymers or nanofibrous scaffolds [82]. Liposome-loaded hybrid scaffolds can sustain therapeutic drug levels at the target site, while reducing toxic effects often related to repeated administration.

Hyaluronic acid based composite scaffolds loaded with liposomes were prepared by Widjaja *et al.* for ocular wound healing application [218]. Hyaluronic acid is well known for its wound healing properties and high biocompatibility, as is a natural component of the extracellular matrix [219, 220]. Latanoprost was encapsulated into egg phosphadityl choline liposomes to localize sustained drug release inside the eye compartment. Hyaluronic acid was chemically modified prior the incorporation of liposomes and, then cross-linked. Longer sustained drug release was observed for composite scaffolds when compared with liposomes or hydrogels alone, suggesting the additional control to drug diffusion and controlled degradation properties [218].

Yu *et al.* produced biphasic drug release nanofibrous multi-layered scaffolds produced by coaxial electrospinning of PVP/Ethyl cellulose core-sheath nanofibers [221]. Ketoprofen was used as model drug, PVP composed the sheath and ethyl cellulose composed the core. Compatibility among polymers and drugs was proved by attenuated total reflectance-Fourier transform infrared spectra. *In vitro* drug release showed an immediate followed by a sustained release. Immediate drug release rate was tailored by adjusting the sheath layer conditions, proving that biphasic novel drug release system can be produced and easily tuned by the adequate selection of polymers and through coaxial electrospinning [222].

SMART SCAFFOLDS

Recently, hybrid smart polymer scaffolds have proven to be able to combine the benefits of different nanocarriers and can also respond to external stimuli such as: temperature, pH, and redox state, allowing for vectorization and control of drug release, which can increase efficiency therapeutic agents and diminish harmful effects to the surrounding tissue.

In such systems, drug release take place as an external signal trigger a major modification on polymer dimensions, physical properties structure or solubility, which leads to a convection-mediated drug release in the target site. This rapid modification is derived from a major change on polymer solubility, alteration of hydrophilic/hydrophobic state, or reversible sol-gel transition [76].

Thus, smart drug delivery systems act not only as temporal controlled drug release devices but also provide on-demand drug release in different environmental conditions, including pH, temperature, light or magnetic field [31, 41, 223]. External stimuli include environmental conditions as pH, temperature, near infrared (NIR) light, magnetic field and ultrasound [14], as shown in Fig. (**11**).

In general, implantable smart scaffolds can be categorized into two types: those preformed prior to implantation and those formed *In situ* upon injection after some external stimuli. Most of the commercially available implantable drug delivery systems are constituted by FDA-approved thermoplastic biopolymers as PCL, PLA, PLGA and hydrogels made from alginate, gelatin, silk *etc.* On the other hand, implantable scaffolds are frequently constituted by thermo or pH-sensitive hydrogels or *In situ* cross-linkable biopolymers [76].

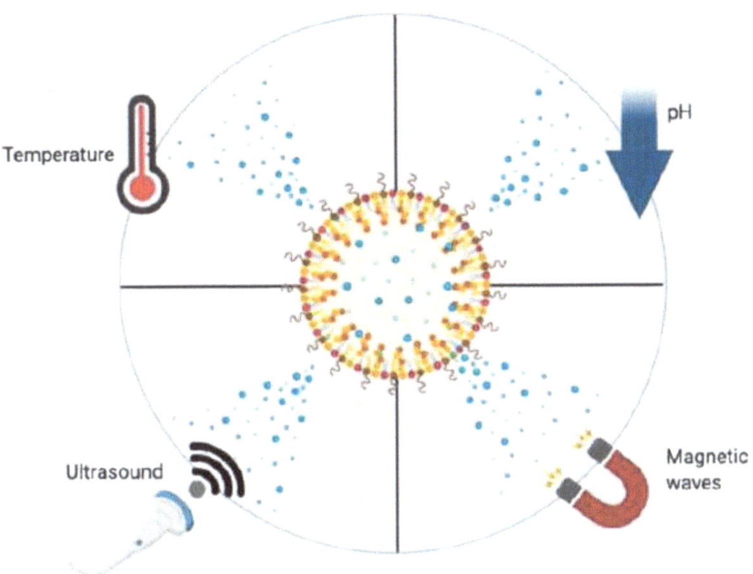

Fig. (11). Schematic representation of different mechanisms of stimuli-responsive drug release. Adapted from [223].

Hybrid smart drug delivery systems can also be produced by incorporation of functional nanocarriers into thermosensitive biopolymer matrix and their mechanism of drug release can comprise three steps: i) heat generation by nanomaterials upon external stimuli; ii) biopolymeric matrix undergo a physical modification; iii) rearrangement of pore structure within the biopolymeric scaffold matrix and resulting in drug release. The type of nanocarrier can dictate of external stimuli that will trigger drug release. Metallic nanoparticles, for instance can be particularly sensitive to electromagnetic waves and magnetic field [12, 76].

Internal stimuli-responsive scaffolds can respond to stimuli generated by the human organism itself, as pH or temperature. In general, thermosensitive scaffolds are polymer materials that can be administered with a minimally invasive technique being stimulated by inner temperature to temporary crosslink through noncovalent interactions [224].

Thermosensitive polymers show low viscosity at room temperature and they comprise polysaccharides, as glycosaminoglycan-based biohybrid hydrogels, elastin and silk-like polypeptides, hydrazide-functionalized poly (N-isopropyl acrylamide) (PNIPAAm), poly (organophosphazene) (PPZ) and Pluronic F127 [224 - 226], among others. Their thermosensitive behavior relies on the self-assembled gelification, usually above 36°C, which make them promising candidates to originate injectable smart scaffolds.

pH-sensitive polymers are those that can undergo physical modifications in different pH levels and the feature pH-dependent solubility. Such materials are water-insoluble at low pH values and become water-soluble at higher pH levels, or vice-versa, resulting in a more porous and permeable matrix. Polysaccharides are commonly used as natural pH-sensitive polymers, such as some natural polymers, such as chitosan, alginate, hyaluronic acid, dextran and their derivatives. The water-soluble polysaccharide derived from *Albizia lebbeck* seeds, for example, is a unique non-ionic polymer often used for the development of pH-sensitive scaffolds. Some of synthetic pH-dependent polymers may include poly(2-dimethylamino) ethylmethacrylate) (PDMAEMA) and poly(acrylic acid) (PAA) [12, 30, 224, 227]. Polyelectrolyte hydrogels are often used due to their similarities to human macromolecules, such as proteins. Besides, they can present volume transitions in response to the environmental variations, such as pH, salt concentration or temperature [228].

pH- and temperature-sensitive polysaccharides, proteins, polymers and copolymers can be exploited as triggers for the double stimuli-controlled drug release. For example, pH-sensitive polymers can be cross-linked or grafted to temperature-sensitive polymers to provide double stimuli-responsive scaffolds [12, 13]. Several authors reported the obtention of both pH and temperature responsive hydrogels based on poly (2-dimethylaminoethyl methacrylate) for biomedical applications. Such polymer shows tertiary amine groups, which can be charged at low pH and uncharged at high pH. Such phenomenon provides a pH dependence and also the existence of both a lower critical solution temperature (LCST) and an Upper critical solution temperature (UCST) [228 - 230].

Nita *et al.* developed stimuli-responsive scaffolds by combining the benefits of natural polymers as carboxymethyl starch and synthetic polymers like poly (2-dimethylaminoethyl methacrylate) for spatial and temporal control of local ibuprofen delivery. Such scaffolds presented a biocompatible hydrogel with a semi-interpenetrating polymer network structure. This material showed a temperature and pH-responsive behavior, adequate mechanical properties and *In vitro* cytocompatibility, being considered promising materials as smart scaffold-based drug delivery systems [228, 230].

Motealleh *et al.* reported the production of implantable pH-responsive scaffolds based on alginate hydrogels and mesoporous organosilica nanoparticles, constituting hybrid smart scaffolds. In this work, mesoporous silica nanoparticles were loaded with doxorubicin, an anti-cancer drug, and then embedded into an alginate network. Nanoparticle has their surface with poly-L-lysine, which was provided pH-responsive drug release due to the different pH-dependent levels of electrostatic interactions between all the charged components of the NC scaffolds. The pH-responsive nanoparticle/alginate hydrogel showed prolonged moderate drug release under physiological and a high dosage under acidic conditions with high cell adhesion. Their results showed that pH-responsive PMO/alginate scaffolds were able to provide local drug delivery to cancer cells than to healthy cells due to the local acidic environment generated by the cancer cells [231].

Magneto-responsive scaffolds are often used as advanced drug delivery systems and tissue regeneration devices. They are obtained by the incorporation of magnetic nanoparticles into biomaterial hydrogel structure. Magnetic nanoparticles are being pointed as advantageous drug delivery nanocarriers as they undergo to chemical and conformational changes in response to magnetic field. On the other hand, although they can be prepared with biomaterials, there are still serious concerns about their clinical application, as their clearance and biocompatibility remains a major limitation [12, 232]. Thus, the introduction of metallic magneto-scaffolds into biocompatible scaffolds can solve several issues. Adedoyin and Ekenseair reviewed the main methods to produce magneto-responsive scaffolds, the techniques to predict and evaluate magneto-responsive biomaterial *in vivo* behavior, and their application as controlled drug delivery systems, tissue engineering scaffolds, and artificial muscles [232].

Magneto-sensitive hydrogels can be implantable scaffolds to local delivery of a bioactive molecule upon an external magnetic signal according to the magnetic field strength, which can lead to tunable pharmacokinetic properties [232]. Casolaro *et al.* reported the production of hybrid pH and magneto-responsive scaffolds constituted by $CoFe_2O_4$ embedded in a N-(acrolyl-L-phenylalanin-)-N-(isopropylacrylamide) copolymer cross-linked with N,N'-ethylen--bisacrylamide. With the increase on ph from 2.9 to 7.4, a sudden increase of drug release was noticed. Moreover, upon an alternating magnetic field provided a pulsatile release of paroxetine, duloxetine and vortioxetine from the nanocomposite scaffold [233].

Photo-/light-responsive materials are attractive materials for the development of scaffolds with biomedical applications. Polymers are photoactive and usually feature a photochromic chromophore as the main moiety. Luminous or UV stimuli are captured by photoactive functional groups and then, polymers undergo significant changes in their physical or chemical characteristics, such as dimerization, isomerization, polymerization or cleavage. Photoactive functional groups as azobenzenes, spiropyrans triphenylmethanes or coumarines, can be introduced to polymer main chain to produce photoresponsive scaffolds [234].

Photoresponsive scaffolds can be prepared by photocrosslinking hydrophilic polymers. UV irradiation enables in-situ polymerization and the production of scaffolds with controllable networks and elasticity. A photoresponsive polymer can be obtained by photo-crossliking dextran with 2-isocyanatoethylmethacrylate and N-isopropylacrylamide, Irgacure® 2959 as the photoinitiating agents. Besides being used as thermorresponsive polymer, poly(N-isopropylacrylamide) (PNIPAM) can also be crosslinked with poly(L-glutamic acid) (PGA) by UV irradiation with a photoinitiator, providing stimuli-responsive scaffolds. Photosensitive scaffolds have been extensively investigated, since UV is considered an unique method to control molecular or cellular behavior with high spatiotemporal precision and minimal invasiveness [224].

APPLICATIONS OF HYBRID/SMART SCAFFOLDS

Tissue Engineering

The creation of functional tissues and assisted cell proliferation are major concerns of tissue engineering science. Hybrid smart scaffolds can deliver bioactive molecules that can provide tissue regeneration and optimized therapeutic efficiency while imitating the complex architecture of natural extracellular matrix [85].

According to the standards parameters recommended by the American Society for Testing and Materials (ASTM), the protocol to be followed to perform appropriated tissue engineering are: (I) selection the biomaterial and fabrication process to produce scaffolds, (II) inoculate the cells in polymer matrix, (III) performing premature tissue growth, (IV) tissue growing in a bioreactor containing the physiological system and (V) implant, as shown in Fig. (**12**) [235].

Recently, hybrid smart scaffolds have emerged as promising materials to be applied in tissue engineering, since they can mimic the nanoscale properties of the extracellular matrix, while delivering bioactive molecules upon an environmental stimulus. In general, compared to self-assembly and phase separation techniques, electrospinning provides a simpler and more cost-effective means to produce scaffolds with an inter-connected porous structure. Highly porous surfaces lead to an increased surface are, which allows cell attachment and provide multiple adhesion anchoring points [146].

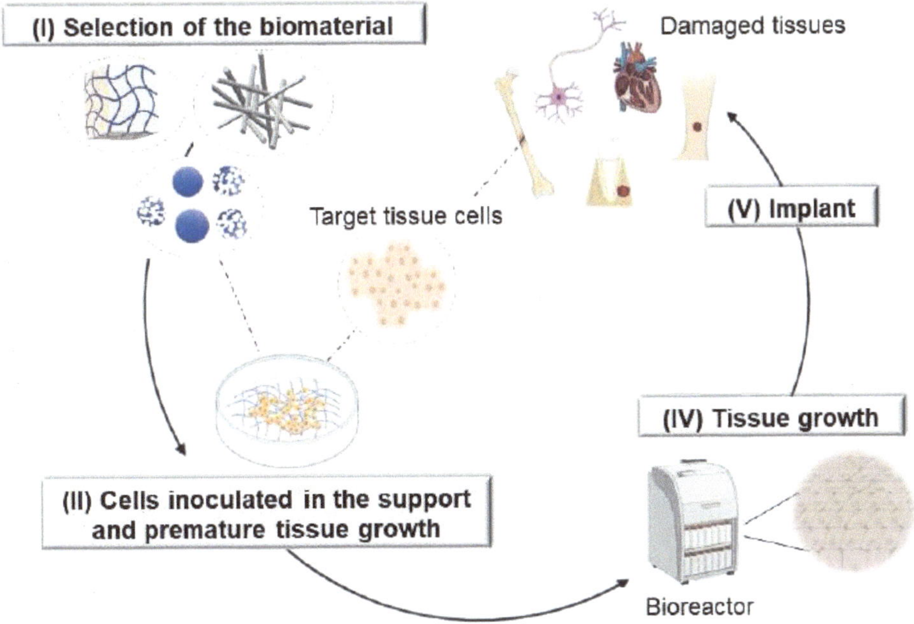

Fig. (12). A brief scheme of the scaffold applications in tissue engineering.

Application in Cardiovascular Tissue Engineering

Cardiovascular tissues are challenging targeting tissues as they constitute thick complex tissues like cardiac muscle and need to be pre-vascularized to provide efficient integration with the biological compartment, maintaining cell viability and also orientating cell growth as tissue regeneration takes place [232]. There are many attempts on the application of scaffolds to develop vascular grafts. Besides, hybrid scaffolds can encapsulate bioactive molecules able to promote angiogenesis, for example.

The electrospinning technique has a great potential to meet the engineering of vascular tissues, however there is still need to make improvements before determining a standard graft for both medium and small vessels [236]. Fleischer *et al*. prepared coiled electrospun fiber scaffolds with gold nanoparticles to improve the performance of engineered cardiac tissues. *In vitro* cell culture results showed that hybrid scaffolds promoted greater organization of cardiac cells, which showed elongated and aligned morphology, essential characteristics to obtaining strong contraction force, high contraction rate and low excitation threshold [237].

Electrically-responsive smart scaffolds have been reported in order to promote the proliferation and differentiation of electrical stimuli responsive cells, such as stem cells, myoblast cells, nerve cells and cardiac cells, thus indicating their ability to act as cardiac repair devices [224]. Smith *et al.* prepared conductive graphene-PEG hybrid scaffolds with micro and nanoparticles with anisotropic electrical conductivity for regeneration of cardiac tissue. Their results showed enhancement of structural properties in myofibrils and sarcomeres with great increase in the expression of cell-cell coupling and calcium handling proteins and greater action potential duration and peak calcium release. Such observations suggested that the lack of electrical conductivity and structural organization often observed in generic scaffolds, which limit their utility for generating physiologically representative models of functional cardiac tissue can be overcome by using graphene-based scaffolds [238].

Bone Tissue Engineering Application

Hydrogels and nanofibers are widely exploited as potential scaffolds for bone repair and grafting as they provide a porous support and proper mechanical properties which allow cell survival, proliferation, biocompatibility and biodegradability [7, 239].

Hydroxyapatite is one of the main inorganic components of bones and, then artificial scaffolds can be formulated with nano or micro hydroxyapatite particles and biopolymers or their blends, including collagen, PCL, chitosan, hyaluronic acid, PLLA, PLGA, collagen-like polypeptide, poly(Pro-Hyp-Gly), alginate, poly(ethylene glycol) (PEG), polyacrylic acid (PAA) and demineralized bone matrix (DBM) and pullulan [224].

Bone graft scaffolds must also feature high resistance to traction, compression and torsion forces, pore size between 100-250 micrometers and ideal porosity greater than 90% [240]. The growth of bone cells can also be favored with the formation of composites as shown by the study carried out Monteiro *et al.*, that reported the encapsulation of dexamethasone in liposomes, which were immobilized on PCL electrospun nanofiber-based scaffolds for osteogenic differentiation of human bone marrow-derived mesenchymal stem cells. The hybrid scaffolds promoted sustained drug release for 21 days with no cytotoxic effect. Moreover, the hybrid scaffolds successfully provided the osteogenic differentiation human bone marrow-derived mesenchymal stem cells [241].

Stimuli-responsive hybrid scaffolds can provide mechanical stimulation to bone cells avoiding the need for expensive biomolecules, such as growth factors [232]. Also, super-paramagnetic responsive systems have been produced with the introduction of y-Fe_2O_3 and hydroxyamatite-loaded nanoparticles into nanofibrous scaffolds. External magnetic stimuli changed the physicochemical properties of the produced scaffolds, which were implanted into rabbits. *In vivo* tests enabled accelerated new bone tissue formation and remodeling phenomenon.

López-Noriega *et al.* developed thermally-responsive collagen-based scaffolds loaded with liposomes for controlled local release of PTHrP 107-111, a pro-osteogenic and antiosteoclastic peptide for bone repair applications. Thermoresponsive liposomes were covalently attached to collagen-hydroxyapatite scaffolds. Their *In vitro* drug release results showed that an external thermal stimulus were able to modify drug release kinetics, without affecting the cell attachment, as indicated by the enhancement of alkaline phosphatase activity, an early osteogenic marker and is correlated with an increased expression of the osteogenic genes osteopontin and osteocalcin [242].

Neural Tissue Engineering Application

Neural tissue feature limited regenerative capacity, as it is not possible to successfully connect nerves directly by surgery, without any damage [243]. Despite this difficulty, it is known that scaffolds can serve as a graft to repair peripheral nerves due to the ability to provide guidance for neural cell growth as well as cell adhesion [244].

Atoufi *et al.* reported the synthesis of a novel biocompatible electrically-responsive scaffold hydrogel based on agarose/alginate-aniline for a tailored electrically controlled dexamethasone local release for neuroregeneration. The novel smart materials showed electroactivity and ionic conductivity of hydrogels against temperature and high biocompatibility and cell proliferation due to its highest ionic conductivity highlighting the fact that electrical stimuli was involved in cell signaling. These results indicate that the newly developed electro-responsive hybrid scaffolds are innovative materials for neuroregenerative medicine [245].

Samudre *et al.* developed xanthan gum-based mucoadhesive composite scaffolds loaded with liposomes for brain delivery of curcumin. Their results showed that the introduction of liposomes into xantan gum scaffolds was able to provide good stability of liposomes and no deleterious effect on nasal mucosa of rats and higher drug distribution in brain, when hybrid scaffolds were administrated through intranasal route [246].

Topical Drug Delivery

Recent efforts to the development of smart composite scaffolds have paved a new path to the design of novel drug delivery systems [7]. Among them, a wide range of applications in drug delivery, wound healing and local cancer therapy are the most investigated [11, 232]. The drug release profile and kinetics can be tailored by the adequate choice of polymer matrix with predictable degradation and erosion rates and proper both polymer and nanocarriers stimuli-responsive properties.

Antitumor Therapy

Postoperative local chemotherapy often relies on anticancer drugs loaded in nanofibrous scaffolds. The most investigated synthetic drugs are doxorubicin, paclitaxel and platinum-based complexes [11]. Nanofibers-based scaffolds have been used for local release of doxorubicin. PVA/Chitosan-based nanofibers were prepared by coaxial electrospinning method and presented a core-shell structure [247]. Chitosan composed the shell layer, which provided highly biocompatible nanofibers, reducing cytotoxicity observed for free doxorubicin. In addition, plain core-shell nanofibers promoted the attachment, proliferation and spreading of human ovary cancer cells, whereas doxorubicin-loaded nanofibers were effective in preventing cancer ovary cells attachment and proliferation [247].

Wang *et al.* produced curcumin-loaded electrospun nanofibers to enhance curcumin bioavailability. *In vitro* drug release experiments showed that PVP-based nanofibers enhanced dissolution and anti-cancer effect of curcumin in comparison with the freely available drug [248].

Resveratrol, a poorly soluble antitumor agent, has been encapsulated into methoxypolyethylene glycol - poly(caprolactone) (mPEG-PCL) block copolymers nanofibers. *In vitro* experiments showed sustained drug release and superior cytotoxicity with apoptosis induction on cancer cells related to the nanofiber-based scaffolds. Local implantation of scaffolds showed great increase in the growth inhibitory effect in comparison with free resveratrol [249].

Wound Healing

Besides being the largest organ in human body, skin barrier function is essential to prevent the infection with pathogens, which could lead to general infections [250, 251]. The management of wounds can be complex and continuous. In that context, the development of wound dressings has been seen as a challenging field for the application of novel materials, such as polymer-based scaffolds.

Modern approaches for managing wound healing are replacing classical bandages, like gauze and tulles. In this context, nanofibrous scaffolds emerge as interesting materials for wound dressing application. They are considered biocompatible, non-irritating systems with proper mechanical properties. Depending on the type of wounds, different material properties are required. For example, wound dressing scaffolds for limited wounds, should basically allow cell migration to the affected site followed by cell proliferation, acting merely as cell support. On the other hand, for larger wounds, cell support alone is not sufficient to cover the whole wound area, and active wound dressing materials are required. In this case, drugs and growth factor-loaded nanofiber scaffolds are useful as they can stimulate and manage cell migration and prevent infections. Exuding wounds demand highly porous or swellable scaffolds to absorb the excess of fluids. Surgical wounds should be addressed with antimicrobial and/or growth factors-loaded scaffolds. Moreover, polymer-based scaffolds require bioreabsorbable materials with rapid drug release profiles, as most of these wound dressings are changed daily. On the other hand, closed wounds require more resistant materials as wound dressing scaffolds with slow drug release rates [252]. Hence, different wound dressing materials are important in maintaining different phases of healing and supporting different types of wounds.

Mohandas *et al.* recently reviewed different nanocomposites Chitosan-based scaffolds containing metal or metal oxide nanoparticles such as Ag, Au, Cu, ZnO or TiO_2 and their application in wound healing and/or infection control due to their antimicrobial properties. The introduction of metallic nanoparticles to chitosan-based scaffolds optimizes the wound healing process, as it favors sustained antimicrobial activity. However, the *in vivo* toxicity of metallic nanoparticles constitutes a major challenge for their clinical application [253].

Chitosan/silk composite scaffolds are prepared by Cai *et al.* for wound dressing application. Their results showed that composite scaffolds feature adequate mechanical properties for wound healing. Moreover, antibacterial activities against *Escherichia coli* and *Staphylococcus aureus* suggested the antibacterial effect of composite scaffolds, which also showed high *In vitro* biocompatibility with human fibroblasts [254].

Several antimicrobial agents can be loaded in nanofibrous scaffolds, also for wound dressing applications. Kataria *et al.* developed drug-loaded PVA/sodium alginate composite scaffolds, used as a patches for controlled and local release of the antibiotic ciprofloxacin [255]. Nanofiber-loaded composite scaffolds promoted wound healing more rapidly, as *in vivo* experiments showed. Moreover, PVA/sodium alginate polymer matrix proved to be a biocompatible and biodegradable hydrophilic basis for the development of wound dressings.

Zahedi *et al*. produced nanofibrous wound dressing scaffolds made from PLA, PCL and their blend (50:50) loaded with tetracycline hydrochloride. The wound healing properties, *In vitro* drug release, water permeability and antibacterial activities of PCL and PLA/PLC blends scaffolds showed better performance compared with the results from Comfeel Plus, a commercial wound dressing product. Water absorption obtained for PLA, PCL, and 50/50 PCL/PLA was higher, which had a direct relation with the hydrophilic properties of these polymers. The 50/50 PCL/PLA blend showed the highest drug-release rate of about 70% in phosphate buffer solution and the most effective antibiotic activity against *S. aureus*.

Scaffolds based on silver-polymer nanocomposites are considered promising materials for wound healing and other infections treatments due to the antibacterial properties attributed to silver-based materials [256]. Silver nanoparticles can penetrate bacteria, fungus or virus and control silver release enhancing the therapeutical effects [66, 257]. Silver nanoparticles when entrapped into polymeric matrixes can combine both improved efficacy and controlled release, resulting in novel and better antibacterial products that can emerge as a solution to the increase of bacterial resistance to common antibiotics. Moreover, scaffold polymeric matrix can mask any toxicity related to silver nanoparticles, as they are composed by biocompatible polymers [258].

Magneto-responsive polymer-based scaffolds are often investigated for hyperthermia applied to cancer therapy, which constitutes the local heating of cancer cells that cannot resist to high temperatures [232]. Xie *et al*. reported the development of a implantable magneto-sensitive smart hybrid scaffold materials by incorporating Fe_3O_4 nanoparticles into a poly(ethylene glycol)-crosslinked chitosan hydrogel for local release of doxorubicin and docetaxel. Both drugs were encapsulated into PLGA polymer nanoparticles. Their results showed self-healing behavior, adequate biocompatibility and controlled release properties. Moreover, hybrid smart scaffolds showed good magnetic field response and induced localized hyperthermia and greatly reduced tumor size in animal models [259].

Topical Delivery of Proteins, DNA, RNA and Growth Factors

Bioactive molecules such as proteins, nucleic acids and growth factors can be incorporated into scaffolds through their encapsulation in drug nanocarriers and electrospun fibers. Moreover, topical delivery of proteins and nucleic is often limited by their relatively short half-life. They represent a challenge in the development of novel materials, as the obtention method and processing conditions must ensure the bioactivity and functional stability, while providing reasonable encapsulation efficiency and homogeneous drug distribution.

Chew *et al.* encapsulated human β-nerve growth factor (NGF) in bovine serum albumin carrier in a copolymer of ε-caprolactone and ethyl ethylene phosphate scaffold. The authors observed a sustained release of NGF for at least 3 months, which was attributed to the successful NGF encapsulation in the scaffold. Besides, NGF bioactivity was confirmed by PC12 neurite outgrowth during the same period [260].

Rubert *et al.* produced highly porous core-shell PCL/PEO nanofibrous scaffolds containing fibroblast growth factor (FGF-2) for local and temporal controlled release. FGF-2 was controlled released for more than 9 days and fibroblast cell adhesion was sustained by PCL/PEO scaffold with enhanced cell viability and proliferation compared to the control group. These results indicated that nanofibrous scaffolds are suitable materials for local sustained protein release, as they were biocompatible and provided prolonged efficacy for connective tissue regeneration [261].

Pinese *et al.* produced hybrid nanofibrous scaffolds containing small interfering RNA (siRNA) encapsulated in silica nanoparticles for long-term gene silencing. Mesoporous silica nanoparticles were used as siRNA carrier due to their biocompatibility and controllable pore size, which enables the obtention of tunable drug delivery. *In vitro* sustained delivery of siRNA was allowed by the introduction of silica nanoparticles in a nanofiber scaffold for at least 30 days. *In vivo* subcutaneous implantation of the hybrid scaffolds showed that siRNA was located up to 290 um from the original site of the implants, proving that local release of siRNA was achieved [262].

Biodegradable tissue regenerative scaffolds were developed by Nelson *et al.* for controlled release of siRNA encapsulated in nanoparticles for local gene silencing for enhancing angiogenesis. Porous polyester urethane scaffolds were used since they are easily tunable and adaptable to achieve a high level of gene silencing. PH-dependent polymeric nanoparticles were produced to escape endosomal inactivation to increase siRNA intracellular bioavailability. Their results indicated that scaffolds showed interconnected pores, which enabled both enhanced drug release and cell infiltration. When implanted subcutaneously, scaffolds promoted angiogenesis *in vivo* [263].

Other recent results showed significant advances in biomedical applications that have been achieved by the development of novel scaffolds designs, which combined nonencapsulated enzymes, nucleic acids and growth factors and biodegradable polymers. Their results were able to provide extended release of entrapped molecules in all cases. More specifically their innovative hybrid scaffolds enabled tunable transfection efficiency [264], to maintain enzymatic activity [265], and to obtain biphasic drug release profile, which can be promising therapeutic approaches where time-dependent cascades of biological signals may be valuable, such as in tissue regeneration [266]. The development of these multifunctional scaffolds can go beyond to simply mimic natural properties of the target tissue, as they also promote one or more therapeutic functions by encapsulating small molecule drugs or peptides or nucleic acids. The research on this field is a rapidly emerging field in the development of innovative devices that combine multiple functionalities to scaffolds materials. In this sense, novel design concepts bring novel challenges and opportunities for deeper investigations regarding the development of scaffolds as drug delivery devices for innovative therapeutic applications.

CONCLUSIONS

Drug nanocarriers and scaffolds feature a significant role in tissue engineering and organ regeneration as they offer controlled delivery of drugs, genes, peptides or growth factors and a porous support that promote accelerated cell growth and attachment. However, it is often difficult to maintain local delivery of bioactive agents when nanoparticles are administrated alone as they can diffuse to other biological compartments. Thus, their incorporation into a scaffold polymer matrix, opens a new perspective to the development of novel scaffolding materials that can be called hybrid scaffolds or composite scaffolds.

Hybrid smart scaffold-based drug delivery systems are considered promising strategies to local treat diseases, since they contain therapeutic agents to be released at the target site. Such properties, combined with the unique characteristics of polymers, as biocompatibility, biodegradability, versatility, and stimuli-responsive tunable properties provide de development of a new generation of scaffolding materials that do not demand surgical removal. Moreover, scaffolds provide unique characteristics as controllable porous size and distribution, which enable cell attachment, bioadhesivity and maintain drug local treatment. The application of biocompatible polymers to produce scaffolds can eliminate the immunologic response to the scaffold.

Tissue engineering continues to expand and it is necessary to improve both the obtention technique and the physical and chemical design of the scaffolds, such as controllable parameters, which allow the production of different types of polymeric scaffolds and the development of devices that more adequately mimic the target tissue. The proper selection of a wide range of polymers, such as of polysaccharides, synthetic polymers, stimuli-sensitive polymer, and protein-based natural polymers that can be used to create new type smart scaffolds can bring new opportunities to treat the most diverse diseases and target drug delivery to the most diverse tissues. Scaffolds may also as a platform for the delivery of small molecules, proteins, and growth factors, providing more clinically relevant tissue engineered scaffolds.

This chapter reported the different scaffolds obtention and characterization techniques, the advantages and application of hybrid smart scaffold-based materials that gather several properties such as scaffolding, drug delivery and stimuli-responsiveness in different environments. The development of such multifunctional materials has several potential application in a wide range of fields, like cancer therapy, bone repair, cardiac tissue regeneration, wound healing and many others.

CONSENT FOR PUBLICATION

Not applicable.

CONFLICT OF INTEREST

The authors declare no conflict of interest, financial or otherwise.

ACKNOWLEDGEMENTS

Declared none.

REFERENCES

[1] Bayat M, Nasri S. Injectable microgel-hydrogel composites "plum pudding gels": New system for prolonged drug delivery. Nanomater Drug Deliv Ther. Elsevier 2019; pp. 343-72. [http://dx.doi.org/10.1016/B978-0-12-816505-8.00001-1]

[2] Yu M, Ma H, Lei M, Li N, Tan F. *In vitro/in vivo* characterization of nanoemulsion formulation of metronidazole with improved skin targeting and anti-rosacea properties. Eur J Pharm Biopharm 2014; 88(1): 92-103. [http://dx.doi.org/10.1016/j.ejpb.2014.03.019] [PMID: 24704200]

[3] Zhu W, Guo C, Yu A, Gao Y, Cao F, Zhai G. Microemulsion-based hydrogel formulation of penciclovir for topical delivery. Int J Pharm 2009; 378(1-2): 152-8. [http://dx.doi.org/10.1016/j.ijpharm.2009.05.019] [PMID: 19463929]

[4] Lima SRM, Junior VF, Christo HB, Pinto AC, Fernandes PD. *In vivo* and *in vitro* studies on the anticancer activity of Copaifera multijuga hayne and its fractions. Phytother Res 2003; 17(9): 1048-53. [http://dx.doi.org/10.1002/ptr.1295] [PMID: 14595585]

[5] Roberts MS, Mohammed Y, Pastore MN, *et al.* Topical and cutaneous delivery using nanosystems. J Control Rel 2017; 247: 86-105. [http://dx.doi.org/10.1016/j.jconrel.2016.12.022] [PMID: 28024914]

[6] Vilar G, Tulla-Puche J, Albericio F. Polymers and drug delivery systems. Curr Drug Deliv 2012; 9(4): 367-94. [http://dx.doi.org/10.2174/156720112801323053] [PMID: 22640038]

[7] Gupta KC, Haider A, Choi YR, Kang IK. Nanofibrous scaffolds in biomedical applications. Biomater Res 2014; 18: 5.

[http://dx.doi.org/10.1186/2055-7124-18-5] [PMID: 26331056]

[8] Rampichová M, Košt'áková Kuželová E, Filová E, *et al.* Composite 3D printed scaffold with structured electrospun nanofibers promotes chondrocyte adhesion and infiltration. Cell Adhes Migr 2018; 12(3): 271-85.
[http://dx.doi.org/10.1080/19336918.2017.1385713] [PMID: 29130836]

[9] Jeong KH, Park D, Lee YC. Polymer-based hydrogel scaffolds for skin tissue engineering applications: a mini-review. J Polym Res 2017; 24: 1-10.
[http://dx.doi.org/10.1007/s10965-017-1278-4]

[10] de Lima Nascimento TR, de Amoêdo Campos Velo MM, Silva CF, *et al.* Current Applications of Biopolymer-based Scaffolds and Nanofibers as Drug Delivery Systems. Curr Pharm Des 2019; 25(37): 3997-4012.
[http://dx.doi.org/10.2174/1381612825666191108162948] [PMID: 31701845]

[11] Hu X, Liu S, Zhou G, Huang Y, Xie Z, Jing X. Electrospinning of polymeric nanofibers for drug delivery applications. J Control Release 2014; 185: 12-21.
[http://dx.doi.org/10.1016/j.jconrel.2014.04.018] [PMID: 24768792]

[12] Franco L, del Valle LJ, Puiggalí J. Smart systems related to polypeptide sequences. AIMS Mater Sci 2016; 3: 289-323.
[http://dx.doi.org/10.3934/matersci.2016.1.289]

[13] Yu S, Zhang X, Tan G, *et al.* A novel pH-induced thermosensitive hydrogel composed of carboxymethyl chitosan and poloxamer cross-linked by glutaraldehyde for ophthalmic drug delivery. Carbohydr Polym 2017; 155: 208-17.
[http://dx.doi.org/10.1016/j.carbpol.2016.08.073] [PMID: 27702506]

[14] Chan A, Orme RP, Fricker RA, Roach P. Remote and local control of stimuli responsive materials for therapeutic applications. Adv Drug Deliv Rev 2013; 65(4): 497-514.
[http://dx.doi.org/10.1016/j.addr.2012.07.007] [PMID: 22820529]

[15] Loomis's Essentials of Toxicology. Elsevier 1996.
[http://dx.doi.org/10.1016/b978-0-12-455625-6.x5000-4]

[16] Hadgraft J. Passive enhancement strategies in topical and transdermal drug delivery. Int J Pharm 1999; 184(1): 1-6.
[http://dx.doi.org/10.1016/S0378-5173(99)00095-2] [PMID: 10425346]

[17] Patel HK, Barot BS, Parejiya PB, Shelat PK, Shukla A. Topical delivery of clobetasol propionate loaded microemulsion based gel for effective treatment of vitiligo: ex vivo permeation and skin irritation studies. Colloids Surf B Biointerfaces 2013; 102: 86-94.
[http://dx.doi.org/10.1016/j.colsurfb.2012.08.011] [PMID: 23000677]

[18] Kathe K, Kathpalia H. Film forming systems for topical and transdermal drug delivery. Asian J Pharm Sci 2017; 12(6): 487-97.
[http://dx.doi.org/10.1016/j.ajps.2017.07.004] [PMID: 32104362]

[19] Boegh M, Foged C, Müllertz A, Nielsen HM. Mucosal drug delivery: barriers, *In vitro* models and formulation strategies I. mucosal drug delivery. J Drug Del Sci Tech (Paris) 2013; 23: 383-91.

[20] Aggarwal G, Verma S, Gupta M, Nagpal M. Local Drug Delivery Based Treatment Approaches for Effective Management of Periodontitis. Curr Drug Ther 2019; 14: 135-52.
[http://dx.doi.org/10.2174/1574885514666190103112855]

[21] Rybak LP, Dhukhwa A, Mukherjea D, Ramkumar V. Local drug delivery for prevention of hearing loss. Front Cell Neurosci 2019; 13: 300.
[http://dx.doi.org/10.3389/fncel.2019.00300] [PMID: 31338024]

[22] Cao FH, OuYang WQ, Wang YP, Yue PF, Li SP. A combination of a microemulsion and a phospholipid complex for topical delivery of oxymatrine. Arch Pharm Res 2011; 34(4): 551-62.
[http://dx.doi.org/10.1007/s12272-011-0405-8] [PMID: 21544720]

[23] Guglielmini G. Nanostructured novel carrier for topical application. Clin Dermatol 2008; 26(4): 341-6. [http://dx.doi.org/10.1016/j.clindermatol.2008.05.004] [PMID: 18691513]

[24] Johal HS, Garg T, Rath G, Goyal AK. Advanced topical drug delivery system for the management of vaginal candidiasis. Drug Deliv 2016; 23(2): 550-63. [http://dx.doi.org/10.3109/10717544.2014.928760] [PMID: 24959937]

[25] T. M, H. CN, R. J.. Novel topical drug delivery systems and their potential use in scars treatment. Ski Ther Lett 2008; 6-8.https://pubmed.ncbi.nlm.nih.gov/18648713/

[26] A.C.W. Marc B. Brown. The art and science of dermal formulation development. Marc B. Brown, Adrian C. Williams - Google Livros. 2019. https://www.taylorfrancis.com/books/art-science-derm-l-formulation-development-marc-brown-adrian-williams/10.1201/9780429059872

[27] Shah P, Goodyear B, Haq A, Puri V, Michniak-Kohn B. Evaluations of quality by design (QbD) elements impact for developing niosomes as a promising topical drug delivery platform. Pharmaceutics 2020; 12(3): E246. [http://dx.doi.org/10.3390/pharmaceutics12030246] [PMID: 32182792]

[28] Lee JH, Yeo Y. Controlled drug release from pharmaceutical nanocarriers. Chem Eng Sci 2015; 125: 75-84. [http://dx.doi.org/10.1016/j.ces.2014.08.046] [PMID: 25684779]

[29] Qu T, Wang A, Yuan J, Gao Q. Preparation of an amphiphilic triblock copolymer with pH- and thermo-responsiveness and self-assembled micelles applied to drug release. J Colloid Interface Sci 2009; 336(2): 865-71. [http://dx.doi.org/10.1016/j.jcis.2009.04.001] [PMID: 19464019]

[30] Kojima C. Design of stimuli-responsive dendrimers. Expert Opin Drug Deliv 2010; 7(3): 307-19. [http://dx.doi.org/10.1517/17425240903530651] [PMID: 20095875]

[31] Fleige E, Quadir MA, Haag R. Stimuli-responsive polymeric nanocarriers for the controlled transport of active compounds: concepts and applications. Adv Drug Deliv Rev 2012; 64(9): 866-84. [http://dx.doi.org/10.1016/j.addr.2012.01.020] [PMID: 22349241]

[32] Guo X, Cheng Y, Zhao X, Luo Y, Chen J, Yuan WE. Advances in redox-responsive drug delivery systems of tumor microenvironment. J Nanobiotechnology 2018; 16(1): 74. [http://dx.doi.org/10.1186/s12951-018-0398-2] [PMID: 30243297]

[33] Peppas N. Chemical and physical structure of polymers as carriers for controlled release of bioactive agents: a review. J Macromol Sci 1983; 23(Part C): 61-126. [http://dx.doi.org/10.1080/07366578308079439]

[34] Sciences H. Review kinetic modeling on drug release from controlled drug delivery systems 2010; 67: 217-23. https://pubmed.ncbi.nlm.nih.gov/20524422/

[35] Frenning G. Modelling drug release from inert matrix systems: from moving-boundary to continuous-field descriptions. Int J Pharm 2011; 418(1): 88-99. [http://dx.doi.org/10.1016/j.ijpharm.2010.11.030] [PMID: 21095224]

[36] N. a Peppas, P. Bures, W. Leobandung, H. Ichikawa, Hydrogels in pharmaceutical formulations. Eur J Pharm Biopharm 2000; 50: 27-46.

[37] Peppas NA, Khare AR. Preparation, structure and diffusional behavior of hydrogels in controlled release. Adv Drug Deliv Rev 1993. [http://dx.doi.org/10.1016/0169-409X(93)90025-Y]

[38] Siepmann J, Peppas NA. Modeling of drug release from delivery systems based on hydroxypropyl methylcellulose (HPMC). Adv Drug Deliv Rev 2001; 48(2-3): 139-57.www.elsevier.com [http://dx.doi.org/10.1016/S0169-409X(01)00112-0] [PMID: 11369079]

[39] Sahu P, Kashaw SK, Jain S, Sau S, Iyer AK. Assessment of penetration potential of pH responsive double walled biodegradable nanogels coated with eucalyptus oil for the controlled delivery of 5-

fluorouracil: *In vitro* and ex vivo studies. J Control Release 2017; 253: 122-36. [http://dx.doi.org/10.1016/j.jconrel.2017.03.023] [PMID: 28322977]

[40] Sivaraman A, Banga AK. Novel *in situ* forming hydrogel microneedles for transdermal drug delivery. Drug Deliv Transl Res 2017; 7(1): 16-26. [http://dx.doi.org/10.1007/s13346-016-0328-5] [PMID: 27562294]

[41] Zhang T, Yang R, Yang S, *et al.* Research progress of self-assembled nanogel and hybrid hydrogel systems based on pullulan derivatives. Drug Deliv 2018; 25(1): 278-92. [http://dx.doi.org/10.1080/10717544.2018.1425776] [PMID: 29334800]

[42] Suvakanta Dash PNMLNPC. 2010.https://pubmed.ncbi.nlm.nih.gov/20524422/

[43] Prow TW, Grice JE, Lin LL, *et al.* Nanoparticles and microparticles for skin drug delivery. Adv Drug Deliv Rev 2011; 63(6): 470-91. [http://dx.doi.org/10.1016/j.addr.2011.01.012] [PMID: 21315122]

[44] Shah PP, Desai PR, Patel AR, Singh MS. Skin permeating nanogel for the cutaneous co-delivery of two anti-inflammatory drugs. Biomaterials 2012; 33(5): 1607-17. [http://dx.doi.org/10.1016/j.biomaterials.2011.11.011] [PMID: 22118820]

[45] Neubert RHH. Potentials of new nanocarriers for dermal and transdermal drug delivery. Eur J Pharm Biopharm 2011; 77(1): 1-2. [http://dx.doi.org/10.1016/j.ejpb.2010.11.003] [PMID: 21111043]

[46] Jafari SM. Nanoencapsulation technologies for the food and nutraceutical industries. Elsevier 2017.

[47] Lim SB, Banerjee A, Önyüksel H. Improvement of drug safety by the use of lipid-based nanocarriers. J. Control. Release 2012. [http://dx.doi.org/10.1016/j.jconrel.2012.06.002]

[48] Cevc G. Lipid vesicles and other colloids as drug carriers on the skin. Adv Drug Deliv Rev 2004; 56(5): 675-711. [http://dx.doi.org/10.1016/j.addr.2003.10.028] [PMID: 15019752]

[49] Rajabi M, Mousa S A. Lipid Nanoparticles and their Application in Nanomedicine n.d. [http://dx.doi.org/10.2174/1389201017666160415155457]

[50] Puri A, Loomis K, Smith B, *et al.* Lipid-based nanoparticles as pharmaceutical drug carriers: from concepts to clinic. Crit Rev Ther Drug Carrier Syst 2009; 26(6): 523-80. [http://dx.doi.org/10.1615/CritRevTherDrugCarrierSyst.v26.i6.10] [PMID: 20402623]

[51] Bilalov A, Olsson U, Lindman B. DNA-lipid self-assembly: Phase behavior and phase structures of a DNA-surfactant complex mixed with lecithin and water. Soft Matter 2011; 7: 730-42. [http://dx.doi.org/10.1039/C0SM00650E]

[52] Montenegro L, Lai F, Offerta A, *et al.* From nanoemulsions to nanostructured lipid carriers: A relevant development in dermal delivery of drugs and cosmetics. J Drug Deliv Sci Technol 2016. [http://dx.doi.org/10.1016/j.jddst.2015.10.003]

[53] Garcês A, Amaral MH, Sousa Lobo JM, Silva AC. Formulations based on solid lipid nanoparticles (SLN) and nanostructured lipid carriers (NLC) for cutaneous use: A review. Eur J Pharm Sci 2018; 112: 159-67. [http://dx.doi.org/10.1016/j.ejps.2017.11.023] [PMID: 29183800]

[54] Kadam Y, Yerramilli U, Bahadur A, Bahadur P. Micelles from PEO-PPO-PEO block copolymers as nanocontainers for solubilization of a poorly water soluble drug hydrochlorothiazide. Colloids Surf B Biointerfaces 2011; 83(1): 49-57. [http://dx.doi.org/10.1016/j.colsurfb.2010.10.041] [PMID: 21123038]

[55] Kataoka K, Harada A, Nagasaki Y. Block copolymer micelles for drug delivery: design, characterization and biological significance. Adv Drug Deliv Rev 2001; 47(1): 113-31. [http://dx.doi.org/10.1016/S0169-409X(00)00124-1] [PMID: 11251249]

[56] Liu S, Li L. Molecular interactions between PEO-PPO-PEO and PPO-PEO-PPO triblock copolymers in aqueous solution. Colloids Surf A Physicochem Eng Asp 2015; 484: 485-97. [http://dx.doi.org/10.1016/j.colsurfa.2015.08.034]

[57] Torcello-Gómez A, Wulff-Pérez M, Gálvez-Ruiz MJ, Martín-Rodríguez A, Cabrerizo-Vílchez M, Maldonado-Valderrama J. Block copolymers at interfaces: interactions with physiological media. Adv Colloid Interface Sci 2014; 206: 414-27. [http://dx.doi.org/10.1016/j.cis.2013.10.027] [PMID: 24268588]

[58] Helgeson ME. Colloidal behavior of nanoemulsions: Interactions, structure, and rheology. Curr Opin Colloid Interface Sci 2016; 25: 39-50. [http://dx.doi.org/10.1016/j.cocis.2016.06.006]

[59] Crucho CIC, Barros MT. Polymeric nanoparticles: A study on the preparation variables and characterization methods. Mater Sci Eng C 2017; 80: 771-84. [http://dx.doi.org/10.1016/j.msec.2017.06.004] [PMID: 28866227]

[60] Douroumis D, Fahr A. Nano- and micro-particulate formulations of poorly water-soluble drugs by using a novel optimized technique. Eur J Pharm Biopharm 2006; 63(2): 173-5. [http://dx.doi.org/10.1016/j.ejpb.2006.02.004] [PMID: 16621482]

[61] Schwarz JC, Weixelbaum A, Pagitsch E, Löw M, Resch GP, Valenta C. Nanocarriers for dermal drug delivery: influence of preparation method, carrier type and rheological properties. Int J Pharm 2012; 437(1-2): 83-8. [http://dx.doi.org/10.1016/j.ijpharm.2012.08.003] [PMID: 22903049]

[62] Buwalda SJ, Vermonden T, Hennink WE. Hydrogels for Therapeutic Delivery: Current Developments and Future Directions. Biomacromolecules 2017; 18(2): 316-30. [http://dx.doi.org/10.1021/acs.biomac.6b01604] [PMID: 28027640]

[63] Zhang H, Zhai Y, Wang J, Zhai G. New progress and prospects: The application of nanogel in drug delivery. Mater Sci Eng C 2016; 60: 560-8. [http://dx.doi.org/10.1016/j.msec.2015.11.041] [PMID: 26706564]

[64] Goyal R, Macri LK, Kaplan HM, Kohn J. Nanoparticles and nanofibers for topical drug delivery. J Control Release 2016; 240: 77-92. [http://dx.doi.org/10.1016/j.jconrel.2015.10.049] [PMID: 26518723]

[65] Verma P, Maheshwari SK. Applications of Silver nanoparticles in diverse sectors. Int J Nanodimens 2019; 10: 18-36.http://www.ijnd.ir/article_661552.html

[66] Kalwar K, Shan D. Antimicrobial effect of silver nanoparticles (AgNPs) and their mechanism – A mini review. Micro & Nano Lett 2018; 13: 277-80. [http://dx.doi.org/10.1049/mnl.2017.0648]

[67] Akash MSH, Rehman K. Recent progress in biomedical applications of Pluronic (PF127): Pharmaceutical perspectives. J Control Release 2015; 209: 120-38. [http://dx.doi.org/10.1016/j.jconrel.2015.04.032] [PMID: 25921088]

[68] Peng LC, Liu CH, Kwan CC, Huang KF. Optimization of water-in-oil nanoemulsions by mixed surfactants. Colloids Surf A Physicochem Eng Asp 2010. [http://dx.doi.org/10.1016/j.colsurfa.2010.08.060]

[69] Bharti C, Nagaich U, Pal AK, Gulati N. Mesoporous silica nanoparticles in target drug delivery system: A review. Int J Pharm Investig 2015; 5(3): 124-33. [http://dx.doi.org/10.4103/2230-973X.160844] [PMID: 26258053]

[70] Vallet-Regí M, Colilla M, Izquierdo-Barba I, Manzano M. Mesoporous silica nanoparticles for drug delivery: Current insights. Molecules 2017; 23(1): E47. [http://dx.doi.org/10.3390/molecules23010047] [PMID: 29295564]

[71] Zhou Y, Quan G, Wu Q, *et al.* Mesoporous silica nanoparticles for drug and gene delivery. Acta

Pharm Sin B 2018; 8(2): 165-77.
[http://dx.doi.org/10.1016/j.apsb.2018.01.007] [PMID: 29719777]

[72] Patel GC, Yadav BK. Polymeric nanofibers for controlled drug delivery applications.Org Mater as Smart Nanocarriers Drug Deliv. Elsevier 2018; pp. 147-75.
[http://dx.doi.org/10.1016/B978-0-12-813663-8.00004-X]

[73] Cho S, Lowe L, Hamilton TA, Fisher GJ, Voorhees JJ, Kang S. Long-term treatment of photoaged human skin with topical retinoic acid improves epidermal cell atypia and thickens the collagen band in papillary dermis. J Am Acad Dermatol 2005; 53(5): 769-74.
[http://dx.doi.org/10.1016/j.jaad.2005.06.052] [PMID: 16243124]

[74] Oscar Robles Vazquez IOAJCSDEH. 2014. http://www.lifescienceglobal.com/pms/index.php/jrups/article/view/3549

[75] Lee KY, Jeong L, Kang YO, Lee SJ, Park WH. Electrospinning of polysaccharides for regenerative medicine. Adv Drug Deliv Rev 2009; 61(12): 1020-32.
[http://dx.doi.org/10.1016/j.addr.2009.07.006] [PMID: 19643155]

[76] Talebian S, Foroughi J, Wade SJ, *et al.* Biopolymers for antitumor implantable drug delivery systems: recent advances and future outlook. Adv Mater 2018; 30(31): e1706665.
[http://dx.doi.org/10.1002/adma.201706665] [PMID: 29756237]

[77] Motealleh A, Kehr NS. Nanocomposite hydrogels and their applications in tissue engineering. Adv Healthc Mater 2017; 6(1)
[http://dx.doi.org/10.1002/adhm.201600938] [PMID: 27900856]

[78] Stamatialis DF, Papenburg BJ, Gironés M, *et al.* Medical applications of membranes: Drug delivery, artificial organs and tissue engineering. J Memb Sci 2008.

[79] Stitzel J, Liu J, Lee SJ, *et al.* Controlled fabrication of a biological vascular substitute. Biomaterials 2006; 27(7): 1088-94.
[http://dx.doi.org/10.1016/j.biomaterials.2005.07.048] [PMID: 16131465]

[80] Zong X, Ran S, Fang D, Hsiao BS, Chu B. Control of structure, morphology and property in electrospun poly(glycolide-co-lactide) non-woven membranes *via* post-draw treatments. Polymer (Guildf) 2003; 44: 4959-67.
[http://dx.doi.org/10.1016/S0032-3861(03)00464-6]

[81] Kim K, Yu M, Zong X, *et al.* Control of degradation rate and hydrophilicity in electrospun non-woven poly(D,L-lactide) nanofiber scaffolds for biomedical applications. Biomaterials 2003; 24(27): 4977-85.
[http://dx.doi.org/10.1016/S0142-9612(03)00407-1] [PMID: 14559011]

[82] Zylberberg C, Matosevic S. Bioengineered liposome-scaffold composites as therapeutic delivery systems. Ther Deliv 2017; 8(6): 425-45.
[http://dx.doi.org/10.4155/tde-2017-0014] [PMID: 28530145]

[83] Dhandayuthapani B, Yoshida Y, Maekawa T, Kumar DS. Polymeric scaffolds in tissue engineering application. RE: view 2011; 2011
[http://dx.doi.org/10.1155/2011/290602]

[84] Rahmani Del Bakhshayesh A, Annabi N, Khalilov R, *et al.* Recent advances on biomedical applications of scaffolds in wound healing and dermal tissue engineering. Artif Cells Nanomed Biotechnol 2018; 46(4): 691-705.
[http://dx.doi.org/10.1080/21691401.2017.1349778] [PMID: 28697631]

[85] Keck M, Haluza D, Lumenta DB, *et al.* Construction of a multi-layer skin substitute: Simultaneous cultivation of keratinocytes and preadipocytes on a dermal template. Burns 2011; 37(4): 626-30.
[http://dx.doi.org/10.1016/j.burns.2010.07.016] [PMID: 20869175]

[86] Cui L, Peng J, Ding Y, Li X, Han Y. Ordered porous polymer films *via* phase separation in humidity environment. Polymer (Guildf) 2005; 46: 5334-40.

[http://dx.doi.org/10.1016/j.polymer.2005.04.018]

[87] Ravichandran R, Sundarrajan S, Venugopal JR, Mukherjee S, Ramakrishna S. Advances in polymeric systems for tissue engineering and biomedical applications. Macromol Biosci 2012; 12(3): 286-311. [http://dx.doi.org/10.1002/mabi.201100325] [PMID: 22278779]

[88] Wu GH, Hsu SH. Review: Polymeric-based 3D printing for tissue engineering. J Med Biol Eng 2015; 35(3): 285-92. [http://dx.doi.org/10.1007/s40846-015-0038-3] [PMID: 26167139]

[89] Xue L, Han Y. Pattern formation by dewetting of polymer thin film. Prog Polym Sci 2011; 36: 269-93. [http://dx.doi.org/10.1016/j.progpolymsci.2010.07.004]

[90] Giulbudagian M, Yealland G, Hönzke S, *et al.* Breaking the barrier - Potent anti-inflammatory activity following efficient topical delivery of etanercept using thermoresponsive nanogels. Theranostics 2018; 8(2): 450-63. [http://dx.doi.org/10.7150/thno.21668] [PMID: 29290820]

[91] Frederiksen K, Guy RH, Petersson K. Formulation considerations in the design of topical, polymeric film-forming systems for sustained drug delivery to the skin. Eur J Pharm Biopharm 2015; 91: 9-15. [http://dx.doi.org/10.1016/j.ejpb.2015.01.002] [PMID: 25595740]

[92] Huang A, Jiang Y, Napiwocki B, Mi H, Peng X, Turng LS. Fabrication of poly(ϵ-caprolactone) tissue engineering scaffolds with fibrillated and interconnected pores utilizing microcellular injection molding and polymer leaching. RSC Advances 2017; 7: 43432-44. [http://dx.doi.org/10.1039/C7RA06987A]

[93] Huang C, Thomas NL. Fabricating porous poly(lactic acid) fibres *via* electrospinning. Eur Polym J 2018; 99: 464-76. [http://dx.doi.org/10.1016/j.eurpolymj.2017.12.025]

[94] Akbarzadeh R, Yousefi AM. Effects of processing parameters in thermally induced phase separation technique on porous architecture of scaffolds for bone tissue engineering. J Biomed Mater Res B Appl Biomater 2014; 102(6): 1304-15. [http://dx.doi.org/10.1002/jbm.b.33101] [PMID: 24425207]

[95] Nam YS, Park TG. Porous biodegradable polymeric scaffolds prepared by thermally induced phase separation. J Biomed Mater Res 1999; 47(1): 8-17. [http://dx.doi.org/10.1002/(SICI)1097-4636(199910)47:1<8::AID-JBM2>3.0.CO;2-L] [PMID: 10400875]

[96] Kasoju N, Kubies D, Sedlačík T, *et al.* Polymer scaffolds with no skin-effect for tissue engineering applications fabricated by thermally induced phase separation. Biomed Mater 2016; 11(1): 015002. [http://dx.doi.org/10.1088/1748-6041/11/1/015002] [PMID: 26752658]

[97] Guo J, Liu X, Lee Miller A II, Waletzki BE, Yaszemski MJ, Lu L. Novel porous poly(propylene fumarate-co-caprolactone) scaffolds fabricated by thermally induced phase separation. J Biomed Mater Res A 2017; 105(1): 226-35. [http://dx.doi.org/10.1002/jbm.a.35862] [PMID: 27513282]

[98] Liu M, Liu S, Xu Z, Wei Y, Yang H. Formation of microporous polymeric membranes *via* thermally induced phase separation: A review. Front Chem Sci Eng 2016; 10: 57-75. [http://dx.doi.org/10.1007/s11705-016-1561-7]

[99] Jing X, Mi HY, Salick MR, *et al.* Morphology, mechanical properties, and shape memory effects of poly(lactic acid)/ thermoplastic polyurethane blend scaffolds prepared by thermally induced phase separation. J Cell Plast 2014; 50: 361-79. [http://dx.doi.org/10.1177/0021955X14525959]

[100] Gay S, Lefebvre G, Bonnin M, *et al.* PLA scaffolds production from Thermally Induced Phase Separation: Effect of process parameters and development of an environmentally improved route assisted by supercritical carbon dioxide. J Supercrit Fluids 2018; 136: 123-35.

[http://dx.doi.org/10.1016/j.supflu.2018.02.015]

[101] Onder OC, Yilgor E, Yilgor I. Critical parameters controlling the properties of monolithic poly(lactic acid) foams prepared by thermally induced phase separation, J Polym Sci Part B Polym Phys 2019; 57: 98-108.
[http://dx.doi.org/10.1002/polb.24762]

[102] Kim JF. Recent progress on improving the sustainability of membrane fabrication graphical abstract keywords. J Membrane Sci Res 2020; 6(3): 241-50.

[103] Wang DM, Lai JY. Recent advances in preparation and morphology control of polymeric membranes formed by nonsolvent induced phase separation. Curr Opin Chem Eng 2013; 2: 229-37.
[http://dx.doi.org/10.1016/j.coche.2013.04.003]

[104] Guillen GR, Pan Y, Li M, Hoek EMV. Preparation and characterization of membranes formed by nonsolvent induced phase separation: A review. Ind Eng Chem Res 2011; 50: 3798-817.
[http://dx.doi.org/10.1021/ie101928r]

[105] Xin Y, Fujimoto T, Uyama H. Facile fabrication of polycarbonate monolith by non-solvent induced phase separation method. Polymer (Guildf) 2012; 53: 2847-53.
[http://dx.doi.org/10.1016/j.polymer.2012.04.029]

[106] Weigel T, Schinkel G, Lendlein A. Design and preparation of polymeric scaffolds for tissue engineering. Expert Rev Med Devices 2006; 835-51.
[http://dx.doi.org/10.1586/17434440.3.6.835]

[107] Venault A, Chang Y, Wang D-M, Bouyer D. A Review on Polymeric Membranes and Hydrogels Prepared by Vapor-Induced Phase Separation Process. Polym Rev (Phila Pa) 2013; 53: 568-626.
[http://dx.doi.org/10.1080/15583724.2013.828750]

[108] Fan H, Peng Y, Li Z, Chen P, Jiang Q, Wang S. Preparation and characterization of hydrophobic PVDF membranes by vapor-induced phase separation and application in vacuum membrane distillation. J Polym Res 2013; 20
[http://dx.doi.org/10.1007/s10965-013-0134-4]

[109] Ismail N, Venault A, Mikkola JP, Bouyer D, Drioli E, Tavajohi Hassan Kiadeh N. Investigating the potential of membranes formed by the vapor induced phase separation process. J Membr Sci 2020; 597: 117601.
[http://dx.doi.org/10.1016/j.memsci.2019.117601]

[110] Felton LA. Mechanisms of polymeric film formation. Int J Pharm 2013; 457(2): 423-7.
[http://dx.doi.org/10.1016/j.ijpharm.2012.12.027] [PMID: 23305867]

[111] Ho AK, Aernouts B, Saeys W, Vankelecom IFJ. Study of polymer concentration and evaporation time as phase inversion parameters for polysulfone-based SRNF membranes. 2013; 442: 196-205.

[112] Soroko I, Makowski M, Spill F, Livingston A. The effect of membrane formation parameters on performance of polyimide membranes for organic solvent nanofiltration (OSN). Part B : Analysis of evaporation step and the role of a co-solvent. J Membr Sci 2011; 381: 163-71.
[http://dx.doi.org/10.1016/j.memsci.2011.07.028]

[113] Dong X, Al-jumaily A, Escobar IC. Investigation of the use of a bio-derived solvent for non-solvent induced phase separation (NIPS) fabrication of polysulfone membranes. Membranes 2018; 8(2): 23.
[http://dx.doi.org/10.3390/membranes8020023]

[114] Xue L, Zhang J, Han Y. Progress in Polymer Science. Prog Polym Sci 2012; 37: 564-94.
[http://dx.doi.org/10.1016/j.progpolymsci.2011.09.001]

[115] Liao CJ, Chen CF, Chen JH, Chiang SF, Lin YJ, Chang KY. Fabrication of porous biodegradable polymer scaffolds using a solvent merging/particulate leaching method. J Biomed Mater Res 2002; 59(4): 676-81.
[http://dx.doi.org/10.1002/jbm.10030] [PMID: 11774329]

[116] Kim JH, Cook M, Park SH, *et al.* A compact and scalable fabrication method for robust thin film composite membranes. Green Chem 2018; 20: 1887-98.
[http://dx.doi.org/10.1039/C8GC00731D]

[117] Trenfield SJ, Awad A, Madla CM, *et al.* Shaping the future: recent advances of 3D printing in drug delivery and healthcare. Expert Opin Drug Deliv 2019; 16(10): 1081-94.
[http://dx.doi.org/10.1080/17425247.2019.1660318] [PMID: 31478752]

[118] Yoon JJ, Song SH, Lee DS, Park TG. Immobilization of cell adhesive RGD peptide onto the surface of highly porous biodegradable polymer scaffolds fabricated by a gas foaming/salt leaching method. Biomaterials 2004; 25(25): 5613-20.
[http://dx.doi.org/10.1016/j.biomaterials.2004.01.014] [PMID: 15159077]

[119] Thadavirul N, Pavasant P, Supaphol P. Development of polycaprolactone porous scaffolds by combining solvent casting, particulate leaching, and polymer leaching techniques for bone tissue engineering. J Biomed Mater Res A 2014; 102(10): 3379-92.
[http://dx.doi.org/10.1002/jbm.a.35010] [PMID: 24132871]

[120] Sempertegui ND, Narkhede AA, Thomas V, Rao SS. A combined compression molding, heating, and leaching process for fabrication of micro-porous poly(ε-caprolactone) scaffolds. J Biomater Sci Polym Ed 2018; 29(16): 1978-93.
[http://dx.doi.org/10.1080/09205063.2018.1498719] [PMID: 30220215]

[121] Song MJ, Amirian J, Linh NTB, Lee BT. Bone morphogenetic protein-2 immobilization on porous PCL-BCP-Col composite scaffolds for bone tissue engineering. J Appl Polym Sci 2017; 134: 1-11.
[http://dx.doi.org/10.1002/app.45186]

[122] Varshney N, Sahi AK, Vajanthri KY, *et al.* Culturing melanocytes and fibroblasts within three-dimensional macroporous PDMS scaffolds: towards skin dressing material. Cytotechnology 2019; 71(1): 287-303.
[http://dx.doi.org/10.1007/s10616-018-0285-6] [PMID: 30603924]

[123] Deen GR, Loh XJ. Stimuli-Responsive Cationic Hydrogels in Drug Delivery Applications. Gels 2018; 4(1): 13.
[http://dx.doi.org/10.3390/gels4010013] [PMID: 30674789]

[124] Deng H, Dong A, Song J, Chen X. Injectable thermosensitive hydrogel systems based on functional PEG/PCL block polymer for local drug delivery. J Control Release 2019; 297: 60-70.
[http://dx.doi.org/10.1016/j.jconrel.2019.01.026] [PMID: 30684513]

[125] Bode C, Kranz H, Siepmann F, Siepmann J. In-situ forming PLGA implants for intraocular dexamethasone delivery. Int J Pharm 2018; 548(1): 337-48.
[http://dx.doi.org/10.1016/j.ijpharm.2018.07.013] [PMID: 29981408]

[126] Wei W, Li J, Qi X, *et al.* Synthesis and characterization of a multi-sensitive polysaccharide hydrogel for drug delivery. Carbohydr Polym 2017; 177: 275-83.
[http://dx.doi.org/10.1016/j.carbpol.2017.08.133] [PMID: 28962769]

[127] Fu X, Hosta-Rigau L, Chandrawati R, Cui J. Multi-Stimuli-Responsive Polymer Particles, Films, and Hydrogels for Drug Delivery. Chem 2018; 4: 2084-107.
[http://dx.doi.org/10.1016/j.chempr.2018.07.002]

[128] He Y, Li J, Turvey ME, Funkenbusch MLT, Hong C. Di.S.S.M. Uppu, H. He, D.J. Irvine, P.T. Hammond, Synthetic Lift-off Polymer beneath Layer-by-Layer Films for Surface-Mediated Drug Delivery. ACS Macro Lett 2017; 6: 1320-4.
[http://dx.doi.org/10.1021/acsmacrolett.7b00584]

[129] Park K, Choi D, Hong J. Nanostructured Polymer Thin Films Fabricated with Brush-based Layer-b--Layer Self-assembly for Site-selective Construction and Drug release. Sci Rep 2018; 8(1): 3365.
[http://dx.doi.org/10.1038/s41598-018-21493-9] [PMID: 29463825]

[130] Sabale AS, Kulkarni AD, Sabale AS. Nasal *In situ* Gel: Novel Approach for Nasal Drug Delivery. J

Drug Deliv Ther 2020; 10: 183-97.
[http://dx.doi.org/10.22270/jddt.v10i2-s.4029]

[131] Madan M, Bajaj A, Lewis S, Udupa N, Baig JA. *In situ* forming polymeric drug delivery systems. Indian J Pharm Sci 2009; 71(3): 242-51.
[http://dx.doi.org/10.4103/0250-474X.56015] [PMID: 20490289]

[132] Kranz H, Bodmeier R. Structure formation and characterization of injectable drug loaded biodegradable devices: *in situ* implants *versus in situ* microparticles. Eur J Pharm Sci 2008; 34(2-3): 164-72.
[http://dx.doi.org/10.1016/j.ejps.2008.03.004] [PMID: 18501569]

[133] Chauhan V, Patel V, Akbari B, Barse R. Development and evaluation of biodegradable polymeric based long acting *In situ* forming microparticles of lhrh agonist goserelin acetate. Indian J Pharm Educ Res 2019; 53: 216-24.
[http://dx.doi.org/10.5530/ijper.53.2.29]

[134] Amini-Fazl MS, Mobedi H. Investigation of mathematical models based on diffusion control release for Paclitaxel from in-situ forming PLGA microspheres containing HSA microparticles. Mater Technol 2020; 35: 50-9.
[http://dx.doi.org/10.1080/10667857.2019.1651549]

[135] Bhardwaj N, Kundu SC. Electrospinning: a fascinating fiber fabrication technique. Biotechnol Adv 2010; 28(3): 325-47.
[http://dx.doi.org/10.1016/j.biotechadv.2010.01.004] [PMID: 20100560]

[136] Chakraborty S, Liao IC, Adler A, Leong KW. Electrohydrodynamics: A facile technique to fabricate drug delivery systems. Adv Drug Deliv Rev 2009; 61(12): 1043-54.
[http://dx.doi.org/10.1016/j.addr.2009.07.013] [PMID: 19651167]

[137] Reneker DH, Yarin AL. Electrospinning jets and polymer nanofibers. Polymer (Guildf) 2008; 49: 2387-425.
[http://dx.doi.org/10.1016/j.polymer.2008.02.002]

[138] Sill TJ, von Recum HA. Electrospinning: applications in drug delivery and tissue engineering. Biomaterials 2008; 29(13): 1989-2006.
[http://dx.doi.org/10.1016/j.biomaterials.2008.01.011] [PMID: 18281090]

[139] Megelski S, Stephens JS, Chase DB, Rabolt JF. Micro- and Nanostructured Surface Morphology on Electrospun Polymer Fibers 2002; 8456-66.

[140] Sridhar R, Lakshminarayanan R, Madhaiyan K, Amutha Barathi V, Lim KH, Ramakrishna S. Electrosprayed nanoparticles and electrospun nanofibers based on natural materials: applications in tissue regeneration, drug delivery and pharmaceuticals. Chem Soc Rev 2015; 44(3): 790-814.
[http://dx.doi.org/10.1039/C4CS00226A] [PMID: 25408245]

[141] Imran YG, Rafaqat S. Electrospun fibers for tissue engineering, drug delivery, and wound dressing 2013; 790-814.
[http://dx.doi.org/10.1007/s10853-013-7145-8]

[142] Min BM, Lee G, Kim SH, Nam YS, Lee TS, Park WH. Electrospinning of silk fibroin nanofibers and its effect on the adhesion and spreading of normal human keratinocytes and fibroblasts *in vitro*. Biomaterials 2004; 25(7-8): 1289-97.
[http://dx.doi.org/10.1016/j.biomaterials.2003.08.045] [PMID: 14643603]

[143] Li D, Xia Y. Electrospinning of nanofibers: Reinventing the wheel? Adv Mater 2004; 16: 1151-70.
[http://dx.doi.org/10.1002/adma.200400719]

[144] Demir MM, Yilgor I, Yilgor E, Erman B. Electrospinning of polyurethane fibers. Polymer (Guildf) 2002; 43: 3303-9.
[http://dx.doi.org/10.1016/S0032-3861(02)00136-2]

[145] Casper CL, Stephens JS, Tassi NG, Chase DB, Rabolt JF. Controlling surface morphology of

electrospun polystyrene fibers: Effect of humidity and molecular weight in the electrospinning process. Macromolecules 2004; 37: 573-8.
[http://dx.doi.org/10.1021/ma0351975]

[146] Pham QP, Sharma U, Mikos AG. Electrospinning of polymeric nanofibers for tissue engineering applications: a review. Tissue Eng 2006; 12(5): 1197-211.
[http://dx.doi.org/10.1089/ten.2006.12.1197] [PMID: 16771634]

[147] Sundaray B, Subramanian V, Natarajan TS, Xiang RZ, Chang CC, Fann WS. Electrospinning of continuous aligned polymer fibers. Appl Phys Lett 2004; 84: 1222-4.
[http://dx.doi.org/10.1063/1.1647685]

[148] Khorshidi S, Solouk A, Mirzadeh H, *et al.* A review of key challenges of electrospun scaffolds for tissue-engineering applications. 2015.
[http://dx.doi.org/10.1002/term]

[149] Deitzel JM, Kleinmeyer J, Harris D, Tan NCB. The effect of processing variables on the morphology of electrospun nanofibers and textiles. 2001; 42: 261-72.

[150] Haghi AK, Akbari M. Trends in electrospinning of natural nanofibers. 2007; 1830-4.
[http://dx.doi.org/10.1002/pssa.200675301]

[151] Liu H, Hsieh Y. Ultrafine fibrous cellulose membranes from electrospinning of cellulose acetate. 2002; 2119-29.
[http://dx.doi.org/10.1002/polb.10261]

[152] Jun Y, Yong H, Hyung K, Chon H, Rae D. Transport properties of electrospun nylon 6 nonwoven mats. 2003; 39: 1883-9.

[153] Cramariuc B, Cramariuc R, Scarlet R, Manea LR, Lupu IG, Cramariuc O. Fiber diameter in electrospinning process. J Electrost 2013; 71: 189-98.
[http://dx.doi.org/10.1016/j.elstat.2012.12.018]

[154] Yuan XY, Zhang YY, Dong C, Sheng J. Morphology of ultrafine polysulfone fibers prepared by electrospinning. Polym Int 2004; 53: 1704-10.
[http://dx.doi.org/10.1002/pi.1538]

[155] Casper CL, Stephens JS, Tassi NG, Chase DB, Rabolt JF. Controlling surface morphology of electrospun polystyrene fibers : effect of humidity and molecular weight in the electrospinning process. Polym Int 2004; 573-8.
[http://dx.doi.org/10.1021/ma0351975]

[156] Luo CJ, Nangrejo M, Edirisinghe M. A novel method of selecting solvents for polymer electrospinning. Polymer (Guildf) 2010; 51: 1654-62.
[http://dx.doi.org/10.1016/j.polymer.2010.01.031]

[157] Cui W, Zhou Y, Chang J. Electrospun nanofibrous materials for tissue engineering and drug delivery. 2016; 6996.
[http://dx.doi.org/10.1088/1468-6996/11/1/014108]

[158] Vasita R, Katti DS. Nanofibers and their applications in tissue engineering. Int J Nanomedicine 2006; 1(1): 15-30.
[http://dx.doi.org/10.2147/nano.2006.1.1.15] [PMID: 17722259]

[159] Hong J, Yeo M, Yang GH, Kim G. Cell-Electrospinning and Its Application for Tissue Engineering 2019.
[http://dx.doi.org/10.3390/ijms20246208]

[160] Liu J, Yan C. 3D printing of scaffolds for tissue engineering. 3D Print, InTech. 2018.
[http://dx.doi.org/10.5772/intechopen.78145]

[161] Hoque ME, Chuan YL, Pashby I, Enamul Hoque M, Leng Chuan Y. Extrusion based rapid prototyping technique: an advanced platform for tissue engineering scaffold fabrication. Biopolymers 2012; 97(2):

83-93.
[http://dx.doi.org/10.1002/bip.21701] [PMID: 21830198]

[162] Trenfield SJ, Awad A, Madla CM, *et al.* Shaping the future: recent advances of 3D printing in drug delivery and healthcare. Expert Opin Drug Deliv 2019; 16(10): 1081-94.
[http://dx.doi.org/10.1080/17425247.2019.1660318] [PMID: 31478752]

[163] An J, Ee J, Teoh M, Suntornnond R, Chua CK. 3D Printing — Review Design and 3D Printing of Scaffolds and Tissues. Engineering 2015; 1: 261-8.
[http://dx.doi.org/10.15302/J-ENG-2015061]

[164] Palo M, Holländer J, Suominen J, Yliruusi J, Sandler N. 3D printed drug delivery devices: perspectives and technical challenges. Expert Rev Med Devices 2017; 14(9): 685-96.
[http://dx.doi.org/10.1080/17434440.2017.1363647] [PMID: 28774216]

[165] Goyanes A, Det-Amornrat U, Wang J, Basit AW, Gaisford S. 3D scanning and 3D printing as innovative technologies for fabricating personalized topical drug delivery systems. J Control Release 2016; 234: 41-8.
[http://dx.doi.org/10.1016/j.jconrel.2016.05.034] [PMID: 27189134]

[166] Tan DK, Maniruzzaman M, Nokhodchi A. Advanced pharmaceutical applications of hot-melt extrusion coupled with fused deposition modelling (FDM) 3D printing for personalised drug delivery. Pharmaceutics 2018; 10(4): E203.
[http://dx.doi.org/10.3390/pharmaceutics10040203] [PMID: 30356002]

[167] Awad A, Gaisford S, Basit AW. Fused deposition modelling: Advances in engineering and medicine. AAPS Adv Pharm Sci Ser 2018; 31: 107-32.

[168] Prasad LK, Smyth H III. 3D Printing technologies for drug delivery: a review. Drug Dev Ind Pharm 2016; 42(7): 1019-31.
[http://dx.doi.org/10.3109/03639045.2015.1120743] [PMID: 26625986]

[169] Beck RCR, Chaves PS, Goyanes A, *et al.* 3D printed tablets loaded with polymeric nanocapsules: An innovative approach to produce customized drug delivery systems. Int J Pharm 2017; 528(1-2): 268-79.
[http://dx.doi.org/10.1016/j.ijpharm.2017.05.074] [PMID: 28583328]

[170] Liu C, Li Y, Zhang L, Mi S, Xu Y, Sun W. Development of a novel low-temperature deposition machine using screw extrusion to fabricate poly(l-lactide-co-glycolide) acid scaffolds. Proc Inst Mech Eng H 2014; 228(6): 593-606.
[http://dx.doi.org/10.1177/0954411914538612] [PMID: 24925551]

[171] Liao CY, Wu WJ, Hsieh CT, Tseng CS, Dai NT, Hsu SH. Design and Development of a Novel Frozen-Form Additive Manufacturing System for Tissue Engineering Applications, 3D Print. Addit Manuf 2016; 3: 217-25.
[http://dx.doi.org/10.1089/3dp.2015.0042]

[172] Norman J, Madurawe RD, Moore CMV, Khan MA, Khairuzzaman A. A new chapter in pharmaceutical manufacturing: 3D-printed drug products. Adv Drug Deliv Rev 2017; 108: 39-50.
[http://dx.doi.org/10.1016/j.addr.2016.03.001] [PMID: 27001902]

[173] Katakam P, Dey B, Assaleh FH, *et al.* Top-down and bottom-up approaches in 3D printing technologies for drug delivery challenges. Crit Rev Ther Drug Carrier Syst 2015; 32(1): 61-87.
[http://dx.doi.org/10.1615/CritRevTherDrugCarrierSyst.2014011157] [PMID: 25746205]

[174] Mathew E, Pitzanti G, Larrañeta E, Lamprou DA. Three-dimensional printing of pharmaceuticals and drug delivery devices. Pharmaceutics 2020; 12: 1-9.
[http://dx.doi.org/10.3390/pharmaceutics12030266] [PMID: 32183435]

[175] Chia HN, Wu BM. Recent advances in 3D printing of biomaterials. J Biol Eng 2015; 9: 4.
[http://dx.doi.org/10.1186/s13036-015-0001-4] [PMID: 25866560]

[176] Jamróz W, Kurek M, Łyszczarz E, *et al.* 3D printed orodispersible films with Aripiprazole. Int J

Pharm 2017; 533(2): 413-20.
[http://dx.doi.org/10.1016/j.ijpharm.2017.05.052] [PMID: 28552800]

[177] Dou Y, Zhang B, He M, Yin G, Cui Y, Savina IN. Keratin/polyvinyl alcohol blend films cross-linked by dialdehyde starch and their potential application for drug release. Polymers (Basel) 2015; 7: 580-91.
[http://dx.doi.org/10.3390/polym7030580]

[178] Ubaid M, Murtaza G. Fabrication and characterization of genipin cross-linked chitosan/gelatin hydrogel for pH-sensitive, oral delivery of metformin with an application of response surface methodology. Int J Biol Macromol 2018; 114: 1174-85.
[http://dx.doi.org/10.1016/j.ijbiomac.2018.04.023] [PMID: 29634962]

[179] Wang K, Zhang Y, Jiang S, *et al.* Surface Charge Reversible Polymeric Micelle-Laden Hydrogels for Drug Delivery and 3D Cell Culture. Macromol Chem Phys 2018; 219: 1-9.
[http://dx.doi.org/10.1002/macp.201800391]

[180] Sadiasa A, Nguyen TH, Lee BT. *In vitro* and *in vivo* evaluation of porous PCL-PLLA 3D polymer scaffolds fabricated *via* salt leaching method for bone tissue engineering applications. J Biomater Sci Polym Ed 2014; 25(2): 150-67.
[http://dx.doi.org/10.1080/09205063.2013.846633] [PMID: 24138179]

[181] Skodje A, Idris SBM, Sun Y, *et al.* Biodegradable polymer scaffolds loaded with low-dose BMP-2 stimulate periodontal ligament cell differentiation. J Biomed Mater Res A 2015; 103(6): 1991-8.
[http://dx.doi.org/10.1002/jbm.a.35334] [PMID: 25231842]

[182] Akduman C, Özgüney I, Kumbasar EPA. Preparation and characterization of naproxen-loaded electrospun thermoplastic polyurethane nanofibers as a drug delivery system. Mater Sci Eng C 2016; 64: 383-90.
[http://dx.doi.org/10.1016/j.msec.2016.04.005] [PMID: 27127068]

[183] Li JJ, Yang YY, Yu DG, Du Q, Yang XL. Fast dissolving drug delivery membrane based on the ultra-thin shell of electrospun core-shell nanofibers. Eur J Pharm Sci 2018; 122: 195-204.
[http://dx.doi.org/10.1016/j.ejps.2018.07.002] [PMID: 30008429]

[184] Zhang X, Tang K, Zheng X. Electrospinning and Crosslinking of COL/PVA Nanofiber-microsphere Containing Salicylic Acid for Drug Delivery. J Bionics Eng 2016; 13: 143-9.
[http://dx.doi.org/10.1016/S1672-6529(14)60168-2]

[185] da Silva TN, Gonçalves RP, Rocha CL, *et al.* Controlling burst effect with PLA/PVA coaxial electrospun scaffolds loaded with BMP-2 for bone guided regeneration. Mater Sci Eng C 2019; 97: 602-12.
[http://dx.doi.org/10.1016/j.msec.2018.12.020] [PMID: 30678947]

[186] Eswaramma S, Reddy NS, Rao KSVK. Phosphate crosslinked pectin based dual responsive hydrogel networks and nanocomposites: Development, swelling dynamics and drug release characteristics. Int J Biol Macromol 2017; 103: 1162-72.
[http://dx.doi.org/10.1016/j.ijbiomac.2017.05.160] [PMID: 28576553]

[187] Pere CPP, Economidou SN, Lall G, *et al.* 3D printed microneedles for insulin skin delivery. Int J Pharm 2018; 544(2): 425-32.
[http://dx.doi.org/10.1016/j.ijpharm.2018.03.031] [PMID: 29555437]

[188] Goyanes A, Buanz ABM, Hatton GB, Gaisford S, Basit AW. 3D printing of modified-release aminosalicylate (4-ASA and 5-ASA) tablets. Eur J Pharm Biopharm 2015; 89: 157-62.
[http://dx.doi.org/10.1016/j.ejpb.2014.12.003] [PMID: 25497178]

[189] Boparai KS, Singh R, Fabbrocino F, Fraternali F. Thermal characterization of recycled polymer for additive manufacturing applications. Compos, Part B Eng 2016; 106: 42-7.
[http://dx.doi.org/10.1016/j.compositesb.2016.09.009]

[190] El-Newehy MH, El-Naggar ME, Alotaiby S, El-Hamshary H, Moydeen M, Al-Deyab S. Preparation

of biocompatible system based on electrospun CMC/PVA nanofibers as controlled release carrier of diclofenac sodium. J Macromol Sci Part A Pure Appl Chem 2016; 53: 566-73. [http://dx.doi.org/10.1080/10601325.2016.1201752]

[191] Singh B, Sharma S, Dhiman A. Acacia gum polysaccharide based hydrogel wound dressings: Synthesis, characterization, drug delivery and biomedical properties. Carbohydr Polym 2017; 165: 294-303. [http://dx.doi.org/10.1016/j.carbpol.2017.02.039] [PMID: 28363552]

[192] Abilova GK, Kaldybekov DB, Ozhmukhametova EK, *et al.* Chitosan/poly(2-ethyl-2-oxazoline) films for ocular drug delivery: Formulation, miscibility, *in vitro* and *in vivo* studies. Eur Polym J 2019; 116: 311-20. [http://dx.doi.org/10.1016/j.eurpolymj.2019.04.016]

[193] Saadatkhah N, Carillo Garcia A, Ackermann S, *et al.* Experimental methods in chemical engineering: Thermogravimetric analysis—TGA. Can J Chem Eng 2020; 98: 34-43. [http://dx.doi.org/10.1002/cjce.23673]

[194] Ford JL, Mann TE. Fast-Scan DSC and its role in pharmaceutical physical form characterisation and selection. Adv Drug Deliv Rev 2012; 64(5): 422-30. [http://dx.doi.org/10.1016/j.addr.2011.12.001] [PMID: 22178405]

[195] Holländer J, Genina N, Jukarainen H, *et al.* Three-Dimensional Printed PCL-Based Implantable Prototypes of Medical Devices for Controlled Drug Delivery. J Pharm Sci 2016; 105(9): 2665-76. [http://dx.doi.org/10.1016/j.xphs.2015.12.012] [PMID: 26906174]

[196] Dalton MB, Halligan SC, Killion JA, *et al.* The Effect Acetic Acid has on Poly(N-Vinylcaprolactam) LCST for Biomedical Applications. Polym Plast Technol Eng 2018; 57: 1165-74. [http://dx.doi.org/10.1080/03602559.2017.1373400]

[197] Moydeen AM, Padusha MSA, Thamer BM. A. Ahamed N, A.M. Al-Enizi, H. El-Hamshary, M.H. El-Newehy, Single-nozzle Core-shell Electrospun Nanofibers of PVP/Dextran as Drug Delivery System. Fibers Polym 2019; 20: 2078-89. [http://dx.doi.org/10.1007/s12221-019-9187-2]

[198] Feng X, Wang G, Neumann K, *et al.* Synthesis and characterization of biodegradable poly(ether-ester) urethane acrylates for controlled drug release. Mater Sci Eng C 2017; 74: 270-8. [http://dx.doi.org/10.1016/j.msec.2016.12.009] [PMID: 28254295]

[199] Ullah K, Ali Khan S, Murtaza G, *et al.* Gelatin-based hydrogels as potential biomaterials for colonic delivery of oxaliplatin. Int J Pharm 2019; 556: 236-45. [http://dx.doi.org/10.1016/j.ijpharm.2018.12.020] [PMID: 30553956]

[200] Alagha A, Nourallah A, Hariri S. Characterization of dexamethasone loaded collagen-chitosan sponge and *In vitro* release study. J Drug Deliv Sci Technol 2020; 55: 101449. [http://dx.doi.org/10.1016/j.jddst.2019.101449]

[201] Klang V, Matsko NB, Valenta C, Hofer F. Electron microscopy of nanoemulsions: an essential tool for characterisation and stability assessment. Micron 2012; 43(2-3): 85-103. [http://dx.doi.org/10.1016/j.micron.2011.07.014] [PMID: 21839644]

[202] Yadollahi M, Farhoudian S, Barkhordari S, Gholamali I, Farhadnejad H, Motasadizadeh H. Facile synthesis of chitosan/ZnO bio-nanocomposite hydrogel beads as drug delivery systems. Int J Biol Macromol 2016; 82: 273-8. [http://dx.doi.org/10.1016/j.ijbiomac.2015.09.064] [PMID: 26433177]

[203] Ye Y, Hu X. A pH-sensitive injectable nanoparticle composite hydrogel for anticancer drug delivery. J Nanomater 2016; 2016 [http://dx.doi.org/10.1155/2016/9816461]

[204] Ribeiro SD, -Rodrigues Filho G, Meneguin AB, *et al.* Cellulose triacetate films obtained from sugarcane bagasse: Evaluation as coating and mucoadhesive material for drug delivery systems.

Carbohydr Polym 2016; 152: 764-74.
[http://dx.doi.org/10.1016/j.carbpol.2016.07.069] [PMID: 27516328]

[205] Sarwar MS, Ghaffar A, Islam A, *et al.* Controlled drug release behavior of metformin hydrogen chloride from biodegradable films based on chitosan/poly(ethylene glycol) methyl ether blend. Arab J Chem 2020; 13: 393-403.
[http://dx.doi.org/10.1016/j.arabjc.2017.05.005]

[206] Yu H, Chen X, Cai J, Ye D, Wu Y, Liu P. Dual controlled release nanomicelle-in-nanofiber system for long-term antibacterial medical dressings. J Biomater Sci Polym Ed 2019; 30(1): 64-76.
[http://dx.doi.org/10.1080/09205063.2018.1549771] [PMID: 30449259]

[207] Matalanis A, Jones OG, McClements DJ. Structured biopolymer-based delivery systems for encapsulation, protection, and release of lipophilic compounds. Food Hydrocoll 2011; 25: 1865-80.
[http://dx.doi.org/10.1016/j.foodhyd.2011.04.014]

[208] Dash M, Chiellini F, Ottenbrite RM, Chiellini E. Chitosan - A versatile semi-synthetic polymer in biomedical applications. Prog Polym Sci 2011; 36: 981-1014.
[http://dx.doi.org/10.1016/j.progpolymsci.2011.02.001]

[209] Thoniyot P, Tan MJ, Karim AA, Young DJ, Loh XJ. Nanoparticle-Hydrogel Composites: Concept, Design, and Applications of These Promising, Multi-Functional Materials. Adv Sci (Weinh) 2015; 2(1-2): 1400010.
[http://dx.doi.org/10.1002/advs.201400010] [PMID: 27980900]

[210] Desfrançois C, Auzély R, Texier I. Lipid nanoparticles and their hydrogel composites for drug delivery: A review. Pharmaceuticals (Basel) 2018; 11(4): E118.
[http://dx.doi.org/10.3390/ph11040118] [PMID: 30388738]

[211] Varaprasad K, Murali Mohan Y, Ravindra S, *et al.* Hydrogel-silver nanoparticle composites: A new generation of antimicrobials. J Appl Polym Sci 2010; 115: 1199-207.
[http://dx.doi.org/10.1002/app.31249]

[212] Song F, Li X, Wang Q, Liao L, Zhang C. Nanocomposite hydrogels and their applications in drug delivery and tissue engineering. J Biomed Nanotechnol 2015; 11(1): 40-52.
[http://dx.doi.org/10.1166/jbn.2015.1962] [PMID: 26301299]

[213] Hoare TR, Kohane DS. Hydrogels in drug delivery: Progress and challenges. Polymer (Guildf) 2008.
[http://dx.doi.org/10.1016/j.polymer.2008.01.027]

[214] Cruz L, Soares LU, Costa TD, *et al.* Diffusion and mathematical modeling of release profiles from nanocarriers. Int J Pharm 2006; 313(1-2): 198-205.
[http://dx.doi.org/10.1016/j.ijpharm.2006.01.035] [PMID: 16503103]

[215] Rossi F, Ferrari R, Castiglione F, Mele A, Perale G, Moscatelli D. Polymer hydrogel functionalized with biodegradable nanoparticles as composite system for controlled drug delivery. Nanotechnology 2015; 26(1): 015602.
[http://dx.doi.org/10.1088/0957-4484/26/1/015602] [PMID: 25490351]

[216] Constantinides PP, Chaubal MV, Shorr R. Advances in lipid nanodispersions for parenteral drug delivery and targeting. Adv Drug Deliv Rev 2008; 60(6): 757-67.
[http://dx.doi.org/10.1016/j.addr.2007.10.013] [PMID: 18096269]

[217] Leung WWF, Hung CH, Yuen PT. Effect of face velocity, nanofiber packing density and thickness on filtration performance of filters with nanofibers coated on a substrate. Separ Purif Tech 2010; 71: 30-7.
[http://dx.doi.org/10.1016/j.seppur.2009.10.017]

[218] Widjaja LK, Bora M, Chan PNPH, Lipik V, Wong TTL, Venkatraman SS. Hyaluronic acid-based nanocomposite hydrogels for ocular drug delivery applications. J Biomed Mater Res A 2014; 102(9): 3056-65.
[http://dx.doi.org/10.1002/jbm.a.34976] [PMID: 24124098]

[219] Neuman MG, Nanau RM, Oruña-Sanchez L, Coto G. Hyaluronic acid and wound healing. J Pharm

Pharm Sci 2015; 18(1): 53-60.
[http://dx.doi.org/10.18433/J3K89D] [PMID: 25877441]

[220] Iacob AT, Drăgan M, Gheţu N, *et al.* Preparation, characterization and wound healing effects of new membranes based on chitosan, hyaluronic acid and arginine derivatives. Polymers (Basel) 2018; 10(6): E607.
[http://dx.doi.org/10.3390/polym10060607] [PMID: 30966641]

[221] Yu DG, Wang X, Li XY, Chian W, Li Y, Liao YZ. Electrospun biphasic drug release polyvinylpyrrolidone/ethyl cellulose core/sheath nanofibers. Acta Biomater 2013; 9(3): 5665-72.
[http://dx.doi.org/10.1016/j.actbio.2012.10.021] [PMID: 23099302]

[222] Madheswaran T, Baskaran R, Yong CS, Yoo BK. Enhanced topical delivery of finasteride using glyceryl monooleate-based liquid crystalline nanoparticles stabilized by cremophor surfactants. AAPS PharmSciTech 2014; 15(1): 44-51.
[http://dx.doi.org/10.1208/s12249-013-0034-2] [PMID: 24222268]

[223] Zabara A, Mezzenga R. Controlling molecular transport and sustained drug release in lipid-based liquid crystalline mesophases. J Control Release 2014; 188: 31-43.
[http://dx.doi.org/10.1016/j.jconrel.2014.05.052] [PMID: 24910192]

[224] Li X, Su X. Multifunctional smart hydrogels: potential in tissue engineering and cancer therapy. J Mater Chem B Mater Biol Med 2018; 6(29): 4714-30.
[http://dx.doi.org/10.1039/C8TB01078A] [PMID: 32254299]

[225] Klouda L, Mikos AG. Thermoresponsive hydrogels in biomedical applications. Eur J Pharm Biopharm 2008; 68(1): 34-45.
[http://dx.doi.org/10.1016/j.ejpb.2007.02.025] [PMID: 17881200]

[226] Gioffredi E, Boffito M, Calzone S, *et al.* Pluronic F127 Hydrogel Characterization and Biofabrication in Cellularized Constructs for Tissue Engineering Applications. Procedia CIRP 2016; 49: 125-32.
[http://dx.doi.org/10.1016/j.procir.2015.11.001]

[227] da Silva DA, Feitosa JPA, Paula HCB, de Paula RCM. Synthesis and characterization of cashew gum/acrylic acid nanoparticles. Mater Sci Eng C 2009.
[http://dx.doi.org/10.1016/j.msec.2008.08.029]

[228] Nita LE, Chiriac AP, Rusu AG, *et al.* Stimuli Responsive Scaffolds Based on Carboxymethyl Starch and Poly(2-Dimethylaminoethyl Methacrylate) for Anti-Inflammatory Drug Delivery. Macromol Biosci 2020; 20(4): e1900412.
[http://dx.doi.org/10.1002/mabi.201900412] [PMID: 32090495]

[229] Rao KM, Rao KS, Ramanjaneyulu G, Rao KC, Subha MCS, Ha C-S. Biodegradable sodium alginate-based semi-interpenetrating polymer network hydrogels for antibacterial application. J Biomed Mater Res A 2014; 102(9): 3196-206.
[http://dx.doi.org/10.1002/jbm.a.34991] [PMID: 24151188]

[230] Nita LE, Chiriac AP, Rusu AG, Bercea M, Diaconu A, Tudorachi N. Interpenetrating polymer network systems based on poly(dimethylaminoethyl methacrylate) and a copolymer containing pendant spiroacetal moieties. Mater Sci Eng C 2018; 87: 22-31.
[http://dx.doi.org/10.1016/j.msec.2018.02.016] [PMID: 29549946]

[231] Motealleh A, De Marco R, Kehr NS. Stimuli-responsive local drug molecule delivery to adhered cells in a 3D nanocomposite scaffold. J Mater Chem B Mater Biol Med 2019; 7: 3716-23.
[http://dx.doi.org/10.1039/C9TB00591A]

[232] Adedoyin AA, Ekenseair AK. Biomedical applications of magneto-responsive scaffolds. Nano Res 2018; 11: 5049-64.
[http://dx.doi.org/10.1007/s12274-018-2198-2]

[233] Casolaro M, Casolaro I. Pulsed release of antidepressants from nanocomposite hydrogels. Biol Eng Med 2017; 3

[http://dx.doi.org/10.15761/BEM.1000132]

[234] Bacelar AH, Cengiz IF, Silva-Correia J, Sousa RA, Oliveira JM, Reisa RL. "Smart" Hydrogels in Tissue Engineering and Regenerative Medicine Applications Biological relevance of hyaluronic acid: high-throughput platforms for molecular and biological studies View project Football medicine View project, Handb. Intell. Scaffolds Tissue Eng Regen Med 2017. [http://dx.doi.org/10.1201/9781315364698]

[235] Morgan ML, Jeffrey R. Tissue engineering methods and protocols. Springer. 1999; 18. https://www.springer.com/gp/book/9781592596027

[236] Novosel EC, Kleinhans C, Kluger PJ. Vascularization is the key challenge in tissue engineering. Adv Drug Deliv Rev 2011; 63(4-5): 300-11. [http://dx.doi.org/10.1016/j.addr.2011.03.004] [PMID: 21396416]

[237] Fleischer S, Shevach M, Feiner R, Dvir T. Coiled fiber scaffolds embedded with gold nanoparticles improve the performance of engineered cardiac tissues. Nanoscale 2014; 6(16): 9410-4. [http://dx.doi.org/10.1039/C4NR00300D] [PMID: 24744098]

[238] Smith AST, Yoo H, Yi H, *et al.* Micro- and nano-patterned conductive graphene-PEG hybrid scaffolds for cardiac tissue engineering. Chem Commun (Camb) 2017; 53(53): 7412-5. [http://dx.doi.org/10.1039/C7CC01988B] [PMID: 28634611]

[239] Censi R, Di Martino P, Vermonden T, Hennink WE. Hydrogels for protein delivery in tissue engineering. J Control Release 2012; 161(2): 680-92. [http://dx.doi.org/10.1016/j.jconrel.2012.03.002] [PMID: 22421425]

[240] Pramanik S, Pingguan-Murphy B, Abu Osman NA. Progress of key strategies in development of electrospun scaffolds: bone tissue. Sci Technol Adv Mater 2012; 13(4): 043002. [http://dx.doi.org/10.1088/1468-6996/13/4/043002] [PMID: 27877500]

[241] Monteiro N, Martins A, Pires R, *et al.* Immobilization of bioactive factor-loaded liposomes on the surface of electrospun nanofibers targeting tissue engineering. Biomater Sci 2014; 2(9): 1195-209. [http://dx.doi.org/10.1039/C4BM00069B] [PMID: 32481891]

[242] López-Noriega A, Ruiz-Hernández E, Quinlan E, Storm G, Hennink WE, O'Brien FJ. Thermally triggered release of a pro-osteogenic peptide from a functionalized collagen-based scaffold using thermosensitive liposomes. J Control Release 2014; 187: 158-66. [http://dx.doi.org/10.1016/j.jconrel.2014.05.043] [PMID: 24878185]

[243] Rajzer I, Menaszek E, Kwiatkowski R, Planell JA, Castano O. Electrospun gelatin/poly(ε-caprolactone) fibrous scaffold modified with calcium phosphate for bone tissue engineering. Mater Sci Eng C 2014; 44: 183-90. [http://dx.doi.org/10.1016/j.msec.2014.08.017] [PMID: 25280695]

[244] Vimal SK, Ahamad N, Katti DS. A simple method for fabrication of electrospun fibers with controlled degree of alignment having potential for nerve regeneration applications. Mater Sci Eng C 2016; 63: 616-27. [http://dx.doi.org/10.1016/j.msec.2016.03.008] [PMID: 27040257]

[245] Atoufi Z, Zarrintaj P, Motlagh GH, Amiri A, Bagher Z, Kamrava SK. A novel bio electro active alginate-aniline tetramer/ agarose scaffold for tissue engineering: synthesis, characterization, drug release and cell culture study. J Biomater Sci Polym Ed 2017; 28(15): 1617-38. [http://dx.doi.org/10.1080/09205063.2017.1340044] [PMID: 28589747]

[246] Samudre S, Tekade A, Thorve K, Jamodkar A, Parashar G, Chaudhari N. Xanthan Gum Coated Mucoadhesive Liposomes for Efficient Nose to Brain Delivery of Curcumin. Drug Deliv Lett 2016; 5: 201-7. [http://dx.doi.org/10.2174/2210303106666160120215857]

[247] Yan E, Fan Y, Sun Z, *et al.* Biocompatible core-shell electrospun nanofibers as potential application for chemotherapy against ovary cancer. Mater Sci Eng C 2014; 41: 217-23.

[http://dx.doi.org/10.1016/j.msec.2014.04.053] [PMID: 24907754]

[248] Wang C, Ma C, Wu Z, *et al.* Enhanced Bioavailability and Anticancer Effect of Curcumin-Loaded Electrospun Nanofiber: *in vitro* and *in vivo* Study. Nanoscale Res Lett 2015; 10(1): 439. [http://dx.doi.org/10.1186/s11671-015-1146-2] [PMID: 26573930]

[249] Zhou H, Liu X, Wu F, *et al.* Preparation, Characterization, and Antitumor Evaluation of Electrospun Resveratrol Loaded Nanofibers. J Nanomater 2016; 2016 [http://dx.doi.org/10.1155/2016/5918462]

[250] Subhas Gupta RPS. 1, Charles Andersen 2, Joyce Black 3, Jean de Leon 4, Caroline Fife 5, John C Lantis Ii 6, Jeffrey Niezgoda 7, Robert Snyder 8, Bauer Sumpio 9, William Tettelbach 10, Terry Treadwell 11, Dot Weir 12, Management of Chronic Wounds: Diagnosis, Preparation, Treatment, and Follow-up - PubMed. Wounds 2017; 29: 19-36.https://pubmed.ncbi.nlm.nih.gov/28862980/

[251] Boateng JS, Matthews KH, Stevens HNE, Eccleston GM. Wound healing dressings and drug delivery systems: a review. J Pharm Sci 2008; 97(8): 2892-923. [http://dx.doi.org/10.1002/jps.21210] [PMID: 17963217]

[252] Leung V, Hartwell R, Yang H, Ghahary A, Ko F. Bioactive Nanofibres for Wound Healing Applications. J Fiber Bioeng Informatics 2011; 4: 1-14. [http://dx.doi.org/10.3993/jfbi04201101]

[253] Mohandas A, Deepthi S, Biswas R, Jayakumar R. Chitosan based metallic nanocomposite scaffolds as antimicrobial wound dressings. Bioact Mater 2017; 3(3): 267-77. [http://dx.doi.org/10.1016/j.bioactmat.2017.11.003] [PMID: 29744466]

[254] Cai ZX, Mo XM, Zhang KH, *et al.* Fabrication of chitosan/silk fibroin composite nanofibers for wound-dressing applications. Int J Mol Sci 2010; 11(9): 3529-39. [http://dx.doi.org/10.3390/ijms11093529] [PMID: 20957110]

[255] Kataria K, Gupta A, Rath G, Mathur RB, Dhakate SR. *In vivo* wound healing performance of drug loaded electrospun composite nanofibers transdermal patch. Int J Pharm 2014; 469(1): 102-10. [http://dx.doi.org/10.1016/j.ijpharm.2014.04.047] [PMID: 24751731]

[256] Wahab MA, Islam N, Enamul Hoque M, James Young D. Recent Advances in Silver Nanoparticle Containing Biopolymer Nanocomposites for Infectious Disease Control – A Mini Review. Curr Anal Chem 2017; 13: 198-202. [http://dx.doi.org/10.2174/1573411013666171009163829]

[257] Boroumand Z, Golmakani N, Boroumand S. Clinical trials on silver nanoparticles for wound healing. Nanomedicine J 2018; 5: 186-91. [http://dx.doi.org/10.22038/nmj.2018.05.00001]

[258] Chandra Babu A, Prabhakar MN, Suresh Babu A, Mallikarjuna B, Subha MCS, Chowdoji Rao K. Development and Characterization of Semi-IPN Silver Nanocomposite Hydrogels for Antibacterial Applications. Int J Carbohydr Chem 2013; 2013: 1-8. [http://dx.doi.org/10.1155/2013/243695]

[259] Xie W, Gao Q, Guo Z, *et al.* Injectable and self-healing thermosensitive magnetic hydrogel for asynchronous control release of doxorubicin and docetaxel to treat triple-negative breast cancer. ACS Appl Mater Interfaces 2017; 9(39): 33660-73. [http://dx.doi.org/10.1021/acsami.7b10699] [PMID: 28901139]

[260] Chew SY, Wen J, Yim EKF, Leong KW. Sustained release of proteins from electrospun biodegradable fibers. Biomacromolecules 2005; 6(4): 2017-24. [http://dx.doi.org/10.1021/bm0501149] [PMID: 16004440]

[261] Rubert M, Dehli J, Li YF, *et al.* Electrospun PCL/PEO coaxial fibers for basic fibroblast growth factor delivery. J Mater Chem B Mater Biol Med 2014; 2(48): 8538-46. [http://dx.doi.org/10.1039/C4TB01258E] [PMID: 32262212]

[262] Pinese C, Lin J, Milbreta U, *et al.* Sustained delivery of siRNA/mesoporous silica nanoparticle

complexes from nanofiber scaffolds for long-term gene silencing. Acta Biomater 2018; 76: 164-77. [http://dx.doi.org/10.1016/j.actbio.2018.05.054] [PMID: 29890267]

[263] Nelson CE, Kim AJ, Adolph EJ, *et al.* Tunable delivery of siRNA from a biodegradable scaffold to promote angiogenesis *in vivo*. Adv Mater 2014; 26(4): 607-614, 506. [http://dx.doi.org/10.1002/adma.201303520] [PMID: 24338842]

[264] Saraf A, Baggett LS, Raphael RM, Kasper FK, Mikos AG. Regulated non-viral gene delivery from coaxial electrospun fiber mesh scaffolds. J Control Release 2010; 143(1): 95-103. [http://dx.doi.org/10.1016/j.jconrel.2009.12.009] [PMID: 20006660]

[265] Mickova A, Buzgo M, Benada O, *et al.* Core/shell nanofibers with embedded liposomes as a drug delivery system. Biomacromolecules 2012; 13(4): 952-62. [http://dx.doi.org/10.1021/bm2018118] [PMID: 22401557]

[266] Wickremasinghe NC, Kumar VA, Hartgerink JD. Two-step self-assembly of liposome-multidomain peptide nanofiber hydrogel for time-controlled release. Biomacromolecules 2014; 15(10): 3587-95. [http://dx.doi.org/10.1021/bm500856c] [PMID: 25308335]

SUBJECT INDEX

A

E

F

K

L

M

N

O

P

R

T

U

V

W

X

Y

www.ingramcontent.com/pod-product-compliance
Lightning Source LLC
LaVergne TN
LVHW070117110826
845147LV00002B/136